AF430628

CLINICAL RESEARCH

Principles, Practices, Perspectives

CLINICAL RESEARCH

Principles, Practices, Perspectives

Dr. Niti Mittal

MD, DM (Clinical Pharmacology) (PGIMER, Chandigarh)
Assistant Professor,
Department of Pharmacology
Pt B D Sharma PGIMS
Rohtak, Haryana, India

Dr. Bikash Medhi

Professor & Additional Medical Superintendent (AMS),
Editor in Chief Indian Journal of Pharmacology (IJP),
Coordinator - PGIMER Pharmacovigilance Centre and Materiovigilance Centre,
Regional Resource and Training & Technical Support Centre for North India.
Regional Co-ordinator, NADA for North Zone,
Ministry of Youth Affairs and Sports, Government of India.
Founder Experimental Pharmacology laboratory and
Neurobehavioral laboratory (NBRL)
Co-Convener India Initiate Programme (IPS)
Ex Secretary Clinical Pharmacology of Indian Pharmacology Society,
Department of Pharmacology, Research Block B, Room No 4043,
PGIMER, Chandigarh, India.

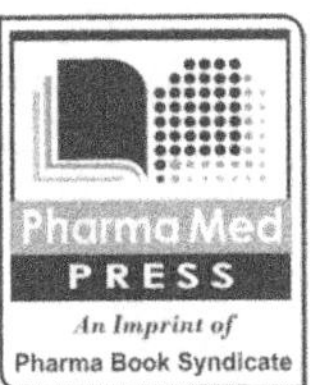

PharmaMed Press
An imprint of Pharma Book Syndicate
A unit of BSP Books Pvt. Ltd.
4-4-309/316, Giriraj Lane,
Sultan Bazar, Hyderabad - 500 095.

Published by

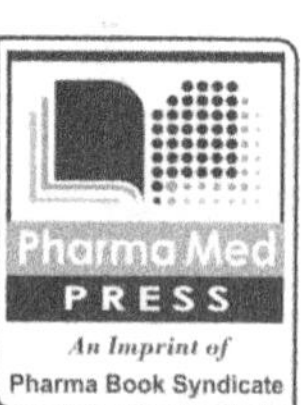

PharmaMed Press
An imprint of Pharma Book Syndicate
A unit of BSP Books Pvt. Ltd.
4-4-309/316, Giriraj Lane, Sultan Bazar, Hyderabad - 500 095.
Phone: 040-23445688, Fax: 91+40-23445611
E-mail: info@pharmamedpress.com
Website: www.bspbooks.net

ISBN: 978-93-89974-44-7 (Hardback)

स्नातकोत्तर चिकित्सा शिक्षा एवं अनुसंधान संस्थान, चण्डीगढ़ – 160012 (भारत)
POSTGRADUATE INSTITUTE OF MEDICAL EDUCATION & RESEARCH, CHANDIGARH-160012 (INDIA)

दूरभाष / Phone (Off.) 0172-2748363, 2755556, फैक्स / Fax : 0172-2745078, 2744401
ई-मेल / E-mail : dpgichd@hotmail.com वैबसाईट / Website : http://pgimer.nic.in, http://pgimer.gov.in

Dr. Jagat Ram
M.S., F. A. M. S.

DIRECTOR
&
PROFESSOR OF OPHTHALMOLOGY

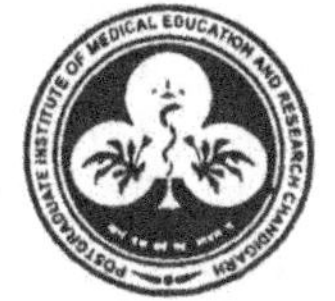

डॉ. जगत राम
एम. एस., एफ. ए. एम. एस.

निदेशक
एवं
प्राचार्य नेत्र विभाग

Foreword

I am delighted to write the foreword for the book entitled "**Clinical Research: Principles, Practice and Perspectives**".

Human experimentation i.e. clinical trials, being the most relevant method at our disposal to explore and establish efficacy and safety of medicines, is the fundamental basis of clinical development programs of healthcare products. Randomized clinical trials form the foundation of evidence based medicine in today's era and are considered as gold standard studies for valuation of healthcare interventions. However, the quality of evidence generated from clinical trials is dependent on the methodological rigor employed at every stage of their execution. Understanding the scientific, methodological and practical concerns involved in this field is a daunting task. Moreover, the past decade has witnessed several changes in the regulatory landscape which have brought numerous changes in the way clinical trials are carried out in the country.

This book lays emphasis on the critical elements of methodological, ethical, scientific, regulatory and practical aspects involved in the entire process of clinical trials. I hope that using this book will assist the readers in learning how to more naturally and quickly identify the various aspects inherent at each step of the research process.

I feel confident that this book will be of immense help to researchers, pharmaceutical companies, drug regulatory authorities, and students of clinical research institutes.

I applaud and commend the enormous efforts directed by authors in bringing out such an extensive and comprehensive book.

I congratulate the authors for the release for the book, which is laudable step in the desired direction.

(Prof. Jagat Ram)

The goal of all patient care goes back to the Hippocrates Oath and the commitment *primum non nocere* (first do no harm). An important step in this direction is the selection of safest and most effective therapy. Clinical research, particularly clinical trials are rightly seen as the key means by which new treatments and interventions are evaluated for their safety and efficacy and therefore provide the cornerstone of evidence-based medicine in current practice. Hence, researchers from a broad range of professional backgrounds need to have a good working knowledge in this area as regards the principles, planning and methodology, ethical and regulatory aspects of clinical research. This book is an admirable venture in that it covers the whole field of clinical research in an elaborative detailed manner. The book is intended both for experienced investigators as well as for those planning to conduct clinical research for the first time. It can serve as a useful teaching aid for clinical trial methodology.

The book's structure, with 44 chapters grouped under 10 different sections, helps the readers to focus on one specific area at a time. At the end of each section, suggested readings are provided to facilitate more elaborate learning. The book also contains a separate section on annexures which includes formats for various documents, detailed step wise process of clinical trial registration etc. for quick and simpler review by the personnel involved in conducting clinical research. The book has been presented in simple English language without undue heavy technicalities or jargons to deliver key practical information in an efficient and effective manner. All the topics have been explained in an easily understandable language that even those with little or no previous knowledge of the subject can follow the content without facing any issues.

We hope that the humble effort made in the form of this book will fulfill the felt needs of not only postgraduate students and students of clinical research institutes but also researchers, pharmaceutical companies and drug regulatory authorities. The valued suggestions from different end users are most welcome to improve the subject content and make it more reader compatible in future editions.

- Niti Mittal

Bikash Medhi

Contents

Niti Mittal (MD, DM) pursued her post-graduation in Pharmacology and DM (Clinical Pharmacology) from the prestigious institute, Postgraduate Institute of Medical Education and Research (PGIMER), Chandigarh. She graduated from Government Medical College and Hospital, Chandigarh. She is currently working as an Assistant Professor in the Department of Pharmacology, Postgraduate Institute of Medical Sciences (PGIMS), Rohtak, Haryana. During her academic career, she has been actively involved in various research, academic, and pharmacovigilance activities. She holds a sound working knowledge in the field of clinical research and has conducted varied types of research including randomized controlled trials, observational studies, Phase 1 study, meta-analysis etc. She has to her credit more than 40 national and international publications in indexed medical journals. She has contributed chapters in Indian books on clinical research, pharmacology and antibiotics. Her research paper was nominated for U.K. Seth award presentation at a conference organized by Indian Pharmacological Society. She is life member of renowned societies like Indian Pharmacological Society (IPS), Association of Physiologists and Pharmacologists of India (APPI), Indian Society of Rational Pharmacotherapeutics (ISRPT), Society of Pharmacovigilance of India (SOPI)and Indian Society of Clinical Research (ISCR). She is among the peer review panel of various national and international indexed journals.

Bikash Medhi is Professor & Additional Medical Ex. Superintendent (AMS) in PGIMER, Department of Pharmacology. His area of expertise is Experimental Pharmacology, Clinical Research, Regulatory Pharmacology, Development of nano-formulations, Pharmacogenetics, Pharmacogenomics and Stem cells etc. He has more than 20 years of teaching and research experience and has owned more than 60 prestigious National and International Awards namely, Dr. D N Prasad memorial award with Gold medal 2009 from Indian Council of Medical Research (ICMR), New Delhi, V K Bhargava Award with a Gold medal from National Academy of Medical Sciences 2013, Col. R N Chopra Oration 2014 by Indian Pharmacology Society (IPS), NN Dutta Award 2016 by Indian Pharmacology Society (IPS), Dr. B N. Ghosh Oration at 43rd Annual Conference of IPS and International Conference on "Pharmacology & Translational Research" He is in core panel of expert for Task Force in IND application & Regulatory Affair, lead GLP Inspector, lead GCP inspector, Principle Assessor for NABH, He is in several committees in DCGI office, ICMR, DBT, DST, CSIR, NBE, MCI etc.

He has authored five books and 80 chapters and published more than 350 articles in National & International journals. Further, he was selected as a member of various central government committees (GOI) and central government funding agencies: in the IND committee, FDC Committee, Compensation Committee, Sub-committee of Drug Regulation, Amendment Committee, Central Working Group Committee for Pharmacovigilance (PvPI), Signal Preview Committee, Member of Biologic Task Force DGCI-DBT committee, Member of GCP inspection team DCGI, Core Training Panel Committee Pharmacovigilance (PvPI), National Formulary Committee (NFI)–IPC, Chairman selection Committee for TA (IPC), Special Invitee for national Advisory board of Hemovigilance programme, Special Invitee for Central Ethics Committee ICMR, member of the committee for evaluation of Spurious Drugs, antimicrobial evaluation committee (ICMR). Basic Medical Sciences Project evaluation Committee (ICMR), HCG Vaccine Committee (ICMR), Member of Apex Technical committee for ICMR institute, Core member for Committee ICMR-NIREH Bhopal, member of ICMR funding to CDRI, Special Invitee - TB Task Force, DBT Task Force member, the Expert member for anti-doping (NADA) and member of Expert group NADA, National Board Examination (NBE), Senate and selection committee member for NIPER, Member of Board of studies of Panjab University, Chandigarh, Working as GLP inspector for GLP monitoring authority (DST, New Delhi), member of Technical committee Department of Health Research (DHR), Ministry of health etc.

Abbreviations

AAHRPP: Association for the Accreditation of Human Research Protection Program

ADME: Absorption Distribution Metabolism Excretion

ADR: Adverse Drug Reaction

AEFI: Adverse Event Following Immunization

AI: Artificial Intelligence

AMS: Accelerator Mass Spectrometry

ANDA: Abbreviated New Drug Application

ASU: Ayurveda, Siddha and Unani

ATC: Anatomical Therapeutic Chemical

AV: Audio Visual

BA: Bioavailability

BE: Bioequivalence

BLA: Biologic License Application

CAPA: Corrective Action and Preventive Action

CDASH: Clinical Data Acquisitions Standards Harmonization

CDER: Center for Drug Evaluation and Research

CDISC: Clinical Data Interchange Standards Consortium

CDL: Central Drugs Laboratory

CDM: Clinical Data Management

CDSCO: Central Drug Standard Control Organization

CFR: Code of Federal Regulations

CIOMS: Council for International Organizations of Medical Sciences

COI: Conflict of Interest

COPE: Committee on Publication Ethics

CPU: Clinical Pharmacology Unit

CRC: Clinical Research Coordinator

CRF: Case Report Form

CRO: Contract Research Organization

CSIR: Council of Scientific and Industrial Research

CT: Clinical Trial

CTCAE: Common Terminology Criteria for Adverse Event

CTD: Common Technical Document

CTRI : Clinical Trial Registry of India

CTS: Clinical Trial Simulation

D & C Act: Drugs and Cosmetics Act

DBT: Department of Biotechnology

DCC: Drugs Consultative Committee

DCG(I): Drug Controller General of India

DDD: Defined Daily Dose

DEC: Designated Ethics Committee

DGFT : Directorate General of Foreign Trade

DGHS: Director General of Health Services

DLT: Dose Limiting Toxicity

DMC: Data Monitoring Committee

DPCO: Drugs Prices Control Order

DRC: Dose Response Curve

DSMB: Data and Safety Monitoring Board

DTAB: Drug Technical Advisory Board

DUR: Drug Utilization Research

EC: Ethics Committee

eCRF: electronic Case Report Form

EDC: Electronic Data Capture

e-IC: electronic Informed Consent

EMA: European Medicines Agency

EMEA: European Medicines Evaluation Agency

EU: European Union

ES cell: Embryonic Stem Cell

FDA: Food and Drug Administration

FERCAP: Forum for Ethics Review Committee in Asia Pacific

FERCI: Forum for Ethics Review Committee in India

FIH: First in Human

GATT: General Agreement on Tariffs and Trade

GCP : Good Clinical Practice

GCTs: Global Clinical Trials

GDP: Good Documentation Practices

GDMP: Good Data Management Practice

GEAC: Genetic Engineering Approval Committee

GLP: Good Laboratory Practice

GMP: Good Manufacturing Practice

GRP: Good Review Practice

HED: Human Equivalent Dose

IB: Investigator's Brochure

IBSC: Institutional Bio Safety Committee

ICD: Informed Consent Document

ICF: Informed Consent Form

ICH: International Conference on Harmonization

ICMJE: International Committee of Medical Journal Editors

ICMR: Indian Council of Medical Research

IC-SCR: Institutional Committee for Stem Cell Research

ICSR: Individual Case Safety Report

IEC: Institutional Ethics Committee

IMP: Investigational Medicinal Product

IND: Investigational New Drug

IndEC: Independent Ethics Committee

IP: Indian Pharmacopoeia

IPC: Indian Pharmacopoeia Commission

IPR: Intellectual Property Rights

iPS cell: induced Pluripotent Stem Cell

IRB: Institutional Review Board

ITT: Intention to Treat

IVRS: Interactive Voice Response System

LAR: Legally Acceptable Representative

LD: Lethal Dose

LOAEL: Lowest Observed Adverse Effect Level

MABEL: Minimal Anticipated Biological Effect Llevel

MAD: Multiple Ascending Dose

MAH: Marketing Authorization Holder

MBDD: Model Based Drug Development

MCCT: Multi Centric Clinical Trial

MDAC: Medical Devices Advisory Committee

MedDRA: Medical Dictionary for Regulatory Authorities

MONARCSi s: MOdified NARanjo Causality Scale for ICSRs

MoHFW: Ministry of Health and Family Welfare

MRSD: Maximum Recommended Starting Dose

MTD: Maximum Tolerated Dose

NABH: National Accreditation Board for Hospitals and Healthcare Providers

NAC-SCRT: National Apex Committee for Stem Cell Research and Therapy

NCE: New Chemical Entity

NDA: New Drug Application

NDAC: New Drug Advisory Committees

NFI: National Formulary of India .

NLEM: National List of Essential Medicines

NME: New Molecular Entity

NOAEL: No Observed Adverse Effect Level

NOEL: No Observed Effect Level

NPPA: National Pharmaceutical Pricing Authority

PBRER: Periodic Benefit Risk Evaluation Report

PD: Pharmacodynamics

PDD: Prescribed Daily Dose

PDUFA: Prescription Drug User Fee Act

PEC: Participating center Ethics Committee

PEM: Prescription Event Monitoring

PET: Positron Emission Tomography

PGDE: Pharmacologically Guided Dose Escalation

PI: Principal Investigator

PK: Pharmacokinetics

PMS: Post Marketing Surveillance

PRO: Patient-Reported Outcome

PSUR: Periodic Safety Update Report

PV: Pharmacovigilance

QA: Quality Assurance

QC: Quality Control

QMS: Quality Management System

R & D: Research & Development

RCGM: Review Committee on Genetic Manipulation

RCT: Randomized Clinical Trial

r-DNA: recombinant Deoxyribonucleic Acid

RECIST: Response Evaluation Criteria in Solid Tumors

RP2D: Recommended Phase 2 Dose

SAD: Single Ascending Dose

SAE: Serious Adverse Event

SAR: Structure Activity Relationship

SEC: Subject Expert Committee

SIDCER: Strategic Initiative for Developing Capacity in Ethical Review

SLA: State Licensing Authorities

SOP: Standard Operating Procedures

SSCs: Somatic Stem Cells

SUSAR: Suspected Unexpected Serious Adverse Reaction

TEAE: Treatment Emergent Adverse Event

TRIPS: Trade Related aspects of Intellectual Property Rights

UMC: Uppsala Monitoring Centre

VAS: Visual Analog Scale

WTO: World Trade Organization

SECTION – A

DRUG DEVELOPMENT: RECENT ADVANCES

CONTENTS

CHAPTER 1

Newer Paradigms in Drug Development

OVERVIEW

Introduction
Approaches to Drug Discovery
Critical Path Initiative
Modeling and Simulation
    Pharmacometrics
    Model Based Drug Development (MBDD)
    Clinical Trial Simulation (CTS)
    Quantitative Pharmacology

Identification and Validation of New Biomarkers
    Pharmacometabolomics
    Toxicogenomics
Streamlining Clinical Trials
Clinical Trial Modernization
Artificial Intelligence in Clinical Trials

INTRODUCTION

Drug discovery is the process of identifying a new drug molecule from the library of various drug candidates screened. After a new drug molecule is discovered, it undergoes various stages of preclinical and clinical testing to become a commercial drug product, this process is called drug development. Huge costs ranging from $ 150 million to several billion are spent to bring a new drug to market. Average time in developing a new drug that reaches market ranges from 10-15 years. Apart from being increasingly expensive and time consuming, pharmaceutical innovation is highly inefficient. Of the total 10,000 candidate compounds screened, only 1 drug molecule succeeds in reaching the market (Figure 1.1). Hence it becomes extremely important for different phases of drug development to be executed in an efficient and effective way to reduce high attrition rates.

APPROACHES TO DRUG DISCOVERY

In ancient times, most drugs were discovered ***serendipitously*** as an observation of potential of certain plant extracts or chemicals to exert physiological or functional alterations in animals

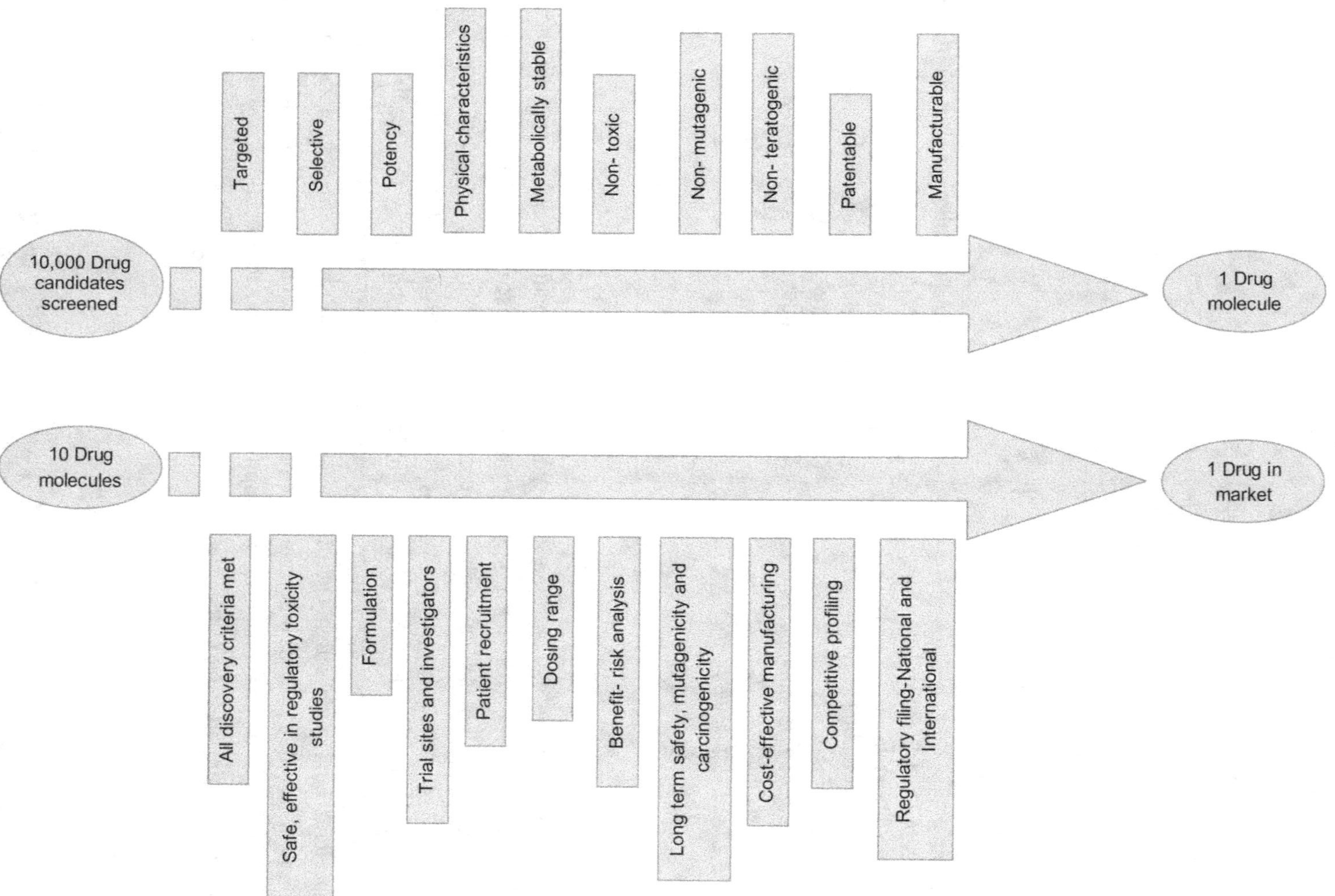

Figure 1.1 Drug discovery and development process.

or humans. Later came the era of ***classical or forward pharmacology***, also called phenotypic drug discovery (PDD). In classical pharmacology, the process of drug discovery moved from functional studies to repeated screenings, towards genomic research (i.e. drug to gene). Various steps involved in classical pharmacology have been outlined in Figure 1.2.

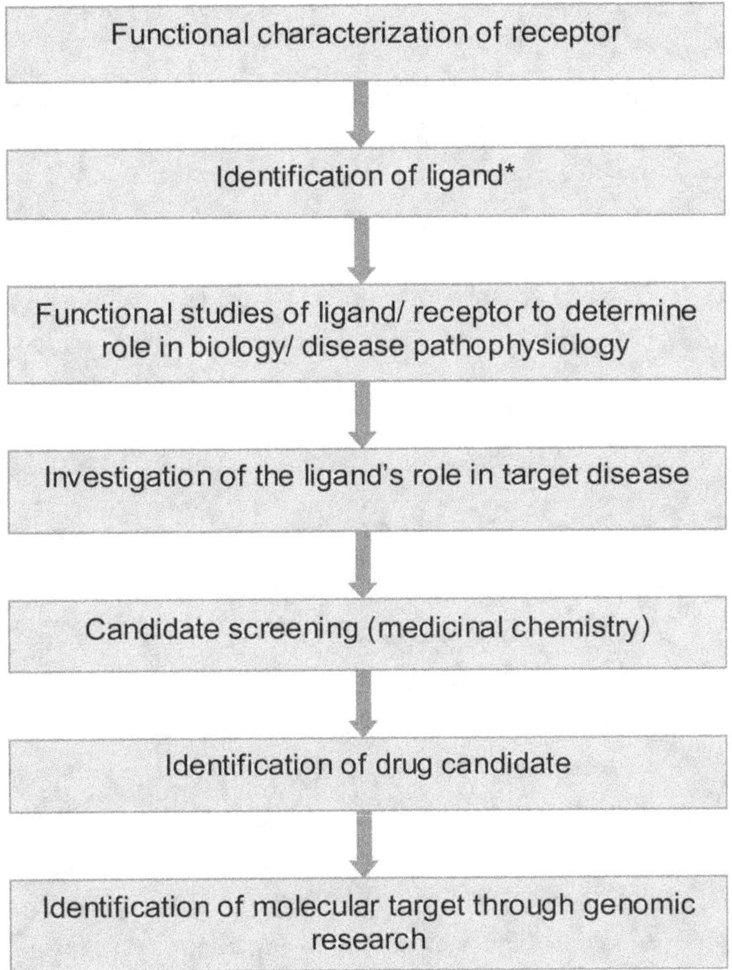

Figure 1.2 Drug discovery steps in classical or forward pharmacology.

*Approaches for ligand identification: (1) *random screening for biological activity of natural sources,* (plants, animals, minerals, microorganisms), *libraries of previously discovered chemical entities, peptides, nucleic acids or other organic molecules*; (2) *random or targeted chemical synthesis* like synthesizing chemical analogues of natural or synthetic compounds having well- defined pharmacological activity; (3) *rational designing of a new drug molecule on the basis of biologic mechanisms and structure of receptor* e.g. computer-assisted design (CAD), combinatorial chemistry, QSAR (Quantitative structure activity relationship) analysis, molecular modeling, biotechnology etc.

Figure 1.3 illustrates an example of the discovery of tamsulosin by classical approach.

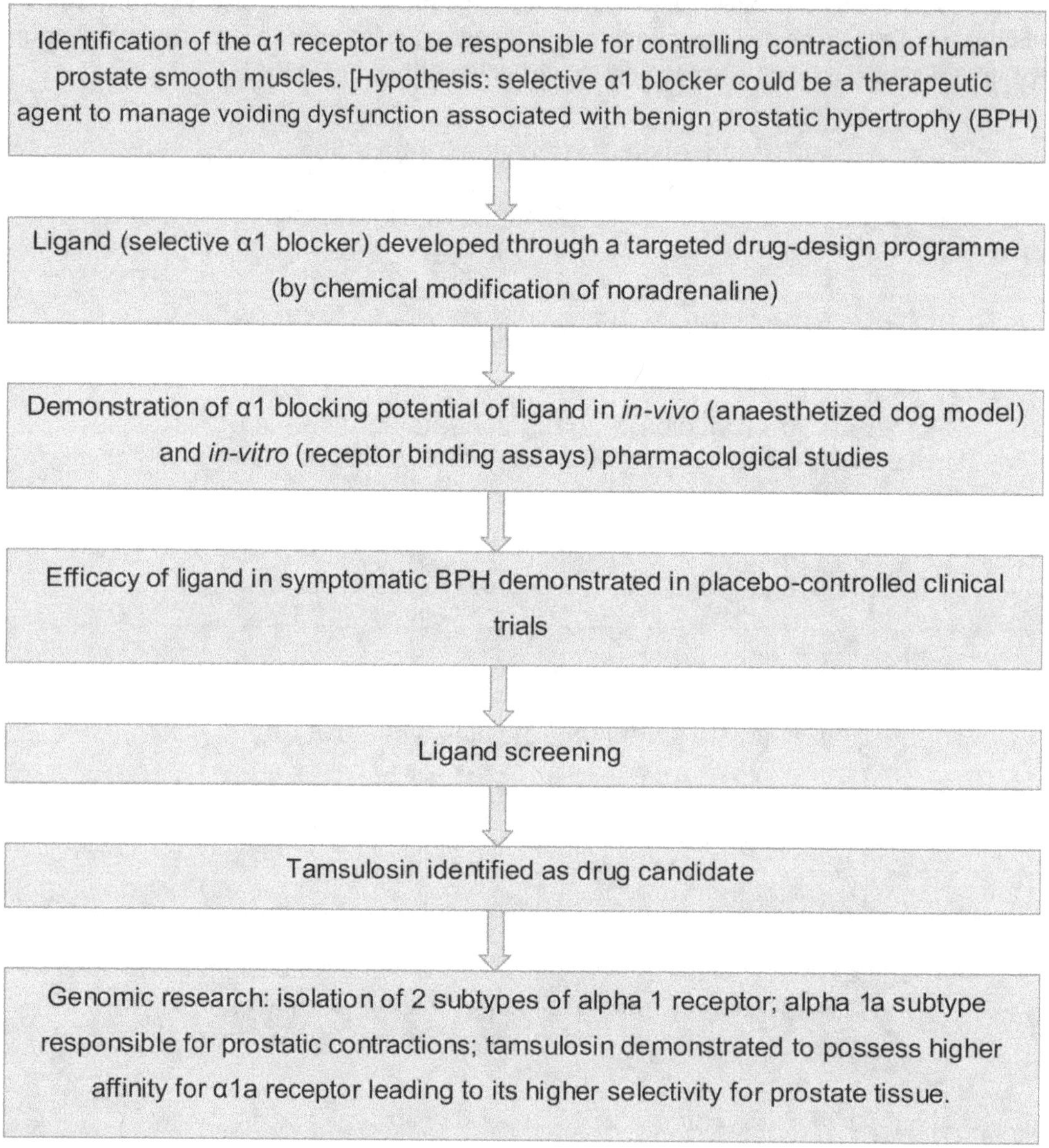

Identification of the α1 receptor to be responsible for controlling contraction of human prostate smooth muscles. [Hypothesis: selective α1 blocker could be a therapeutic agent to manage voiding dysfunction associated with benign prostatic hypertrophy (BPH)

↓

Ligand (selective α1 blocker) developed through a targeted drug-design programme (by chemical modification of noradrenaline)

↓

Demonstration of α1 blocking potential of ligand in *in-vivo* (anaesthetized dog model) and *in-vitro* (receptor binding assays) pharmacological studies

↓

Efficacy of ligand in symptomatic BPH demonstrated in placebo-controlled clinical trials

↓

Ligand screening

↓

Tamsulosin identified as drug candidate

↓

Genomic research: isolation of 2 subtypes of alpha 1 receptor; alpha 1a subtype responsible for prostatic contractions; tamsulosin demonstrated to possess higher affinity for α1a receptor leading to its higher selectivity for prostate tissue.

Figure 1.3 History of discovery of tamsulosin by classical pharmacology approach.

Nowadays, most of the drug discovery is carried out by ***reverse pharmacology***, also called target based drug discovery (TDD). In reverse pharmacology, drug discovery process starts with genomic research followed by repeated screenings and finally functional studies (i.e. gene to drug). The stepwise approach followed in reverse pharmacology is depicted in figure 1.4.

Understanding the disease patho-physiology and mechanisms involved

↓

Bioinformatics/ Molecular genetics: Identification of proteins/ genes responsible for disease causation as potential targets for drugs i.e. *Target identification*

↓

Validation of targets i.e. confirming the actual involvement of potential targets in disease causation and checking their ability to bind to drug/s

↓

Identification of hits: High throughput screening (HTS)* of compound libraries against the purified protein target to identify hits (compound/s having the greatest potential to successfully interact with the potential target).

↓

Hit to lead: Evaluation of hits (in various assays for target selectivity, physical/chemical properties, ADME, in vitro efficacy and with respect to predicted ease of synthesis, cost, scalability, potency, ability to create and protect intellectual property etc.) to identify leads

↓

Lead optimization: series of complex steps (*in vivo* efficacy assays, functional studies, ADME, physical/chemical assays) to improve the druggability of identified leads

↓

Candidate seeking: further evaluation of safety (cytotoxicity assays), ADME, formulation liabilities etc. to identify the candidate/s for formal preclinical and clinical development

Figure 1.4 Steps in the process of drug discovery by reverse pharmacology.

*High throughput screening (HTS): HTS is the process by which large compound libraries are screened for activity against biological targets by means of automation, miniaturized assays, automated robotic techniques and highly sensitive detectors. A key component of HTS is micro-titer plate with 96 (or multiples of 96) wells containing test items. Compared to conventional screening methods, HTS has been demonstrated to be 1,000 times faster and utilizing 1 millionth cost allowing efficient and less time consuming screening.

Drug discovery through reverse pharmacology approach takes about 2-3 years on an average which is time effective as compared to classical pharmacology approach which usually takes more than 5 years to discover a new drug molecule.

CRITICAL PATH INITIATIVE

"Critical Path Initiative" was launched by the US Food and Drug Administration (FDA) in 2004 with an aim to enhance the efficiency of drug development process by the adoption of certain modern scientific technologies. Critical Path has been defined as the whole process of new drug molecule identification and its development through various stages till it is launched as a therapeutically active drug product (Figure 1.5).

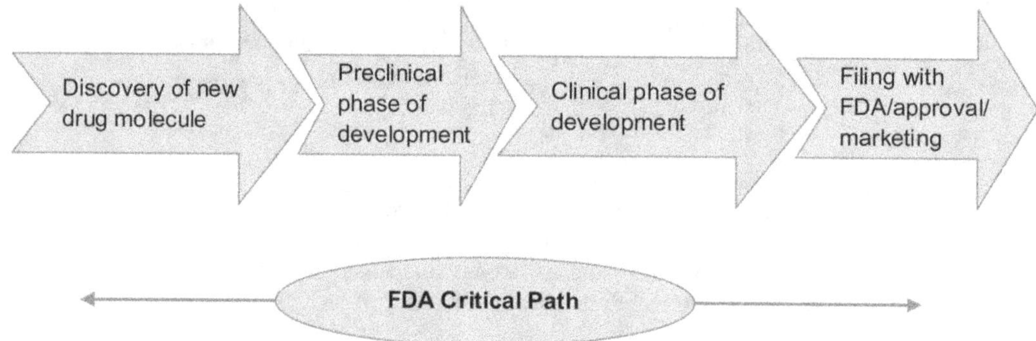

Figure 1.5 The FDA Critical Path for development of new medicinal products.

During its path to marketing, a new candidate drug emerging out of the drug discovery phase has to go through rigorous series of evaluations for its potential efficacy and safety. Besides, it should also be amenable to production on a large scale. Figure 1.6 represents various activities in different dimensions which need to be successfully completed along the critical path.

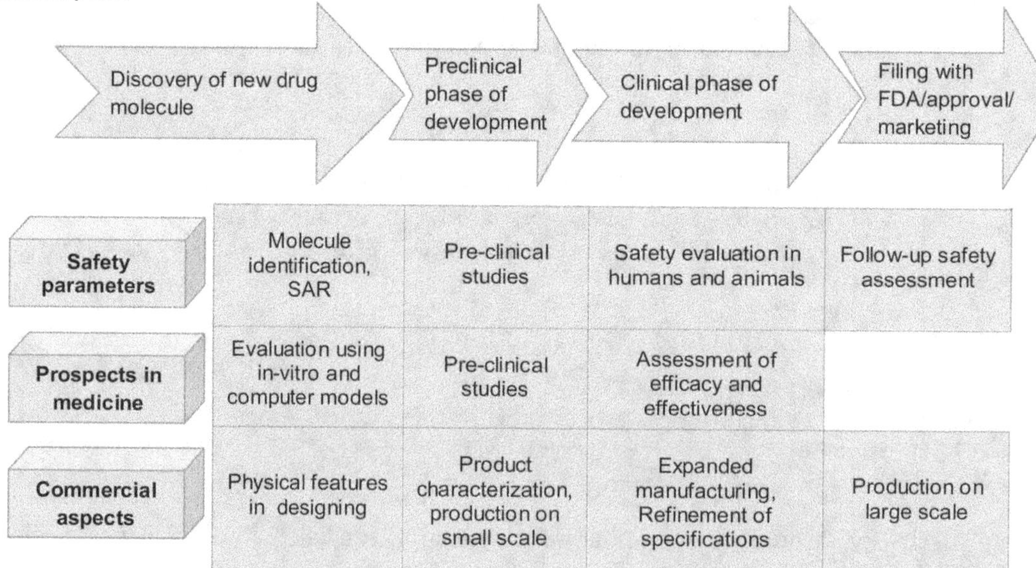

Figure 1.6. Activities in three dimensions in the Critical Path (SAR: Structure Activity Relationship).

Various strategies described in FDA Critical Path Initiative which can be incorporated during the drug development process include:

❖ Novel strategies like modeling and simulation.

❖ Identification and validation of new biomarkers.

❖ Streamlining clinical trials.

❖ Embracing adaptive designs in clinical trials. (For detailed discussion on adaptive designs, kindly refer to the chapter on "Designs used in clinical trials").

❖ Clinical trial modernization.

MODELING AND SIMULATION

As addressed in the critical path initiative, adoption of model-based approaches has great potential in increasing the efficiency of drug development process. Modeling is the process of building mathematical constructs/models by using available data, information and knowledge to describe the aspects of a system. Simulation is building upon these models by incorporating random variability in an attempt to understand its long-term impact.

Uses of modeling and simulation

❖ The advanced developments in the field of modeling and simulation are helpful in determining a dose and dosage regimen which attains the desired clinical benefit and has minimal disagreeable side effects. In this context, biological and pharmacological modeling are usually applied. *Biological modeling* is the application of various genetic, biochemical, physiological and pathological processes involved in the underlying disease condition and its pharmacotherapy. *Pharmacological modeling* provides guidance on clinical trial design, appropriate dose selection and drug development approach. An example of a case scenario using modeling for dose regimen selection is given in box 1.1.

❖ Modeling and simulation techniques can be applied to understand the dose and time relationship of efficacy and toxicity endpoints.

❖ Combined with Bayesian methods, these techniques have been extremely helpful in providing a persistent surge of knowledge across various drug development phases. For instance, the data from preclinical studies can be utilized to build models and predict clinical parameters in advance.

❖ Modeling also enables the utilization of external information to determine variables of interest in the population. For instance, values of safety parameters at baseline from data can be incorporated with information from external sources to increase the efficiency of detection of safety signals.

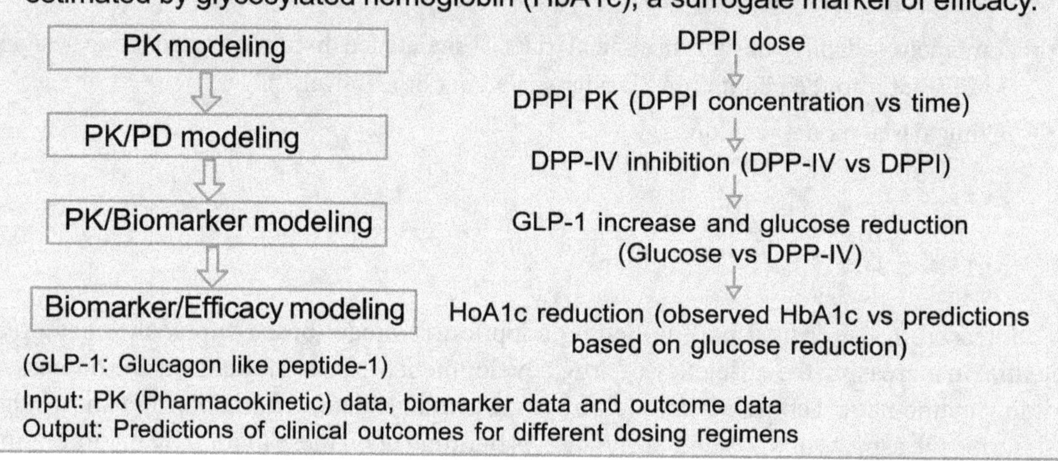

Modeling and simulation hold crucial importance in various stages of the drug development process (Table 1.1).

Table 1.1 Role of modeling and simulation in different stages of drug development.

Preclinical development

- Development of mechanism based models
- Evaluation of potency, efficacy and intrinsic activity in -vivo
- Compartmental modeling
- Development of biomarkers/ surrogates and pre-clinical models for efficacy and safety parameters
- Refinement of dosage form and dosage regimen
- Extrapolation of data from preclinical studies to humans
- Allometric scaling

Clinical development

- Selection of initial dose /dose escalation
- Description of dose-concentration-response relationships
- Evaluation of dosage forms and administration pathways
- In vivo estimation of active metabolites
- Study food effects, gender based effects
- Drug-drug/ drug-disease interactions
- Evaluation of drug analogues
- Disease progression models
- Population PK/PD
- Simulations to predict PK/PD
- Trial forecasting
- Post marketing PK/PD

PHARMACOMETRICS

This is the scientific discipline which relies on the application of mathematical models built on the basis of disease, biology, pathophysiology, and pharmacology for quantification of various interactions between pharmacological therapies and patients. Different models in pharmacometrics on the basis of their application include "exposure–response models," "disease models," "trial execution models" etc.

Pharmacokinetic–Pharmacodynamic Modeling (PK–PD modeling) or Exposure–Response Modeling

This approach is based on mathematical models linking the drug's pharmacokinetics (PK) i.e. concentration-time relationship to its pharmacodynamics (PD) i.e. relationship between effective concentration at target site and magnitude of effect. The integrated PK-PD models, thus obtained, provide an illustration of the entire time course of the effect intensity after administration of a given dosing regimen. Many softwares are available for PK-PD modeling e.g. Phoenix, Winnolin, Pmetrics, etc.

Translational PK-PD modeling

This approach employs the integration of data from in-silico, in vitro, and animal or in-vivo preclinical studies with models constructed on the basis of mechanism to predict the effects of new therapies in humans and across various biological levels (Figure 1.7). Such translational models have various applications in drug development process like identification of lead molecules and their optimization, estimation of starting dose for first in man studies, selection of designs of exploratory and proof-of-concept clinical trials of new drugs and their combinations.

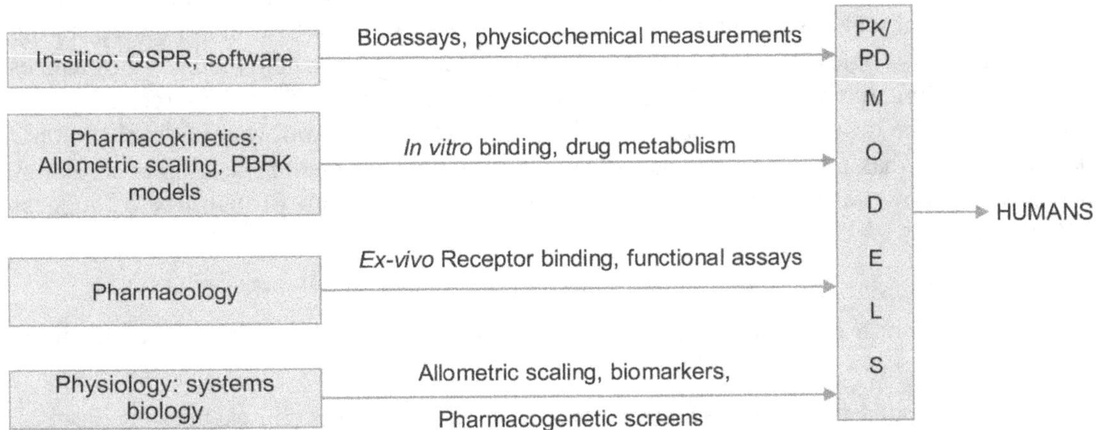

Figure 1.7 Components of PK-PD models for translating pre-clinical data to clinical pharmacology data (QSPR- Quantitative structure PK/PD relationships; PBPK-Physiologically based pharmacokinetic).

MODEL BASED DRUG DEVELOPMENT (MBDD)

It is defined as the development and implementation of pharmacological and statistical models from preclinical and clinical data to predict efficacy and safety of pharmacological interventions with an aim to enhance decision-making in the drug development process. MBDD employs the integration of mathematical as well as statistical approaches to build, validate and apply drug exposure-response and pharmacometric models along with disease models to enhance the quality and efficiency of drug development program.

MBDD is a relatively newer concept embracing the whole drug development process from discovery of a new molecule to its launch as a commercial product. It involves model-based data analysis and simulation at discrete isolated events throughout the development process. MBDD provides a data-driven model framework enhancing the meticulous establishment of a scientific knowledgebase by means of continuously integrating knowledge gained through the development program, and serving as a valuable decision-making tool.

Traditional vs. Model Based Drug Development

As discussed previously, the traditional/ conventional process of drug development makes use of modeling and simulations through different phases of drug development; hence it can be termed as "model- aided drug development". However, the concept of MBDD is quite distinct. Table 1.2 enlists the key differences between model-aided and model-based drug development.

CLINICAL TRIAL SIMULATION (CTS)

CTS is the utilization of simulation techniques like Monte-Carlo simulation in drug development program with an aim to increase the probability of getting favorable results in clinical trials. CTS makes it possible to test varying scenarios simultaneously, predicting potential end results for each and finally choosing the most suitable study design. Prior to study conduct, testing different methodologies by means of such simulation techniques can help increase the chances of success in clinical trials. It also facilitates pooling of data from different sources like prior studies with same drug and external data which may serve as an informative tool to attain superior decision-making. Hence, simulation plays important role in guiding development strategy by clarifying how various study designs influence outcome and probability of success (Table 1.3).

Challenges for CTS

- ✓ Relatively new concept; there is a need for good understanding of the concept and its uses.
- ✓ Requires extensive trainings for pharmacokineticists as well as clinical pharmacologists.
- ✓ Need to educate the pharmaceutical community regarding the applications and limitations of simulation.
- ✓ Willingness of pharmaceutical industry to adopt and consider simulation technology as a component of drug development process.

Table 1.2 Comparison of model-aided drug development with model based drug development.

Model aided drug development	Model based drug development
Models are largely empirical	Both empirical and mechanistic models are developed and applied
Model function formats are driven by observed trend in data	Function formats are elucidated by underlying treatment, disease condition and pathophysiological mechanisms involved
Difficulties in linking models across experiments, response types, developmental stage and compounds	Models include a good knowledge, data and scientific background from various applicable aspects and are regularly upgraded.
Model quality is restricted by data quality and quantity	Rich prior knowledge alleviates the dependence on data quality and quanity
Limited predictability for future studies	Predictability is the major parameter for model's performance
Models are mostly developed in PK/PD during late stages of drug development	Models in different disciplines are developed at various preclinical and clinical development stages of drug development
Models (PK/PD) are used for quantifying response levels in exposure, biomarkers & end points, sources of variation and covariate effects.	Models are used for characterizing candidate attributes, disease mechanisms, competitor knowledge and trial management strategies.
Models are used to confirm decisions	Models facilitate quantitative decisions
The focus of models is on few individual attributes.	Models reflect all known attributes
Models generally do not influence the decision making process.	Models are developed prospectively and are a necessity for decision making

Table 1.3 Applications of Clinical Trial Simulations in various phases of drug development.

Phase I

♦ Estimation of starting/ initial dose for administration in humans

♦ Prediction of pharmacokinetic parameters in multiple-dose study from data of single-dose study

♦ Influence of any drug interactions on pharmacodynamics and pharmacokinetic parameters

♦ Potential effect of renal and/or hepatic disorder on pharmacodynamics and pharmacokinetic parameters

Phase II/III

♦ Dose selection for Phase II/III trials

♦ Estimation of number of subjects required to attain an acceptable power

♦ Dosage required to achieve therapeutic concentration at target site

♦ Choice of statistical test to achieve maximum power under test conditions

♦ Differentiation of alternative clinical trial designs

Phase IV

♦ Comparability of drug to other competing products in market

♦ Influence of any drug interactions on pharmacodynamics and pharmacokinetic parameters

- ✓ Need to have superior biomarkers/ surrogates for drug effect.
- ✓ Depends on a good background knowledge of the link between pharmacokinetics and pharmacodynamics.
- ✓ Better understanding of compliance patterns.
- ✓ Doubtful financial benefit.
- ✓ Cost effectiveness of techniques and beneficial results not guaranteed.

QUANTITATIVE PHARMACOLOGY

This is a multidisciplinary avenue in drug development program which depends on the collaboration of associations between pathological disorder, attributes of pharmacological treatment, and individual variation in response across different drug developmental phases. It involves a continual quantitative integration of data through different phases of drug development.

IDENTIFICATION AND VALIDATION OF NEW BIOMARKERS

The development of newer biomarkers has been identified as one of the highest priorities in the field of drug development. Various innovative technologies like genomics, proteomics, metabolomics, gene expression assays using animal or whole cell systems and advanced imaging methods bear huge potential for developing new biomarkers which can have utility in reflecting the health or disease state at molecular level. These technologies can also be used to compare the effects of new drug candidate to other drugs in its class or other groups of drugs used for similar indications. The newer biomarkers are particularly helpful in improving diagnosis, defining subsets of disease showing differences in response to treatment, defining individual variations in the drug targets at molecular level, and predicting drug response at an early stage. For example, molecular assays employing assessment of target status within tumor cells can be exploited to anticipate response to a targeted molecule like transtuzumab, imatinib etc. In this context, the role of upcoming technologies like metabolomics and toxicogenomics in drug development has been discussed below.

PHARMACOMETABOLOMICS

Metabolomics (metabonomics) is the quantitative measurement of how the living systems respond dynamically to multiple parameters including external stimuli or genetic modification. It studies all small molecular metabolites (whether intermediates and/or obtained as final products of various cellular processes) present in cells, tissues, or organs and hence provides a detailed overview of the metabolic state of an individual.

Pharmacometabolomics, initially termed "Pharmacometabonomics" is defined as the process of predicting a drug's or xenobiotic's outcome (e.g. efficacy or safety) in an individual on the basis of a mathematical model using metabolite signatures prior to intervention. It is a novel approach combining the application of chemo-metrics and metabolite profiling to create models and predict various parameters like drug targets, pharmacodynamics, pharmacokinetics and toxicity on individual as well as population basis.

Pharmacometabolomics complements proteomic, genomic, transcriptomic and epigenomic "systems biology" approaches to new drug development and helps in an extensive and comprehensive understanding of effects of drugs by keeping into consideration both intrinsic (e.g. age, gender, genetic makeup, ethnicity) and extrinsic (e.g. environment factors like diet, lifestyle, use of other medications, gut microbiome) factors determining interindividual variation in drug response (Figure 1.8).

Pharmacometabolomics provides a constructive and economical approach to assess drug efficacy and toxicity and might prove to be instrumental in making personalized medicine practical and realistic from scientific as well as financial perspectives.

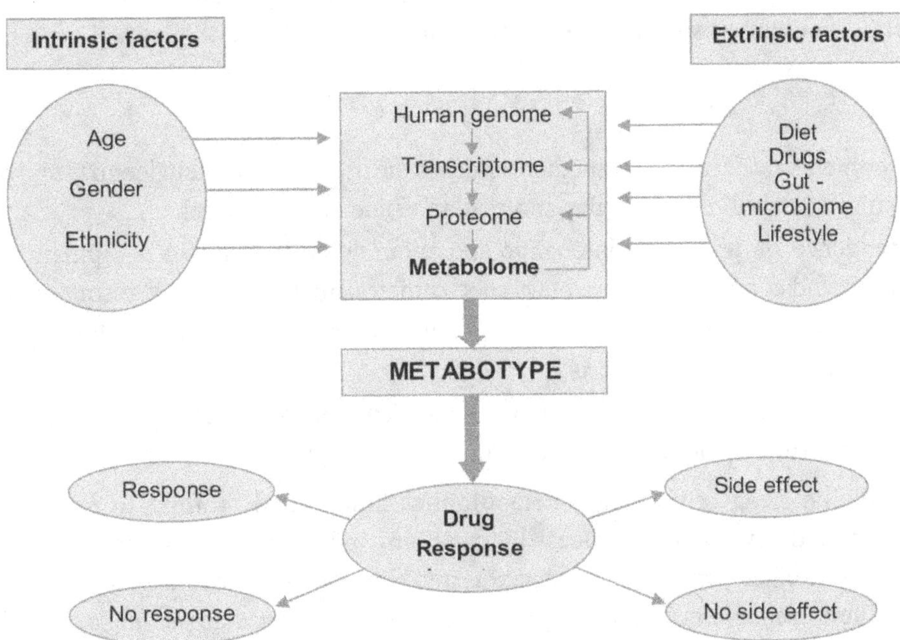

Figure 1.8 Pharmacometabolomic approach for drug response phenotyping.

Role of Pharmacometabolomics in drug development

- *Reducing inter-individual variation in clinical trials: Metabolic profiling to evaluate response phenotype.*

In clinical drug development, the major role of pharmacometabolomics is to reduce inter-individual variability in response to therapy by differentiating patients into responder or non-responder groups. Pharmacometabolomics identifies various characteristics of response to drug or xenobiotic interventions on the basis of individual's metabotype. The "metabotype" is the entirety of person's characteristics which govern disease heterogeneity and response to therapy. In addition to reflecting the individual's constitution and disease impact, it also takes into consideration the product of exposure to environmental factors and effects of any concurrent or past treatments that have influenced the organism. Metabotype, hence, provides a distinctive and holistic profiling of an individual's constitution. Metabotype signatures at baseline (prior to drug exposure) and post exposure to therapeutic intervention can have potential applications in defining mechanisms involved in producing variation in therapeutic response.

♦ *Prediction of therapeutic outcomes: identification of biomarkers*

A major advantage of pharmacometabolomics is a quicker, more reliable and efficient prediction of therapeutic outcomes. This application relies on successful identification and utilization of metabolomic components as intermediate biomarkers or surrogate end points of long term or delayed clinical outcomes such as toxicity, remission, mortality etc.

Challenges for Pharmacometabolomics

- The cornerstone of pharmacometabolomics is the need to accurately identify and quantify the small metabolites at cellular, molecular, tissue or organ level.
- Dependence on proper maintenance and accurate calibration of equipments used in analyses and computations e.g. mass spectrometry, nuclear magnetic resonance (NMR).
- In order to confirm the results of pharmacometabolomics, there should be large enough sample size of selected cohorts.
- Special emphasis needs to be given to the statistical methodologies to avoid false positive/ negative results in metabolomics and allied experiments.

Despite the challenges, pharmacometabolomics holds great promise to improve future drug discovery and development process by providing individual-specific information about drug efficacy and toxicity, revealing new insights into pharmacokinetics and pharmacodynamics, discovery of new biomarkers, identifying novel therapeutic targets and playing a critical role in the movement towards personalized medicine.

TOXICOGENOMICS

Toxicogenomics is the discipline that studies relationship between the structure and function of genome (the cellular complement of genes) and undesired biological effects of exogenously administered agents. Toxicogenomics, as a new risk assessment tool during the drug development program, can prove to be strongly instrumental in increasing our knowledge of the molecular mechanisms (gene and protein expression) and DNA polymorphisms involved in the manifestation of efficacy and toxicity of xenobiotics,

The major principle behind toxicogenomics (TGx) is that "compounds having identical toxicity mechanisms and consequences should perturb the transcriptome in a similar manner and these perturbations could be exploited to serve as biomarkers predicting downstream toxicity outcome." Figure 1.9 shows a flowchart explaining the concept of toxicogenomics.

Genetic response to external factors

Gene and protein expression show discrete responses to environmental/ external stimulants such as disease states or exposure to xenobiotics; a better understanding of biological/ physiological systems and how they respond to toxic insults is facilitated by corresponding 'genomics' and 'proteomics' technologies

↓

Transcriptomes - gene expression signature or fingerprint

Transcripts that are modified as a response to xenobiotic exposure, demonstrate a peculiar 'gene expression profile' or 'fingerprint' or 'molecular signature' of the xenobiotic effect

↓

Predictive biomarkers of efficacy or toxicity outcome

The characteristic 'gene expression profile' or 'molecular signature' serves as a potential biomarker for diagnosing or predicting xenobiotic's effect or toxicity

↓

Predictive Toxicology- Gene expression profiling (by DNA microarray technology) for prediction of toxicity of unknown compounds

Recognition of gene expression profiles associated with toxicity and speculating the toxic potential of new compounds by contrasting their gene-expression profiles with molecular signatures of known, related compounds (reference/model compounds with well-characterized pharmacological and toxicity endpoints).

↓

Mechanistic Toxicology- hypothesis generation on underlying mechanisms of toxicity

Assessment of modifications in gene expression profiles after exposure to drugs can be helpful in understanding the mechanisms of toxicity especially for compounds not having standard, validated biomarkers or not altering the morphology significantly

Figure 1.9 The concept of Toxicogenomics.

TGx is the unique combination of conventional toxicology with emerging "omics" technologies like genomics and bioinformatics. For the implementation of TGx as a predictive tool, it is absolutely essential to have a prior knowledge of patterns of gene expression involved in manifestation of toxicity. Hence, this approach hinges on the accessibility of a standard gene expression database.

The application of global gene expression analysis in TGx has provided considerable quantity of data on already recognized toxicants like hepatotoxins in animal models, allowed classification of compounds according to their mechanism of toxicity and helped in understanding cellular pathways involved in activation of macrophages, proliferation of peroxisomes, causation of oxidative stress or formation of reactive metabolites etc. In recent times, the applications TGx have expanded to evaluate the nephrotoxic, genotoxic and testicular toxicity potential of compounds as well.

Advantages of Toxicogenomics

- TGx serves as a substantial tool for classifying compounds and for detecting novel, functional, responsive and specific markers for the toxicity mechanisms under consideration.

- Higher sensitivity of toxicogenomics (gene expression profiling and predictive biomarkers) than the conventional toxic endpoints, thereby increasing the clinical prediction of toxicity.

- Enables the rapid development of newer compounds with good safety profile while bringing down the cost involved and need for animal experiments.

- Gene expression analysis techniques, by enhancing our knowledge of the molecular mechanisms leading to toxicity, provide a deeper understanding of species-specific factors responsible for response to drugs. This will in turn facilitate a more accurate extrapolation of data across species e.g extrapolation of disease conditions in man from observations in animals.

Challenges for Toxicogenomics

- Technical validation i.e. issues like data comparability and use of standardized methods. For this, various areas like quality control, gene annotations, and data analysis need to be carefully addressed.

- Questionable significance of the findings in biological and toxicological fields due to lack of clear knowledge of any relationship between gene expression and causation of dose-dependent toxicity at present.

- Inability to predict the idiosyncratic adverse drug events.

However, appropriate utilization of toxicogenomics, along with current technologies like proteomics and metabolomics could offer a huge competitive advantage to drug discovery and development industry.

STREAMLINING CLINICAL TRIALS

One of the major critical path priority for the FDA as well as other stakeholders is streamlining and improving the predictive value of clinical trials. The strategies recommended for streamlining the clinical trials include:

- ✓ Design, use and interpretation of active controlled trials, i.e. trials designed to show that a product candidate is not inferior to an existing treatment (rather than superior to placebo as in traditional trial design).

- ✓ Need for transparent rules on deciding the time points to make amendment/s in clinical trial protocol on the basis of results from early or interim data.

- ✓ Application of adequate statistical techniques to increase the reliability of pre-clinical data.

- ✓ Appropriate approaches to handle missing data from subjects lost to follow up.

- ✓ Better methods for evaluating multiple end-points in a single trial.

- ✓ Development of consensus trial designs for specific therapeutic areas.

- ✓ Enhancing the methodologies to measure drug responses in subjects e.g. evaluation of pain and other subjective endpoints.

- ✓ Standardization of forms and methods for recording and reporting clinical trials data.

CLINICAL TRIAL MODERNIZATION

This area as included in critical path initiative comprises

- ❖ Establishment of standard guidelines for handling and managing the data in clinical trials. In this context, the Clinical Data Interchange Standards Consortium (CDISC) has contributed significantly in standardizing the data management. An initiative of CDISC called Clinical Data Acquisitions Standards Harmonization (CDASH) is actively involved in this process and has laid standards for drafting case report forms.

- ❖ Use of automatic techniques during the process of clinical trials and data management;

- ❖ Enhancing the quality management systems;

- ❖ Implementation of modern technologies to facilitate oversight of the trial process by regulatory authorities.

ARTIFICIAL INTELLIGENCE IN CLINICAL TRIALS

Artificial Intelligence (AI), also called machine intelligence, is the ability of a machine or computer or computer- controlled robot to imitate intelligent human behavior such as speech recognition, statistical learning, image processing, translation between languages, processing natural languages, motion and manipulation, pattern recognition, decision-making etc. In other words, it is mechanical intelligence in contrast to natural intelligence exhibited by man and other animals.

The goal of AI is to develop systems and softwares which can function independently and intelligently like human brain. Crucial elements for AI are:

- huge amounts of data,
- advanced algorithms, and
- high performance processors

AI has become an integral component of many industries e.g. automotives (driverless cars), video games, military (lethal autonomous weapons) etc.

Applications of AI in clinical trials

Artificial intelligence and allied technologies e.g. machine learning (ML) and natural language processing (NLP) are increasingly making their way into clinical trials. The existing applications of AI and emerging technologies in clinical trials include:

Patient recruitment. A major challenge faced by clinical trial industry is patient recruitment. It is reported that around 80 percent trials fail in meeting the recruitment timelines while one third of Phase 3 trials are terminated due to recruitment challenges. Also. patients are unable to find appropriate clinical trials in the absence of recommendations from physicians and difficulty in navigating the clinical trial databases (e.g. clinicaltrials.gov).

AI can help address this issue by extracting pertinent information from medical records and comparing it to the inclusion/ exclusion criteria of ongoing trials, thus identifying more effectively and efficiently the appropriate patients for enrollment.

Clinical trial design. AI algorithms and deep learning techniques can help in designing protocols making the clinical trials more intelligent in a number of ways:

- Analyzing historical operational data
- Measuring drug responses
- Predicting site performance
- Monitoring trial risks preemptively
- Centralized trial monitoring
- Enabling voice assisted technologies
- Enabling virtual trials
- Monitoring adherence to therapy
- Providing additional predictive data to determine outcomes, patient drop out etc.

Applying these AI driven techniques and predictive algorithms, risks associated with trials can be mitigated well in advance which would be helpful to enhance the clinical trials success rates.

Clinical trial optimization. The AI-machine learning (ML) models can prove to be helpful in predicting which patients are at risk of dropping out of clinical trials by utilizing the real world evidence (RWE) from medical claims, prescription and other data. This would allow the clinical personnel to intervene and take appropriate steps to preserve trial validity.

Patient centric clinical trial designs. AI-enabled trial management technologies like digital reporting applications, wearable devices, telehealth, smart phone applications etc. are changing the conduct of clinical trials in a number of ways:

- patients can send feedback on their symptoms and manage intake of medications.
- patients can share information with researchers reducing the frequency of visits to trial sites.
- create opportunities for patients to respond immediately to symptomatic or biometric changes.
- automatic and continuous communication of patient- specific trial data to investigators and clinical trial databases etc; this in turn ensures data integrity by eradicating delays in transfer, eliminating transcription errors and reducing the incomplete/missing data.

Hence, such patient centric clinical trial designs allow real time engagement of patients in their own care which in turn can profoundly benefit in improving patient adherence and persistence in trials.

Table 1.4 enlists some AI softwares along with their applications.

Table 1.4 Examples of various AI softwares and their applications.	
Name of software	**Applications**
Antidote (2010) London, England	*Patient recruitment*: uses machine learning (ML) to connect patients to medical research studies through its clinical trial matching platform
Deep 6 AI (2015) Pasadena, California	*Patient recruitment*: uses natural language processing (NLP) to better match patients to clinical trials
Trials.AI (2015) San Diego, California	*Clinical trial design*: uses NLP to help researchers manage clinical trial workflows in an efficient manner
Bullfrog AI (2017) Annapolis, Maryland	*Clinical trial design*: uses platforms which conduct data mining to identify correlations and patterns with large, complex data and generates predictive models
Brite health (2015) Palo Alto, California	*Clinical trial optimization*: uses an algorithm trained on millions of clinical data points; identifies the key markers correlating with patient

Hence, AI offers potential in solving many major challenges encountered by clinical trial industry by assisting and augmenting human intelligence, maximizing patient recruitment and retention, leveraging data, improving clinical trial designs, making predictions of trends, risks and outcomes etc. By improving data quality, reducing trial durations and cutting sky- rocketing costs of developing new drugs, AI can accelerate new drug development. AI applications hold huge promise in dramatically shortening the time to market life saving drugs.

CONTENTS

CHAPTER 2

International Drug Regulations

OVERVIEW

Introduction
The Food and Drug Administration (FDA): Drug Regulatory Authority in USA
Responsibilities of FDA
History of Evolution of Drug Regulations in US
Organization of FDA
Code of Federal Regulations (CFR)
Types of Drug Applications Submitted to FDA
Prescription Drug User Fee Act (PDUFA)
Good Review Practice (GRP)

Procedures for Early/Expanded Access to Unapproved INDs
Expedited Programs for NDA under US-FDA
European Medicines Agency (EMA): Drug Regulatory Agency in European Union
Organization of EMA
Ministry of Health, Labour and Welfare (MHLW): Drug Regulatory Agency in Japan
International Council for Harmonization (ICH)
Common Technical Document (CTD)
Council for International Organizations of Medical Sciences (CIOMS)

INTRODUCTION

Drug regulatory authority/ agency is any government agency/public authority comprising of experts from scientific and administrative background and having the authority to regulate drug research and use.

Table 2.1 enlists the names of various drug regulatory authorities functioning in different countries.

Table 2.1 Various drug regulatory authorities worldwide.

Country/Region	Name of the drug regulatory authority
USA	The Food and Drug Administration (FDA)
Europe	European Medicines Agency (EMA)
UK	Medicines and Healthcare Products Regulatory Agency (MHRA)
Australia	Therapeutic Goods Administration (TGA)
India	Central Drug Standard Control Organization (CDSCO)
Japan	Ministry of Health, Labour and Welfare (MHLW), Pharmaceuticals and Medical Devices (PMDA)
Canada	Therapeutic Products Directorate (TPD), Health Canada
Switzerland	Swiss Agency for Therapeutic Products (Swiss medic)
Russia	Ministry of Health of the Russian Federation

Principal functions of a Drug Regulatory authority (Figure 2.1).

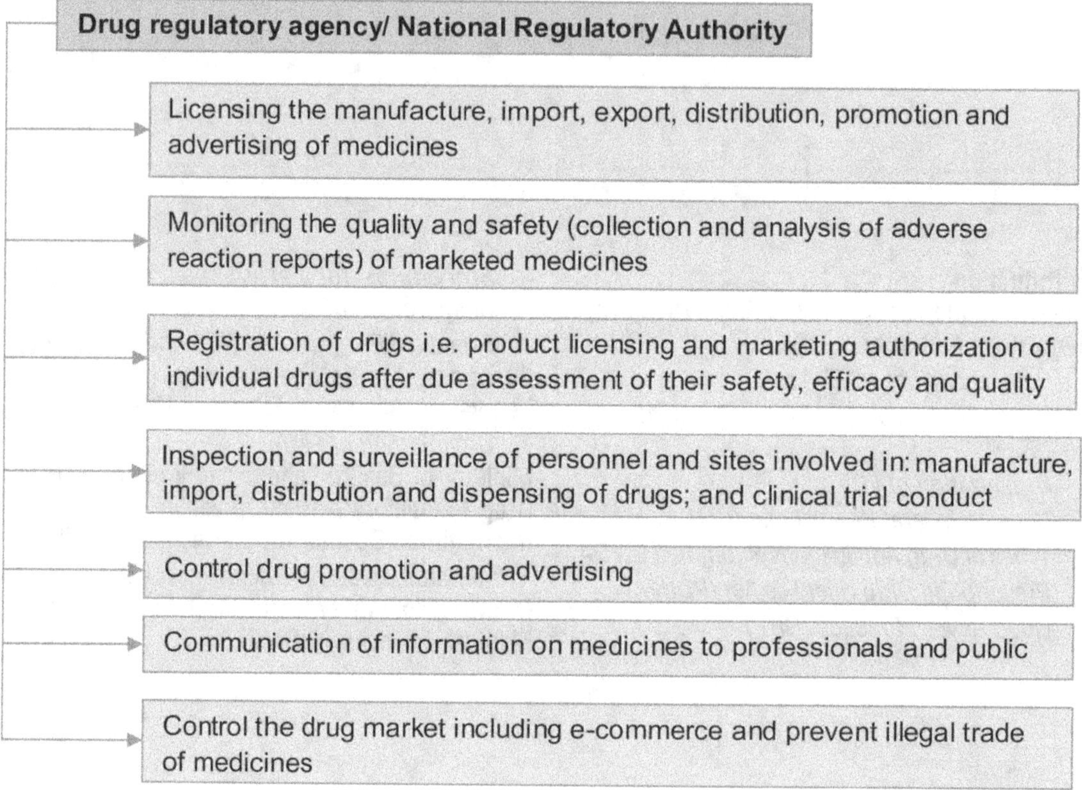

Figure 2.1 Principal functions of a Drug Regulatory authority.

THE FOOD AND DRUG ADMINISTRATION (FDA): DRUG REGULATORY AGENCY IN USA

The Food and Drug Administration (FDA) is a regulatory body within the U.S. Department of Health and Human Services and has its headquarters at Silver Spring, Maryland.

RESPONSIBILITIES OF FDA

- Safeguarding the public health by ensuring that food products are safe, wholesome, clean and appropriately labeled; drugs intended for use in humans and animals, and vaccines, other biological products and medical devices intended for human use are safe and effective;
- Assuring the protection of public from electronic product radiation;
- Ensuring safety and proper labeling of cosmetics and dietary supplements;

- Regulating tobacco products;
- Promoting public health by encouraging the development of new and advanced products.

HISTORY OF EVOLUTION OF DRUG REGULATIONS IN US

Figure 2.2 depicts various milestones in the history of drug regulations in US.

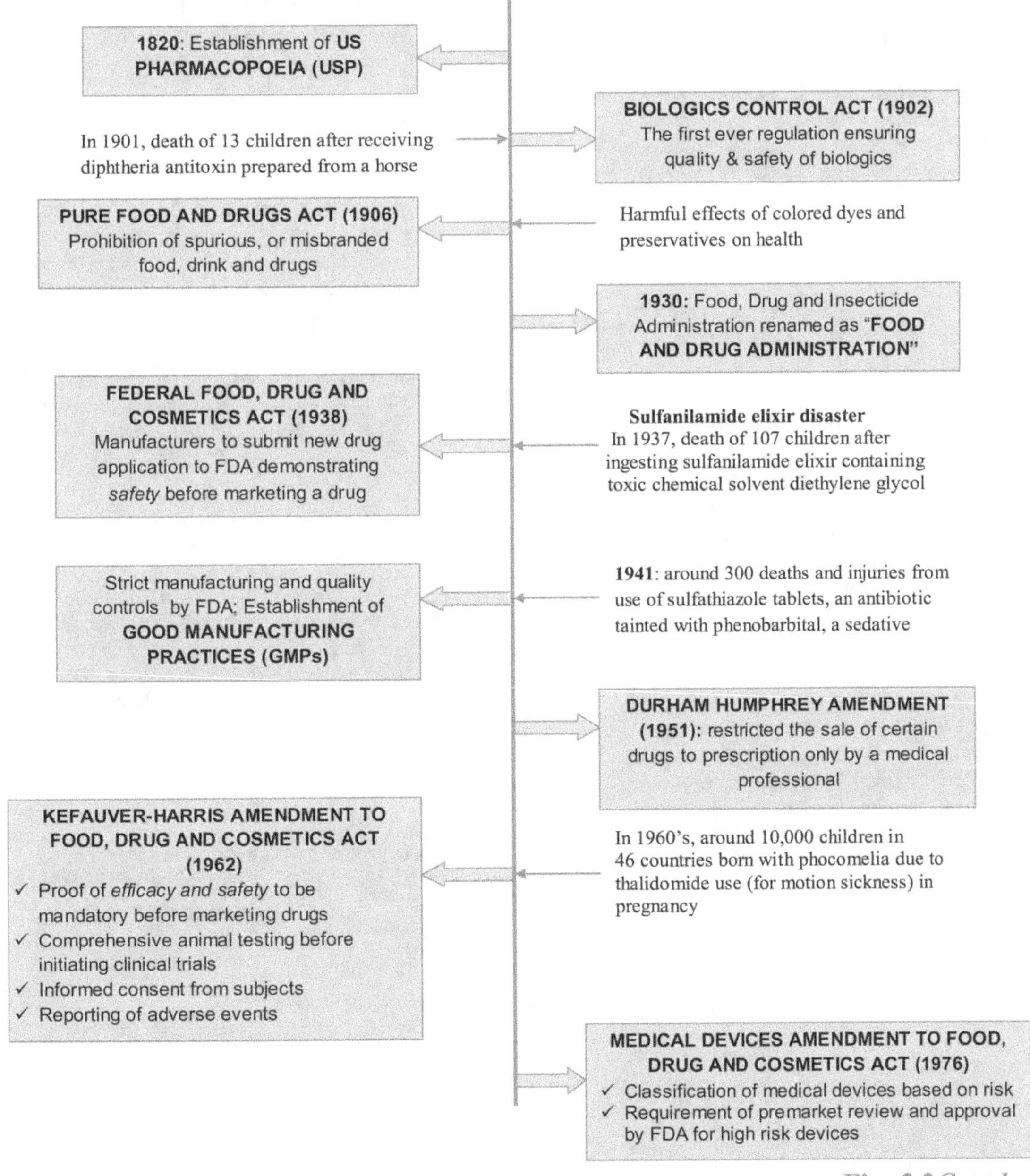

Fig. 2.2Contd...

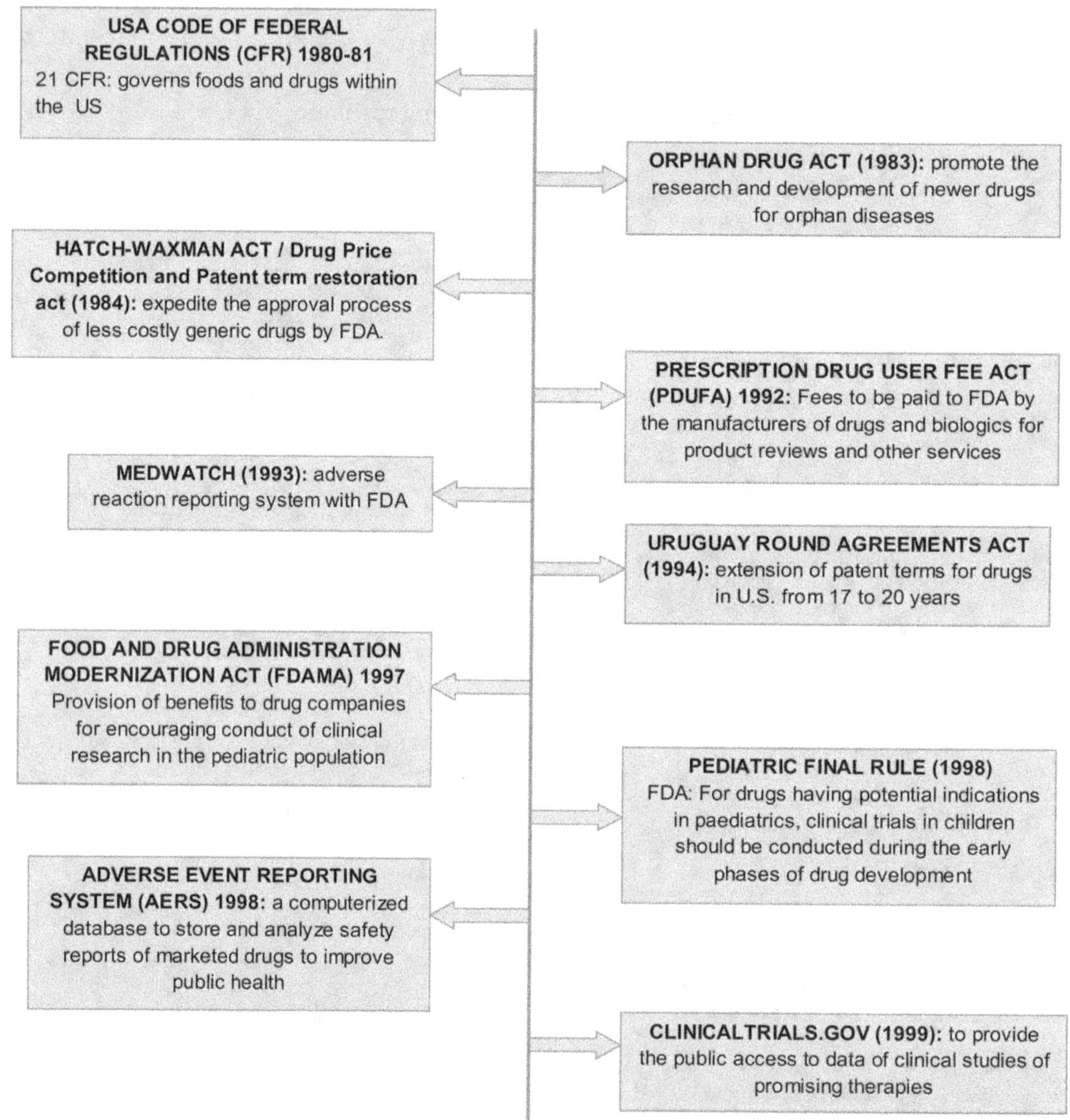

Figure 2.2 Important milestones in the history of drug regulations in US.

ORGANIZATION OF FDA (FIGURE 2.3)

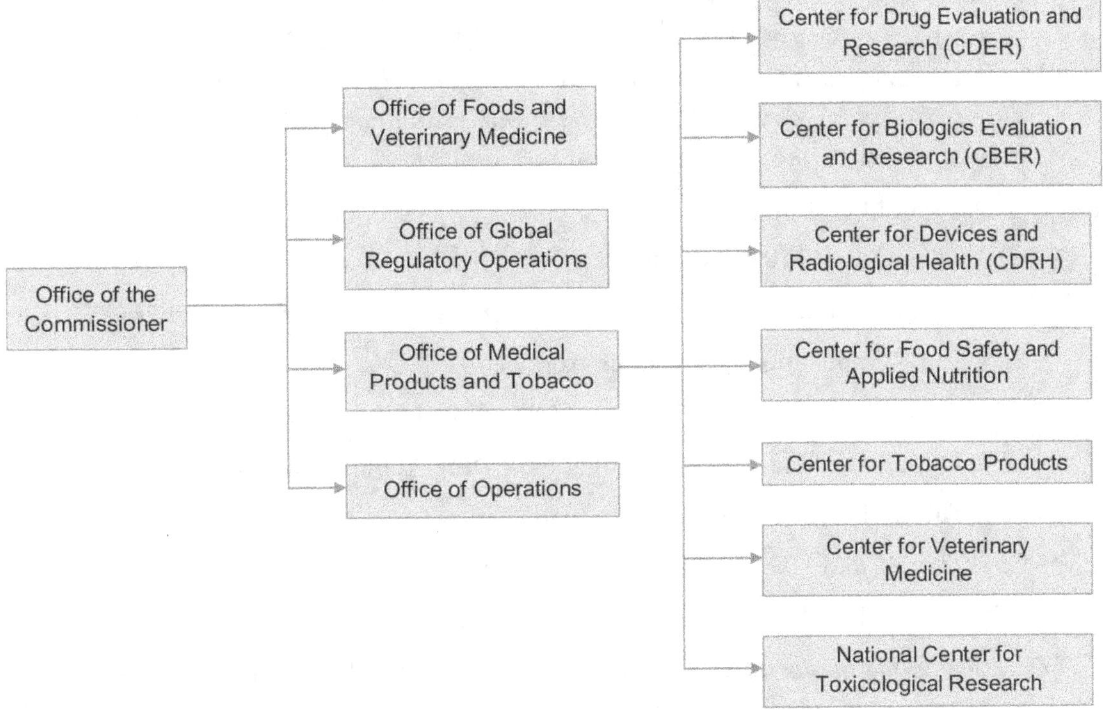

Figure 2.3 Organization of FDA.

The ***Center for Drug Evaluation and Research (CDER)*** is the chief office in the FDA for handling drugs from IND to NDA evaluation for approving or rejecting marketing authorization of the product. It also evaluates safety information of the products during post marketing period. There are more than 20 offices in CDER focusing on different areas including biotechnology, new drug evaluation, pediatric drug development, generic drugs, compliance and drug safety. In 2005, the FDA established the new *Drug Safety Oversight Board (DSB)*, which renders advice to the CDER on issues related to drug safety.

CODE OF FEDERAL REGULATIONS (CFR)

The ***Code of Federal Regulations (CFR)*** is the set of general rules and regulations published in the Federal Register by the executive agencies of the federal government of the United States. ***Title 21*** of CFR governs food and drugs within the United States. It is divided into three chapters and 1499 parts-

- Chapter I: Food and Drug Administration, (Parts 1-1299)

- Chapter II: Drug Enforcement Administration, department of justice (Parts 1300-1399)-*combating drug smuggling and use within the United States.*
- Chapter III: Office of National Drug Control Policy (Parts 1400 to 1499)-*establish policies, priorities, and objectives to eradicate illicit drug use, manufacturing, and trafficking, drug-related crime and violence, and drug-related health consequences in the U.S.*

Important parts of title 21 include:

- ◆ CFR Title 21 Part 310 New drugs
- ◆ CFR Title 21 Part 314 - Applications for FDA approval to market a new drug

  Subpart B - Applications (New Drug Application: NDA)

  Subpart C - Abbreviated Applications (Abbreviated New Drug Application: ANDA)
- ◆ CFR Title 21 Part 312 - Investigational New Drug Application (IND)
- ◆ CFR Title 21 Part 600 Biological products
- ◆ CFR Title 21 Part 803 - Medical device reporting
- ◆ CFR Title 21 Part 11 - Electronic records; electronic signatures

FDA issues **guidance documents** on various topics like clinical trials, biologics, combination products, drugs, food, medical devices, tobacco products etc. which contain the FDA's preferences on laws and regulations and reflect the FDA's opinion on a particular area.

TYPES OF DRUG APPLICATIONS SUBMITTED TO FDA

- Investigational New Drug (IND)
- New Drug Application (NDA)
- Abbreviated New Drug Application (ANDA): containing the data for review and approval of generic drug products.
- Biologic License Application (BLA): comprised of pertinent information regarding the synthesis, chemical structure, pharmacological and clinical pharmacological aspects and the efficacy of biological products.
- Drug applications for over-the-counter drugs

Various steps involved in the review of a new drug molecule by US FDA and its approval are shown in Figure 2.4.

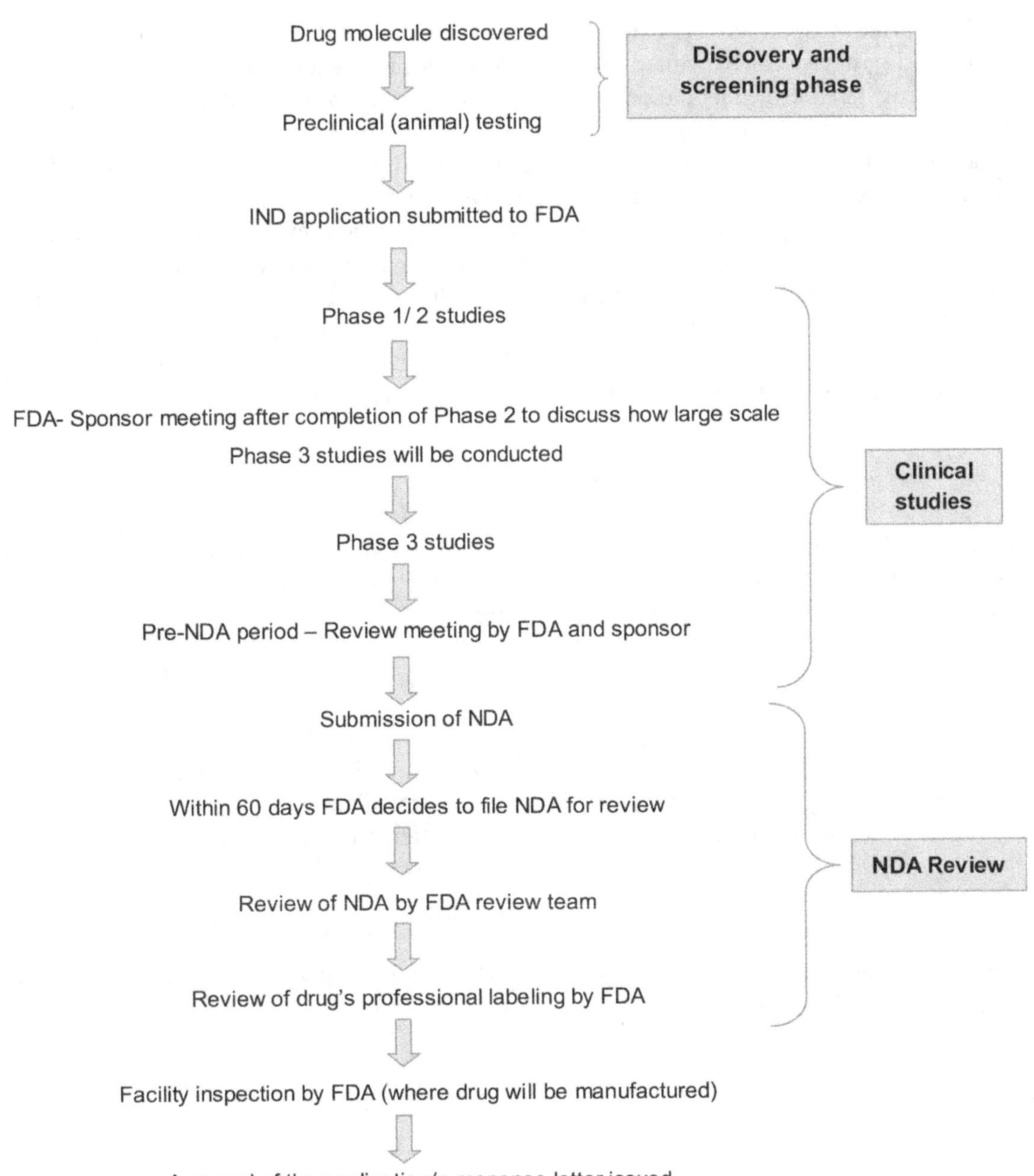

Figure 2.4 Drug review and approval process at US FDA.

Abbreviated New Drug Application (ANDA)

The Drug price competition and Patent term restoration act 1984 (Hatch-Waxman Act) under Section 505 (j) devised an expedited approval process for lower cost generic drugs i.e. ANDA. Generic drugs are defined as the ones which are analogous to innovator or reference listed drug as defined in FDA Orange book enlisting approved drug products with demonstrated therapeutic equivalence. As per the act, pharmaceutical companies manufacturing generic drugs need to submit an ANDA to the regulatory authorities for getting marketing approval. The applications for generic drugs approval are termed as "abbreviated" due to abbreviated or lesser data requirements as compared to NDA approval process e.g. no need to conduct repeated testing of drugs in preclinical and clinical studies as the reference or branded drugs have already been tested and approved for safety and efficacy. The generic drugs must, however, demonstrate bioequivalence with the reference listed drug. Generic drugs are manufactured after the expiry of patent and other exclusivity rights.

PRESCRIPTION DRUG USER FEE ACT (PDUFA)

Under this, the drug manufacturing companies pay fees to FDA in order to boost the FDA's resources and facilitate timely review of applications. PDUFA has enabled faster access to new drugs while maintaining the same review process.

GOOD REVIEW PRACTICE (GRP)

It is defined as the "documented best practice" discussing the various aspects pertaining to the procedure, design, content, conduct and management of a product review. The main aim of GRP is to assure quality reviews and improve the standards of review management.

PROCEDURES FOR EARLY/EXPANDED ACCESS TO UNAPPROVED INDS

Various provisions under FDA to facilitate an early or expanded access to unapproved INDs are described in detail in box 2.1.

> ## Box 2.1 US FDA Procedures for early/expanded access to unapproved INDs.
>
> **EMERGENCY IND.** It is the use of an unapproved investigational drug or biologic in emergency situation. The routine process for obtaining it is by contacting the manufacturer and determining the availability of drug or biologic for emergency use under the manufacturer's IND. Under such circumstances, FDA may allow shipment of test drug prior to IND submission.
>
> Emergency use IND is applied by treating physician. There is no need to obtain prior approval from IRB, however, the physician should notify the IRB within a period of 5 working days after using test drug (*As per USFDA regulations, there is no provision for expedited IRB/IEC approval under emergency circumstances*).
>
> It is mandatory to obtain informed consent of the subject/ patient or his legally authorized representative (LAR). However, in certain circumstances the need to obtain informed consent can be waived off provided the investigator or treating physician certify that:
>
> - the subject/ patient is suffering from a life-threatening condition mandating the administration of test article;
> - legally effective informed consent could not be taken because communication with subject was not possible;
> - insufficient time for obtaining informed consent from the subject's LAR;
> - non-availability of an alternative proven therapy having equal or greater efficacy in decreasing mortality in the concerned condition.
>
> **TREATMENT IND.** This is a means of making available investigational drugs to subjects suffering from serious and life-threatening conditions having no alternative/ approved treatments with proven efficacy. A treatment IND may be permitted on the basis of data demonstrating the drug to be effective and having no undesirable risks.
>
> Requirements to be fulfilled before issuing a treatment IND:
>
> - the drug is indicated in a serious or life-threatening illness;
> - there is non- availability of a proven efficacious alternative therapy;
> - the drug is being investigated, or clinical phases of drug development have been completed and
> - the pharmaceutical company is seeking regulatory approval for launching the drug.
>
> Treatment IND requires IRB review in advance and informed consent. Treatment INDs are for pharmaceutical companies and are not covered by insurance companies

Box 2.1 Contd...

COMPASSIONATE USE IND (EXPANDED ACCESS IND). This is the use of an investigational medicinal product beyond the purview of a clinical trial (i.e. not yet approved by USFDA). This provision allows an expanded access of investigational drug in subjects/ patients who could not be included in a clinical trial (owing to reasons like non-eligibility, or no ongoing trials evaluating the investigational drug) but for whom the treating physician holds opinion that the drug may be beneficial in improving morbidity/ mortality. Expanded access can be made under three categories:

♦ for individual patients,

♦ for medium-size patient populations, and

♦ for extensive general use.

CONTINUED ACCESS IND. USFDA may grant permission to continue recruitment of subjects after the completion of controlled clinical trial to enable access to the investigational drug while the marketing application is under preparation by the pharmaceutical company or under review by FDA.

EXPEDITED PROGRAMS FOR NDA UNDER US-FDA

Fast track designation. This is granted for
- a drug indicated for a serious disease condition AND
- the drug is assumed to potentially address unmet clinical need based on its preclinical and clinical data.

Breakthrough therapy designation. This is applicable in cases where
- a drug is indicated for a serious disease condition AND
- drug has the potential to show significantly greater beneficial effect on a clinical endpoint/s over existing treatments based on preliminary clinical data.

Priority review designation. This is granted for
- a drug intended for treating a serious disease condition AND
- the drug on approval would offer a substantial improvement in efficacy and safety clinically.

In the three expedited programs mentioned above, the FDA needs to respond within 60 calendar days of receipt of the application.

Accelerated approval pathway. This is considered in cases where
- a drug is intended to treat a serious condition AND
- usually offers a therapeutic benefit over existing treatments AND
- affects a biomarker or surrogate end point in a manner that likely correlates with clinical end point which can be evaluated at an earlier point of time than irreversible morbidity or mortality (IMM) and which apparently correlates with effect on IMM or other clinical benefit (i.e. an intermediate clinical endpoint)

The timeline for FDA response is not specified in this program.

Generating Antibiotic Incentives Now (GAIN). Under this program, there is provision to grant incentives to the pharmaceutical manufacturers developing antibacterial and antifungal drugs indicated for serious and life threatening infections. In this program, a drug on fulfilling certain predefined criteria is designated as a *qualified infectious disease product (QIDP),* which then becomes entitled for fast track designation and priority review.

A comprehensive guidance document released by FDA in 2014 describes in details the features of each of these four expedited programs for NDA (Guidance for Industry. Expedited Programs for Serious Conditions – Drugs and Biologics. Available at

http:// www.fda.gov/downloads/drugs/guidance compliance regulatoryinformation/guidances/ucm358301.pdf).

EUROPEAN MEDICINES AGENCY (EMA): DRUG REGULATORY AGENCY IN EUROPEAN UNION

European Medicines Evaluation Agency (EMEA) was created in 1995 which was later renamed as European Medicines Agency (EMA) in 2004.

The major role of EMA is to safeguard human and animal health by means of the evaluation and supervision of drug products throughout the European Union. The EMA regulates medicinal products for human and veterinary use (but not food, unlike the FDA).

ORGANIZATION OF EMA

EMA, headed by the Executive Director has seven scientific committees and a number of working groups which manage the scientific tasks of the Agency.
- CHMP: Committee for medicinal products for human use, formerly Committee for Proprietary Medicinal Products (CPMP)
- PRAC: Pharmacovigilance risk assessment committee
- CVMP: Committee for medical products for veterinary use
- COMP: Committee for orphan medical products
- HMPC: Committee for herbal medical products
- PDCO: Pediatric committee
- CAT: Committee for advanced therapies

The CHMP plays a pivotal part in regulating drugs in the European Union (EU). It is also accountable for various post-approval pursuits like any variations (extensions or withdrawl) to an existing marketing authorisation. Additionally, along with its groups, CHMP contributes to the development of drugs and their regulation, by:
- offering *advice on scientific matters* to pharmaceutical companies involved in research and development of new drugs;

- drafting *scientific guidelines and regulatory guidance* to guide pharmaceutical companies in preparing marketing authorisation applications for human medicines;
- collaborate with *international organizations* for coordinating various regulatory requirements.

MINISTRY OF HEALTH, LABOUR AND WELFARE (MHLW): DRUG REGULATORY AGENCY IN JAPAN

The drug regulatory agency in Japan, MHLW, was set up by the merger of Ministry of Labour and Ministry of Health and Welfare (MHW) in 2001. The major tasks of the agency are promotion and safeguard of general public health, social welfare and social security. The major policy areas under the agency are:

- Health and medical care
- Children and child bearing
- Long term care, health and welfare services
- Employment security, labour
- Pension
- Other policy areas like international affairs, war victim's relief, budget.

The organization comprises of ministry proper, affiliated institutions, councils, regional and external bureaus.

In the Ministry, ***Pharmaceutical Safety and Environmental Health Bureau*** is mainly responsible for regulating the pharmaceuticals and related products. It has various divisions like Pharmaceutical Evaluation Division, Medical Device Evaluation Division, Pharmaceutical Safety Division, Compliance and Narcotics Division, Blood and Blood Products Division, Food Safety Standards and Evaluation Division, Food Inspection and Safety Division, etc.

INTERNATIONAL COUNCIL FOR HARMONIZATION (ICH)

The International Council for Harmonization of Technical Requirements for Pharmaceuticals for Human Use (ICH), formerly the International Conference on Harmonization (ICH) was established in 1990 in Brussels at a meeting held by European Federation of Pharmaceutical Industries and Associations (EFPIA) and attended by representatives of the regulatory authorities and pharmaceutical associations of Europe, Japan and the US. The formation of the Council was an aftermath of the International Conference of Drug Regulatory Authorities (ICDRA; organized by WHO in Paris in 1989) during which the need to harmonize the requirements related to new innovative drugs was discussed.

The major goal of ICH is to attain higher coordination or harmonization internationally to ensure the development and registration of safe, efficacious and good quality drugs in the most efficient manner. For this, ICH has developed various guidelines in consensus with experts from regulatory and pharmaceutical background. These guidelines include:

Quality (Q): relating to areas like conduct of stability studies, approach to pharmaceutical quality, determining thresholds for impurities testing etc. There are 14 quality guidelines viz. Q1 to Q14 e.g.

- Q1A to Q1F: Stability
- Q4 – Q4B: Pharmacopoeias
- Q7: Good Manufacturing Practice
- Q9: Quality Risk Management.

Safety (S): aiming to uncover potential risks with the help of data generated in *in-vitro* and *in-vivo* preclinical studies. There are 12 safety guidelines viz. S1 to S12 e.g.

- S1A - S1C: Carcinogenicity studies,
- S2: Genotoxicity studies,
- S3A - S3B: Toxicokinetics and Pharmacokinetics
- S5: Reproductive toxicology
- S7A - 7B Pharmacology studies
- S8: Immunotoxicology studies

Efficacy (E): related to planning, execution and dissemination of clinical trials; also including biotechnology derived drugs and use of pharmacogenetics/ pharmacogenomics techniques. There are 18 efficacy guidelines viz. E1 to E12, E14 to E19 e.g.

- E6: Good Clinical Practice
- E8: General considerations for Clinical Trials
- E10: Choice of control group in clinical trials
- E17: Multi-regional clinical trials
- E18: Genomic sampling

Multidisciplinary (M): including overlapping areas not fitting into any of the above 3 categories. There are 11 multidisciplinary guidelines viz. M1 to M11 e.g.

- M1: MedDRA terminology
- M2: Electronic Standards for the Transfer of Regulatory Information (ESTRI)
- M4: Common Technical Document
- M8: electronic Common Technical Document (eCTD)
- M11: Clinical electronic Structured Harmonised Protocol (CeSHarP)

COMMON TECHNICAL DOCUMENT (CTD)

CTD provides a common pattern for gathering all the quality, safety and efficacy information for registration of new medicines in ICH and other countries (such as Canada, Switzerland and Australia) enabling implementation of good review practices. From July 2003, CTD is considered as the compulsory format for NDAs submitted in EU and Japan, and strongly recommended format for NDAs in US.

The CTD triangle depicts the 5 modules organized within CTD.

Module 1 (region specific): Regional administrative information   } Not part of CTD

Modules 2-5 (common to all regions).

Module 2:

- Quality overall summary
- Non- clinical overview
- Non-clinical summary
- Clinical overview
- Clinical summary

Module 3: Quality

Module 4: Non- clinical study reports

Module 5: Clinical study reports

Part of CTD

An electronic version of CTD **(eCTD)** can be produced using information from the eCTD Implementation working group.

COUNCIL FOR INTERNATIONAL ORGANISATIONS OF MEDICAL SCIENCES (CIOMS)

CIOMS is an international, non-government, non-profit organization set up jointly by WHO and UNESCO in 1949. CIOMS is mainly governed by an Executive Committee (Secretary General and his team) at the Secretariat based in Geneva, Switzerland. The main goal of CIOMS is to promote public health by means of issuing guidances on various healthcare research areas like bioethics, pharmacovigilance and medical product development.

CIOMS WORKING GROUPS

CIOMS has many specialized international working groups which publish reports on topics related to safe use of medicines, research ethics and drug development.

- CIOMS/ WHO Working group on Vaccine Pharmacovigilance.
- CIOMS VIII: CIOMS Working group on signal detection.
- CIOMS IX: CIOMS Working group on Practical considerations for development and application of a toolkit for medicinal product risk management.
- CIOMS X: CIOMS Working group on considerations for applying good meta-analysis practices to clinical data within the biopharmaceutical regulatory process.
- CIOMS Working group XI: Patient involvement in the development and safe use of medicines.
- CIOMS Working group on vaccine safety.
- CIOMS Working group on Drug induced liver injury.
- CIOMS Working group on Clinical research in resource limited settings.
- CIOMS Implementation Working group on MedDRA.
- CIOMS Working group to revise CIOMS ethical guidelines for biomedical research.

IMPORTANT LINKS

1. The Food and Drug Administration, official website https://www.fda.gov/
2. European Medicines Agency, official website https://www.ema.europa.edu
3. The International Council for Harmonization, official website https://www.ich.org/
4. CIOMS, official website https://cioms.ch/

Contents

CHAPTER 3

Evolution of Drug Regulations in India

OVERVIEW

INTRODUCTION

The history of drug regulations in India predates to pre-independence era when the manufacture of drugs in the country was almost non-existent and the drugs were mainly imported to meet

---

Box 3.1 Gigantic Quinine fraud.

In 1907, a rapid surge in the number of 'quinine failures' owing to adulteration of drug supplies was reported by Dr John Megaw in Calcutta. On testing, he discovered that the stock solutions were massively under-strength. However, despite the publication of his initial report in Indian Medical Gazette, no response was observed. Later, it was estimated that around sixty percent of quinine and cinchona products prescribed and sold in India were adulterated e.g there was deliberate substitution of quinine with less potent cinchona alkaloids, use of adulterants such as chalk and flour mixed with a cheaper antifebrile compound etc. These findings forced the Government to take actions including establishment of committees to revise British Pharmacopoeia and Drug Enquiry Committee.

---

local demands. However, due to lack of any strict legislation, qualified pharmaceutical personnel, well-equipped laboratories etc., the market was largely thronged with spurious and contaminated drugs. No control was exercised over the production, sale and distribution of drugs according to the Indian Medical Gazette (Box 3.1).

INDIAN DRUG REGULATIONS DURING 19TH AND EARLY 20TH CENTURY

Some regulations controlling the drugs in India during 19th and early 20th century were:

Indian Penal Code (IPC), 1860: Adulteration of any drug rendering it 'noxious' or 'lessening its efficacy' was punishable under the provisions of IPC.

The Opium Act, 1878: Regulated the cultivation of poppy, and the possession, manufacture, sale, transport etc. of opium.

Indian Merchandise Act, 1889: prohibited the misbranding of goods in general.

The Indian tariff Act, 1894 and **The Sea Customs Act, 1898:** concerned with providing levy of customs duty on goods including drugs, medicines, chemicals etc. imported to and exported from India.

The Poisons Act, 1919: regulated the import, possession and sale of poisons.

The Cantonment Act, 1920: The cantonment authorities were empowered to enter into any shop and seize any drug or medicine found to be 'adulterated'.

The Dangerous Drugs Act, 1920: regulated the cultivation, possession, manufacture, sale, import, export etc. of dangerous drugs like coca, hemp, opium etc.

Establishment of Drug Enquiry Committee (Chopra Committe), 1930 (Box 3.2).

Box 3.2 Drug Enquiry Committee (Chopra Committee) Report, 1931.

In August 1930, the Government of India constituted the **"Drug enquiry committee"** (**Chopra Committee**) under the chairmanship of Sir Ram Nath Chopra with an aim to:

- Enquire and check the imported, manufactured and sold drugs for their quality
- Suggest remedial measures to prevent adulteration.

Recommendations by the Drug Enquiry (Chopra) Committee in its report submitted in 1931:

- Need of a central legislation (e.g. drugs and/or pharmacy act) to control drugs and pharmacy.
- Establishment of a central biochemical standardization laboratory to test domestically manufactured and imported medicines

Box 3.2 *Contd...*

- Compilation of Indian Pharmacopoeia with monographs on commonly used drugs and pharmaceuticals
- Creation of a drug advisory board.

Major regulatory developments based on the recommendations of the Chopra Committee

1937:   '*Import of Drugs Bill*' introduced by the Government but later withdrawn due to criticism.

1940 : '*Drug Bill*' introduced to regulate the import, manufacture, sale and distribution of drugs in India during British rule; later adopted as '***Drugs Act 1940***'.

1945 : '*Drug Rules*' published under the 'Drugs Act 1940'.

1947:   1ˢᵗ April "Drugs and Cosmetics Act" came into effect.

1962 : Incorporation of Cosmetics within the purview of Drugs Act; adopted as '***Drugs and Cosmetics Act 1940***'.

1948 : ***The Pharmacy Act***

1937 : Establishment of '***Biochemical Standardization Laboratory***' at Calcutta; later renamed as 'Central Drugs Laboratory'.

1941 : Constitution of the first '***Drug Technical Advisory Board***'.

1946 : The *Indian Pharmacopoeial List*, a prelude to Indian Pharmacopoeia published as an Indian supplement to the British Pharmacopoeia 1932.

1955:   Publication of first edition of ***Indian Pharmacopoeia***.

INDIAN DRUG REGULATIONS DURING LATE 20ᵀᴴ CENTURY

Few regulations related with drugs during late 20ᵗʰ century were:

The Drug and Magic Remedies (Objectionable Advertisement) Act, 1954: regulates the advertising of drugs in India. As per the Act,

- advertisements of drugs and remedies which claim to have magical properties is prohibited and considered as a cognizable offence. Examples include drugs to induce miscarriage or prevent conception in women; to improve or maintain the capacity of humans for sexual pleasure; to correct menstrual disorder in women; to diagnose, heal, alleviate, treat or avoid any disorder, disease or condition specified in the Schedule.

- misleading advertisements relating to drugs are prohibited. e.g. advertisements which contain matter giving erroneous feeling about the true character of drug, making incorrect assertion/s about the drug, which is otherwise incorrect or deluding in any context.

Medicinal and Toilet Preparations (Excise duties) Act, 1955. This act made provisions for the imposition and gathering of excise duties on medicinal and toilet preparations consisting of alcohol, opium, Indian hemp or other narcotic drug or narcotic.

Constitution of the Hathi Committee, 1974 (Box 3.3).

The Narcotic Drugs and Psychotropic substances Act (NDPS Act), 1985. An act to prohibit the production/ manufacture/ cultivation, possession, sale, purchase, transport, storage and/ or consumption of any narcotic drug or psychotropic substance.

Box 3.3 Hathi Committee Report, 1975.

The Government of India constituted the Hathi Committee under the Chairmanship of Shri Jaisukhlal Hathi in 1974.

Various recommendations made by the Committee in its report submitted in 1975:

- ✓ Establishment of a **National Drug Authority (NDA)**, a central organization to coordinate the policies for manufacturing, sale and distribution of basic drugs and formulations in public sector units.
- ✓ States to hold the leading role for **production and distribution** of drugs and pharmaceuticals.
- ✓ The **manufacture of bulk drugs** in the Indian sector to be encouraged; Government should impose ban on the import of such items.
- ✓ Highest priority to be accorded to **centrally-directed research** aimed at discovering newer drugs for the treatment of tropical diseases like malaria, filariasis etc. Also, a need to accelerate research in the fields of metabolic, cardiovascular disorders and anti-conceptives.
- ✓ Introduction of a **medical service of rudimentary nature in remote villages** to make available packings containing common household remedies for common cold, fever etc.
- ✓ **Indian drug manufacturing companies** should be given preference over foreign companies.
- ✓ The **prices of imported bulk drugs, raw materials and intermediates** to be screened by NDA which can bring the prices down if deemed excessive.
- ✓ Encourage the improvement of technology through **Research & Development activities** to increase productivity in a rationalized manner.
- ✓ **Rationalizing the costs of basic drugs and formulations** and reduce the drug costs for consumers. For price control of drugs, a vital step would be curtailing the cost of packing; hence emphasis needs to be given to standardization and economy in the use of packing materials.
- ✓ Proposed few **amendments to D & C Act** like addition of a separate definition of "spurious drugs", changes in the penalty for manufacture, sale etc. of misbranded, adulterated drugs and cosmetics etc.
- ✓ Steps need to be taken to provide **essential drugs** to general public specially rural aras.

Pharmaceutical Research & Development Committee (PRDC) was appointed under the expert leadership of Dr. R.A.Mashelkar, Director, Council of Scientific and Industrial Research (CSIR), to provide recommendations on the strategies needed to intensify research and development in the Indian pharmaceutical industry (Box 3.4).

Box 3.4 Mashelkar Committee (PRDC) Report, 1999.

The committee focused on the holistic assessment of Research & Development (R & D) through SWOT analysis (Strengths/Weakness /Opportunities/Threats) and gave recommendations as:

- ✓ ***Provision of intellectual capital*** to make accessible safe, cost-effective, and good quality therapeutics to Indian population in order to curtail morbidity and mortality.

- ✓ ***Prioritization of R & D***: initiate new drug development for conditions relevant in Indian set up.

- ✓ Basic ***changes in the legislation*** e.g. legal status of IECs, allowing import of animals and contract research.

- ✓ Establishment and functioning of an authority to monitor ***Good Manufacturing Practice (GMP), Good Clinical Practice (GCP) and Good Laboratory Practice (GLP).***

- ✓ Comprehensive ***strengthening of CDSCO*** (e.g. well equipped and professionally managed).

- ✓ ***Funding R & D***: mandatory contribution of 1% of MRP of all formulations sold to a fund called "Pharmaceutical R & D Support fund".

- ✓ ***Strengthening the IPR (Intellectual Property Rights) system***: TRIPS compatible IPR legislation.

In **2003**, an expert committee was appointed under Dr. R.A.Mashelkar to do an exhaustive evaluation of various issues pertaining to drug regulation including the trouble of spurious/ substandard drugs (Box 3.5).

Box 3.5 Mashelkar Committee Report, 2003.

Recommendations of the Committee:

- ✓ ***Strengthen the existing drug control infrastructure at the Central and State level.*** CDSCO to be granted the position of Central drug Administration (CDA). A detailed proposal to enhance the state level regulatory apparatus (e.g. provision of additional personnel, infrastructure and adequate resources etc) with complimentary roles of Centre and the States was recommended by the Committee.

Box 3.5 *Contd...*

✓ *Recommendations regarding problem of spurious drugs:*

- o use of scientifically valid methodology to evaluate and quantify the extent of problem.

- o all offences connected to spurious drugs must be cognizable and non-bailable.

- o In addition to penalties of life imprisonment and fines, death penalty should be there in cases resulting in loss of life or grievous body harm.

- o provision of speedy trials of cases concerning offences involving spurious drugs.

- o involvement of police authorities in addition to Drugs Inspectorates.

- o amendments in the D & C Act to give effect to the recommendations given regarding spurious drugs.

An expert committee was constituted by Ministry of Health and Family Welfare in 2013 under the chairmanship of Prof. Ranjit Roy Choudhury with an aim to formulate policy, SOPs and guidelines applicable to new drug appprovals including biologicals, clinical trials and banning of drugs (Box 3.6).

Box 3.6 Prof. Ranjit Roy Choudhury Expert Committee Report, 2013.

Recommendations by the Committee:

✓ Accreditation of Institutional Ethics Committees, Principal Investigators and clinical trial sites by a Central Accreditation Council.

✓ The existing 12 New Drug Advisory Committees (NDACs) to be substituted by a single Technical Review Committee (TRC) to enhance faster and efficient review of clinical trial applications.

✓ Requirements of clinical trials on Indian populations:

- o For NCEs developed in India- need to conduct all clinical trial phases (I-IV) in India.

- o For NCEs developed outside India- Phase I trials not mandatory in Indian population provided they have been conducted in the country of origin.

- o For NCEs under clinical trials outside India, parallel Phase II and III trials can be conducted in India.

- o In Global Clinical Trials (GCTs) if Indians have been included in sufficient numbers with adequate ethnic distribution and safety data is satisfactory, Phase III or bridging studies may be omitted and permission for direct marketing may be granted subject to (i) strict Post Marketing Surveillance (PMS) for 4-6 years (ii) careful scrutiny of data by TRC.

Box 3.6 *Contd...*

o Drugs marketed in well-regulated countries with good PMS (US, UK, European union, Canada, Japan etc.) for more than 4 years may be given direct marketing permission in India after bridging studies or strict PMS for 4-6 years. In case of generics and biosimilars, abbreviated trials to be conducted prior to marketing permission.

✓ Provision of expedited/ abbreviated clinical trials for:

o drugs for HIV/AIDS, life threatening diseases like cancer, new emerging diseases e.g. H1N1

o drugs for Graft versus host disease (GVHD) crisis in organ transplantation

o only available therapy in severe or rare disease

✓ Drug regulatory system to be robust, accountable and transparent (by use of newer technological innovations).

✓ Changes in guidelines for BA/BE studies:

o For NCEs or their generics to be launched in India, BA/BE studies to be conducted as part of the clinical trial.

o Generics manufactured in India- BE studies to be done comparing the generics with the innovator product.

o Bio-waivers to be granted for (i) subsequent generics of same drug with good oral absorption (high solubility and high permeability) and similar in vitro release rate (ii) immediate release solid oral dosage forms with high solubility and low permeability.

✓ Strengthening of IECs by means of accreditation and audit (internal audits, audits by sponsors and regulatory inspections).

✓ Joint / regional IECs i.e. one IEC affiliated to more than 1 institution – for restricting the number of IECs across the country.

✓ Clinical trials conducted at state institutions – monitored at the state level by

o training of state drug regulatory personnel

o joint monitoring with CDSCO personnel

✓ Setting up of a Special Expert Committee to oversee marketed drugs for therapeutic efficacy and/or any associated hazards and provide recommendations on removal of drugs from market.

✓ Provision of a phased programme for drug withdrawal: (i) drugs to be removed immediately (ii) drugs for slow phase out (iii) a list of drugs for restricted use.

Box 3.6 *Contd...*

✓ Management of SAEs and compensation in clinical trials:

  o SAEs during clinical trials- sponsor /investigator responsible for providing medical treatment and compensation.

  o Compensation not payable in proven unrelated causes e.g. road side accident, building collapse etc.

  o Subject's nominee name to be included in informed consent form for compensation purposes.

  o Interim compensation (immediately, preferably within a period of 15 days of the information of SAE) to the participant/legal heirs/ nominee in the event of unresolved SAE, death, disablement or serious consequences.

  o No compensation payable in case of therapeutic inefficiency.

  o CTs involving subjects with terminal illnesses compensation not to be paid for primary end point of death but may be paid if (i) there is increase in SAEs, which may be irreversible, compared to standard treatment (ii) life expectancy is severely curtailed.

✓ Academic research to be approved by IEC.

✓ A fund should be set by central and state Governments and institutions in order to encourage academic and clinical research.

✓ Measures need to be taken to reorganize, upgrade and strengthen the CDSCO and its functioning.

Kokate committee was constituted by CDSCO under the chairmanship of Prof. C.K.Kokate, former Vice-chancellor, KLE University, Belgaum, Karnataka to examine the safety and efficacy of fixed dose combinations (FDCs) which were licensed by state drug controllers without prior approval of DCGI (Box 3.7).

Box 3.7 Kokate Committee Report, 2013.

Recommendations by the Committee:

Out of 418 applications of FDCs examined by the committee, 324 were considered as "irrational" and the committee recommended that manufacture and marketing of the same should be banned in India. As per the committee report, "The FDCs identified as irrational need to be prohibited under the D & C Act, 1940 as safer alternatives to these combinations are available".

EVOLUTION OF DRUGS & COSMETICS ACT AND RULES AND VARIOUS AMENDMENTS

1940: 'Drugs Act 1940'.

1945 : *'Drug Rules'* published under the 'Drugs Act 1940'.

1947: 1ˢᵗ April "Drugs and Cosmetics Act" came into effect.

1962 : Incorporation of Cosmetics within the purview of Drugs Act; adopted as *'Drugs and Cosmetics Act 1940'*.

1964 : Amendment in Drugs & Cosmetics Act; provisions expanded to bring *"Ayurvedic (including Siddha) and Unani drugs"* under its purview.

1988: **SCHEDULE Y** (First ever guideline for conduct of clinical trials in India) added to Drugs and Cosmetics Rules:

Key features of Schedule Y:

- Included specifications for requirements and guidelines for clinical trials in India
- Phase 3 trials to be conducted in India prior to registering new drugs
- *Phase Lag*: any clinical trial conducted in India to be one phase earlier compared to global phase (Box 3.8).

Box 3.8 Implications of Phase Lag.

- ♦ Global Phase III trial data could not be used in the NDA for a new drug in India.
- ♦ In the absence of product patent in India, an Indian drug company could conduct Phase III in Indian population and market its generic brand; this served as a vital *boost to the expansion of Indian generic pharma industry.*

2005 : **Major amendments in SCHEDULE Y, Drugs and Cosmetics Rules:**

Features of Amended Schedule Y, 2005:

- ✓ Included practical definitions for phase 1 to phase 4 trials
- ✓ Post-marketing study (Phase 4) mentioned
- ✓ Specified the responsibilities of Ethics committee (EC), investigator and sponsors
- ✓ Included the layouts for important documents e.g. consent, protocol, EC approval, study report, serious adverse event reports etc.
- ✓ Obliteration of earlier phase lag; conduct of concurrent Phase II and III trials in India permitted
- ✓ Guidelines for studies in special populations: geriatric, pediatric, pregnant.
- ✓ Removal of the limits on the number of subjects and centres in early phases of trials as in older Schedule Y; numbers depend on study requirements.

2005: D & C Act : Devices such as cardiac stents, heart valves, orthopedic implants, catheters, intravenous cannulas and internal prosthetic replacements specified as "drugs" .

2008: D & C Act Amendment : The penalty for manufacturing and selling spurious drugs was enhanced with imprisonment not less than 10 years which can be stretched to life imprisonment and would be liable to a fine of minimum 10 lakh rupees.

2013

- ❖ **Drugs and Cosmetics (first amendment) Rules** *(G.S.R. 53 (E), dated January 30, 2013)*
  - ✓ Provisions for compensation in case of injury/death during clinical trial **(Rule 122 DAB)** (For details, please refer to Chapter 16)
  - ✓ Analysis of Serious Adverse Events (SAEs)
  - ✓ Expansion of responsibilities of sponsor, investigator and Ethics Committee
  - ✓ Amendment in informed consent form (For details, please refer to Chapter 15)
  - ✓ Insertion of Appendix XII in Schedule Y
    - • Compensation in case of injury or death during clinical trial.

- ❖ **Drugs and Cosmetics (second amendment) Rules** *(G.S.R. 63 (E), dated February 1, 2013)*

  Insertion of **"Rule 122 DAC"** after rule 122 DAB which deals with:
  - ✓ Conditions for conduct of clinical trials
  - ✓ Clinical trial inspections
  - ✓ Actions in case of non-compliance
  (For details, please refer to Chapter 5)

- ❖ **Drugs and Cosmetics (third amendment) Rules** *(G.S.R. 72 (E), dated February 8, 2013)*
  - ✓ Registration of Ethics Committees **(Rule 122 DD)** (For details, please refer to Chapter 14).

2015: Drugs and Cosmetics Rules 2015 (8th amendment): "Phytopharmaceutical drug" defined as a new class of drugs (Box 3.9).

Box 3.9 Phytopharmaceutical drug.

As defined in D & C Rules (8th amendment) 2015; "***Phytopharmaceutical drug*** includes purified and standardised fraction with defined minimum four bio-active or phyto-chemical compounds (qualitatively and quantitatively assessed) of an extract of a medicinal plant or its part, for internal or external use in human beings or animals for diagnosis, treatment, mitigation or prevention of any disease or disorder but does not include administration by parenteral route".

2017:   A **revised version of The Drugs and Cosmetics Act and Rules** (as amended upto 31ˢᵗ December 2016) released by CDSCO in February 2017.

The inclusion of **"Biopharmaceutical Classification System"** as a means to classify drugs on the basis of solubility and permeability in the 9ᵗʰ amendment to Drugs and Cosmetics Rules *(G.S.R. 327 (E) dated April 3, 2017).*

2019: New Drugs and Clinical Trials Rules, 2019

New Drugs and Clinical Trials Rules, 2019

The New Drugs and Clinical Trials Rules, 2019 were notified by the Ministry of Health and Family Welfare (MoHFW), India on 25ᵗʰ March 2019 *(Reference document: Ministry of Health GSR notification #227 dated 19 March 2019).*

The rules apply to:
- ✓ all new drugs,
- ✓ investigational new drugs for human use,
- ✓ clinical trial,
- ✓ bioavailability study, bioequivalence study and
- ✓ Ethics Committee.

These rules have been laid down as supersession (replacement) of Part XA and Schedule Y of Drugs and Cosmetics Rules 1945. In case of any discrepancy between these rules and any other rule/s made under D & C Act and Rules, the provisions laid under these rules shall take precedence (Box 3.10).

Box 3.10 Structure of the New Drugs and Clinical Trials Rules, 2019.

The New Drugs and Clinical Trials Rules, 2019 are comprised of 13 chapters and 8 schedules:

Chapter I: Preliminary

Chapter II: Authorities and officers

Chapter III: Ethics committee for clinical trial, bioavailability and bioequivalence study

Chapter IV: Ethics committee for biomedical and health research

Chapter V: Clinical trial, bioavailability and bioequivalence study of new drugs and investigational new drugs

    Part A: Clinical trial

    Part B: Bioavailability and bioequivalence study

Chapter VI: Compensation

---

*Box 3.10 **Contd...***

Chapter VII: Bioavailability and bioequivalence study centre

Chapter VIII: Manufacture of new drugs or investigational new drugs for clinical trial, bioavailability or bioequivalence study or for examination, test and analysis

Chapter IX: Import of new drugs and investigational new drugs for clinical trial or bioavailability or bioequivalance study or for examination, test and analysis

Chapter X: Import or manufacture of new drug for sale or for distribution

Chapter XI: Import or manufacture of unapproved new drug for treatment of patients in government hospital and government medical institution

Chapter XII: Amendments of drugs and cosmetics rules, 1945

Chapter XIII: Miscellaneous

FIRST SCHEDULE: General principles and practices for clinical trial

SECOND SCHEDULE: Requirements and guidelines for permission to import or manufacture of new drug for sale or to undertake clinical trial

THIRD SCHEDULE: Conduct of clinical trial

FOURTH SCHEDULE: Requirements and guidelines for conduct of bioavailability and bioequivalence study of new drugs or investigational new drugs

FIFTH SCHEDULE: Post market assessment

SIXTH SCHEDULE: Fee payable for licence, permission and registration certificate

SEVENTH SCHEDULE: Formulae to determine the quantum of compensation in the cases of clinical trial related injury or death

EIGHTH SCHEDULE: Forms (form CT-01 to CT-27)

Various additions and modifications included in the New Drugs and Clinical Trials Rules, 2019, India have been discussed under relevant topics through different sections of the book.

Important rules of D & C Act and Rules (Box 3.11).

Box 3.11 Important Rules of D & C Act and Rules.	
Rule 122-A	Application for permission to import new drug.
Rule 122-B	Permission to manufacture new drug
Rule 122-D	Permission to import Fixed Dose Combination (FDC)
Rule 122-DA	Application for permission to conduct clinical trials for new drug /IND
Rule 122-DAA	Definition of "clinical trial"
Rule 122-DAB	Compensation in case of injury or death during clinical trial
Rule 122-DAC	Permission to conduct clinical trial
Rule 122-DD	Registration of Ethics Committee
Rule 122-E	Definition of "new drug"

OTHER IMPORTANT DRUG REGULATORY ACTIONS IN INDIA DURING 21ˢᵗ CENTURY

2014

❖ **Norms for CT sites**
  ✓ Office order from CDSCO to limit the number of trials undertaken by Investigators simultaneously. The limit for maximum number of trials which can be conducted by investigators simultaneously was fixed as 3.
  ✓ No clinical trial to be conducted at sites with <50 beds.
  ✓ Mandatory to include at least 50% government sites in most of the studies.

❖ **Clinical trial waiver** for new drugs approved outside India under certain specified conditions like national/ extreme urgency, drugs for diseases with no proven therapy, orphan drugs and epidemic situations. *(File no 12-01/14-DC Pt 47, dated 3rd July, 2014)*

❖ **Medical devices:** Phase 1 studies not mandatory for medical devices. Clinical trial of medical devices will follow the same approval process as drugs and vaccines. *File no 12-01/14-DC Pt 47, dated 3rd July, 2014*

❖ **Placebo-controlled trials:** As per DCGI notification, the trial design in placebo-controlled studies should be appropriate, ethical and efficient. *(File no 12-01/14-DC Pt 47, dated 3rd July, 2014).*

2016

❖ **Revised norms for CT sites**
  ✓ The clauses of not more than 3 trials per investigator at a time and minimum 50 bedded hospital to be a CT site were revoked. Changes implemented under the revised norms were:
  o IECs given the power to decide the suitability of clinical trial site irrespective of the number of beds. However, it was suggested that sites must have emergency rescue and care arrangements.
  o IECs empowered to determine the limit for number of trials per investigator on the basis of complexity and requirements of the particular study and facilities at the site.
  ✓ For addition/deletion of site/s and investigators, only IEC permission would be required. Sponsor needs to inform about any such addition/deletion and obtain no objection certificate from DCGI.

❖ **Academic research studies** *(G.S.R. 313 (E), dated March 16, 2016):* Steps taken to facilitate the conduct of genuine academic research:
  ✓ For clinical trial with an approved drug formulation tested for a new indication or new route of administration, only IEC approval is mandatory and no permission from DCGI is required and the data obtained is not intended to be submitted to DCGI.

✓ IECs are required to pass the information to DCGI regarding the cases approved and potential overlap between academic and regulatory clinical trials. If no comments received from DCGI within 30 days of receipt of notification, it is presumed that no permission from DCGI is required.

❖ **Launch of SUGAM by CDSCO** Since October 2016, a new tool "SUGAM" has been made effective by CDSCO for online clinical trial applications. This tool will help in increasing the accountability and transparency. Moreover, the efficiency of review/approval is expected to increase due to simplification of the process which in turn will enable the conduct of more number of clinical trials in India.

2017

❖ **Medical devices rules 2017** released by CDSCO *(G.S.R 78 (E) dated January 31, 2017).*

2018

❖ Online submission of applications pertaining to recombinant DNA derived products through SUGAM portal made mandatory w.e.f. February 2018; no offline applications to be accepted thereafter. *(Notice issued by CDSCO (X- 11026/08/2018-BD); 15 January, 2018)*

CHAPTER 4

Drug Regulatory Framework in India

OVERVIEW

Introduction
Central Drug Standard Control
Organization (CDSCO)
  Organization of CDSCO
  Roles of CDSCO
  Functioning of CDSCO
Central Drugs Laboratory (CDL), Kolkata
Indian Council of Medical Research (ICMR)

Indian Pharmacopoeia Commission (IPC)
Department of Biotechnology (DBT)
Ministry of AYUSH
National Pharmaceutical Pricing Authority (NPPA)
  Drug Pricing Mechanisms in India
Intellectual Property Rights
State Licensing Authorities (SLA)

INTRODUCTION

In India, Drugs and Cosmetics Act (D & C Act 1940) and Rules (1945) govern all regulatory aspects related to import, manufacture, distribution and sale of drugs and cosmetics as well as medical devices and diagnostics. The main aim of the Act is to make provisions for supply of safe, effective and quality drugs to population.

The D & C Act prohibits the manufacture, sale or distribution or stock or exhibit or offer for sale of;

- any drug or cosmetic which is misbranded or spurious or having substandard quality
- any patent drug not bearing on the label its actual composition or list of active constituents along with their quantities
- any drug which by the inclusion of any information associated with it or by any other methods proposes or assures to prevent, treat and /or alleviate diseases and ailments notified under Schedule J
- any cosmetic having some constituent posing potential risk to users
- any drug the manufacture of which is prohibited under the Act
- any drug or cosmetic manufactured in violation of the provisions laid down in D&C Act and Rules.

Figure 4.1 depicts the organization of drug regulatory framework in India.

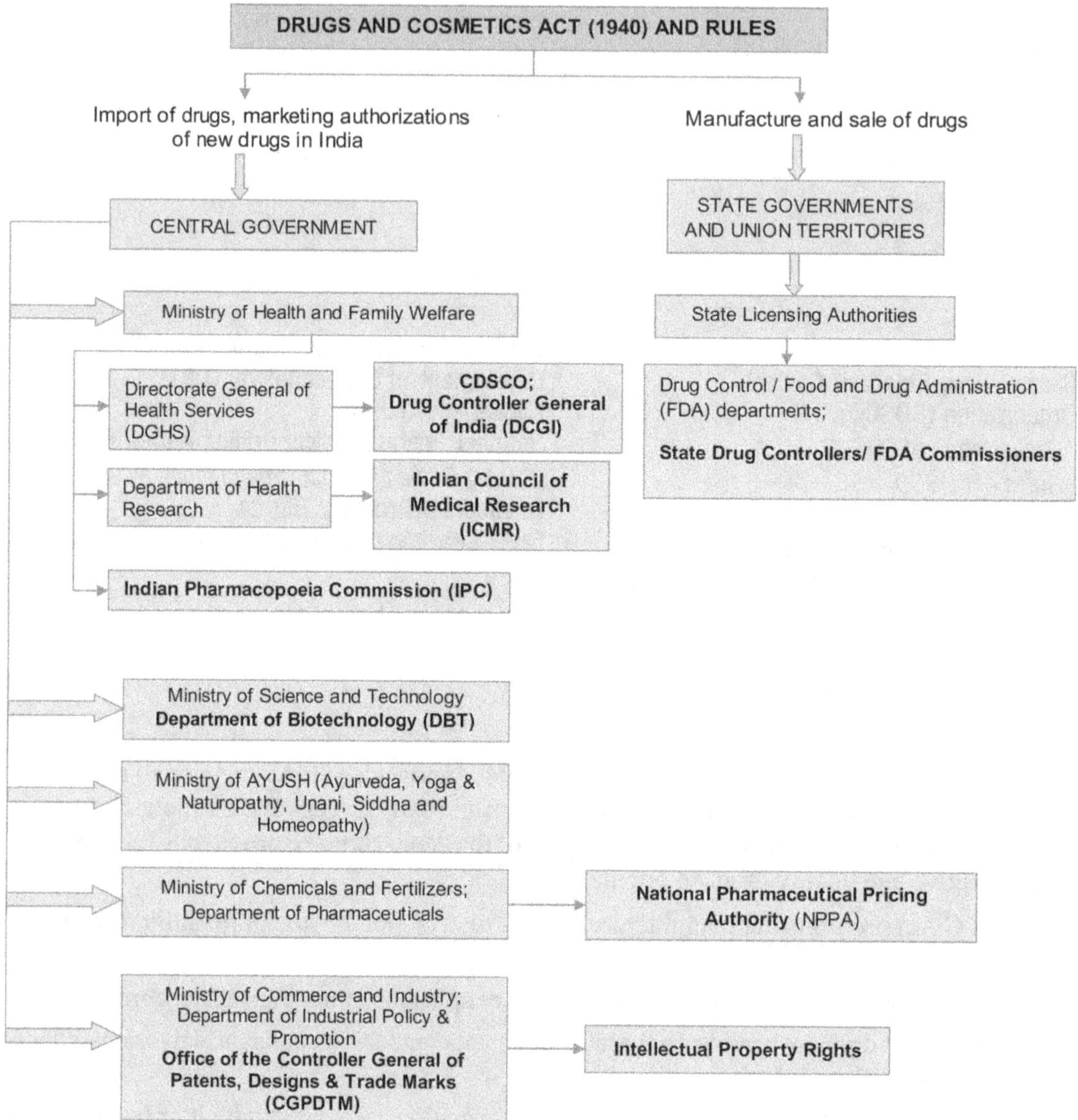

Figure 4.1 Framework of drug regulatory set-up in India.

CENTRAL DRUG STANDARD CONTROL ORGANIZATION (CDSCO)

Under D & C Act, CDSCO headed by DCGI is the National Regulatory Authority (NRA) of India.

ORGANIZATION OF CDSCO (FIGURE 4.2)

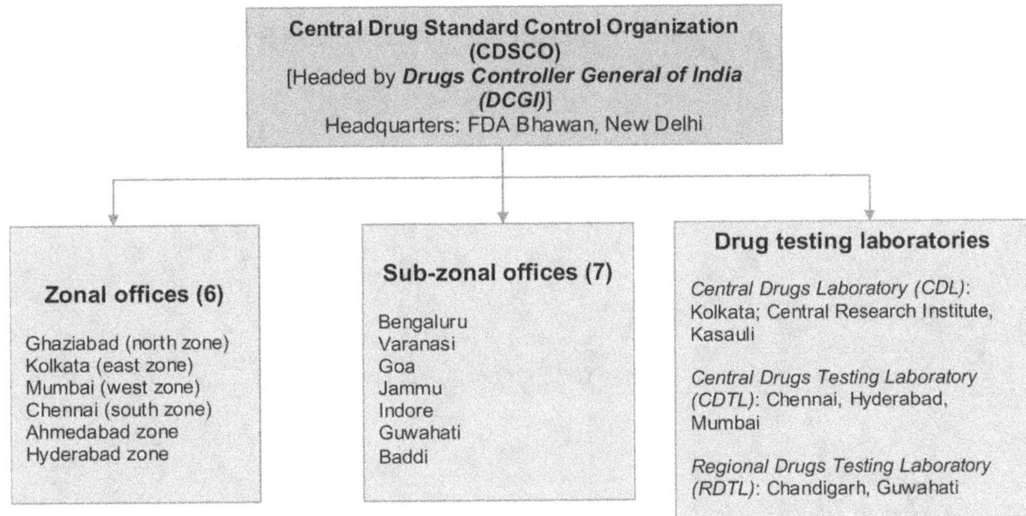

Figure 4.2 Organization of CDSCO.

ROLES OF CDSCO (BOX 4.1)

Box 4.1 Roles of CDSCO.

- ✓ Grant marketing authorization to new drugs
- ✓ Grant approval to conduct clinical trials including global clinical trials in India
- ✓ Regulations related to import of drugs
- ✓ Registration of ethics committees (ECs) and clinical research organizations (CROs)
- ✓ Licensing of blood banks, large volume parenterals (LVPs), vaccines, recombinant DNA products and some medical devices (CLAA scheme)*
- ✓ Conduct of clinical trial inspections to ensure Good Clinical Practice (GCP) compliance
- ✓ Grant of test license, personal license and no objection certificates (NOCs) for exports
- ✓ Laying down regulatory standards by making timely amendments to D&C Act and Rules
- ✓ Providing standards for drugs, cosmetics, medical devices and diagnostics
- ✓ Regulatory decisions related to marketed drugs on the basis of emerging safety data e.g. banning, issuing black box warnings etc.
- ✓ Providing guidance to state governments and union territories on various regulatory issues.

*Central Licensing Approving Authority

FUNCTIONING OF CDSCO

Various committees play important roles in all the matters related to functioning of CDSCO (figure 4.3).

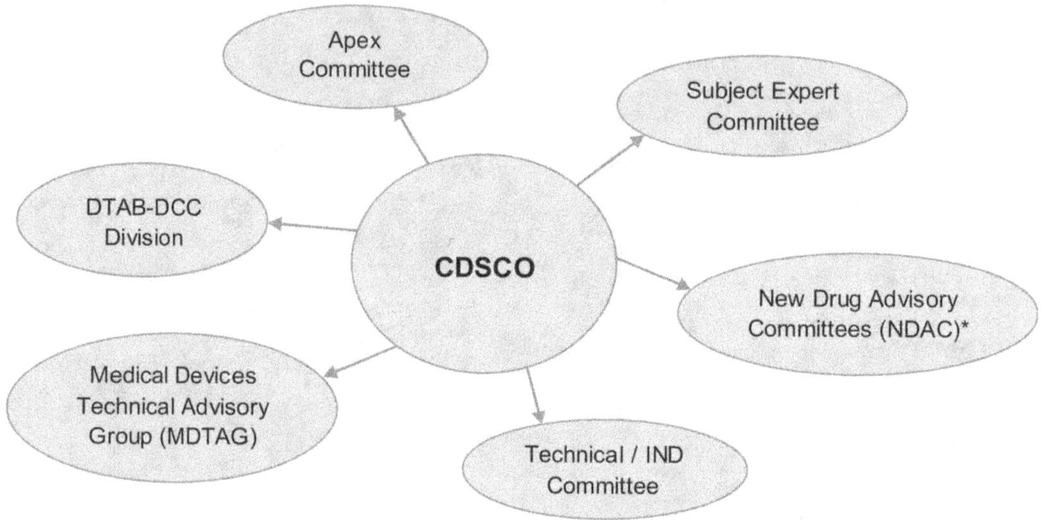

NDACs replaced by SEC since 2014.

Figure 4.3 Various committees under CDSCO.

DTAB-DCC Division. This division of CDSCO deals with organizing and convening meetings of "Drug Technical Advisory Board (DTAB)" and "Drugs Consultative Committee (DCC)".

DTAB and DCC are important statutory bodies constituted under the Drugs and Cosmetics Act. DTAB has Director General of Health Services (DGHS) as its *exofficio* Chairman and DCG(I) as its Member Secretary. DTAB advises governments at central and state level on all technical issues related to drug regulation and plays a crucial role in the amendment, omission or making of new rules in the D & C Act. DCC has DCG(I) as its Chairman and all the State Drug Controllers as its members. It renders advice to central and state Governments and DTAB on issues relating to implementation of D & C Act and Rules throughout India.

Subject Expert Committee (SEC). SEC comprises of 8 experts (7 medical specialists and 1 Pharmacologist) drawn from the 25 teams of experts belonging to various therapeutic domains endorsed by MoHFW through CDSCO. Important functions of SEC are:

- to make essential statements and advice DCG(I) on upcoming clinical trials, drugs and medical devices,
- to examine different types of applications related to clinical trials, drug products and medical devices

The **Technical (IND) Committee** and **Apex Committee** receive the recommendations of SECs on clinical trial protocols, review them and further pass their recommendations to DCGI.

Medical Devices Technical Advisory Group (MDTAG) advices DCGI on matters related to regulation of medical devices.

CENTRAL DRUGS LABORATORY (CDL), KOLKATA

CDL, Kolkata was the first quality control laboratory set up under the Drugs and Cosmetics Act, 1940. It is also the statutory laboratory of the central government for ensuring quality control of drugs and cosmetics.

FUNCTIONS OF CDL, KOLKATA

Statutory functions

- Analytical quality control of most of the drugs imported in India.
- Analytical quality control of various drugs and cosmetics manufactured in India under central and state drug control.
- Acts as an appellate authority in cases of conflicts related to drugs quality.

Other functions

- To assemble, store and distribute various international reference standard preparations of pharmaceutical substances.
- To develop and preserve national reference standards of pharmaceutical substances.
- To preserve microbial cultures used in drug analysis; distribute the standards and cultures to state quality control laboratories and drug manufacturing organizations.
- To train drug analysts and fellows from various state drug control laboratories and abroad on advanced drug analytical techniques.
- To advise the central drug control administration on quality and safety of drugs with pending licence.
- To develop analytical specifications for monographs for the Indian Pharmacopoeia (IP) and the Homoeopathic Pharmacopoeia of India.
- To conduct research on standardizing the analytical techniques for drug and cosmetics.
- To analyse the cosmetics obtained as survey samples from CDSCO.
- To analyse various life saving drugs on national basis obtained from national survey of quality of essential drug programme from zonal offices of CDSCO.
- To collaborate with WHO for preparation of international standards and specifications for International Pharmacopoeia.
- To undertake collaborative studies on behalf of the Indian Pharmacopoeia Commission.

INDIAN COUNCIL OF MEDICAL RESEARCH (ICMR)

ICMR, headquartered in New Delhi, is the key medical research body in India involved in planning, coordinating, implementing and promoting biomedical research.

The missions of ICMR are to:

- Increase focus on health research in vulnerable and disadvantaged sections of society.
- Promote academic research in medical institutions and other health care organizations by nourishing research facilities and resources.
- Encourage innovations and methods associated with diagnosis, prevention and management of diseases.
- Harness the applications of advanced biological technologies to address the healthcare needs of the country.
- Generate and disseminate new health and research related knowledge.

ICMR has 14 divisions dealing with different areas of medical research:

- Reproductive biology and maternal health, child health
- Nutrition
- Basic medical sciences
- International health
- Non- communicable diseases
- Epidemiology and communicable diseases
- Socio-behavioral and health systems research
- Indian journal of medical research unit
- Human resource planning and development
- Research methodology cell
- Research management, policy, planning and coordination
- Informatics, system and research management (ISRM)

ICMR BIOETHICS UNIT

This is located at National Centre for disease informatics and research (NCDIR), Bengaluru. The aim of this unit is to foster and support initiatives towards ethical conduct of biomedical and health research in India.

INDIAN PHARMACOPOEIA COMMISSION (IPC)

IPC, headquartered in Ghaziabad, Uttar Pradesh, is an autonomous institution under the MoHFW, Government of India. The main objective of IPC is to develop standards for pharmaceuticals in the country.

Functions of IPC:

- Providing regular update of the standards of drugs used in the treatment of commonly prevalent diseases.
- Publication of official documents like Indian Pharmacopoeia (IP), National Formulary of India (NFI).
- Issues IP Reference Substances (IPRS), which are the official standards serving as finger prints for the detection of a test product and evaluation of its quality as specified in IP.

❖ Indian Pharmacopoeia (IP)

IP is an official, authoritative and legally enforceable book of standards of drugs manufactured and/or marketed in India. IP contains an assemblage of certified methods of analysis and specifications of drugs for their identity, purity and strength.

IP is regularly published by IPC in fulfillment of the requirements of the D & C Act and Rules. The first edition of IP was published in 1955. The latest, 8th edition of IP, was published in 2018 (Box 4.2).

Box 4.2 Indian Pharmacopoeia 2018/ 8th edition: Salient features.

- ✓ Contains 220 new monographs, 366 revised monographs and 7 omissions.
- ✓ Pyrogen test (carried out in rabbits) can be substituted by bacterial endotoxin test or monocyte activation test (conducted in test tubes).
- ✓ Abnormal toxicity test (carried out in guinea pigs and mice) can be waived if compliance certificate is obtained from National Control Laboratory.
- ✓ 53 new FDCs (fixed drug combinations) monographs included, out of these 25 are not included in any pharmacopoeia.
- ✓ Up-gradation of most of the existing assays and related substances, test methods to harmonize with other International Pharmacopoeias.
- ✓ An index incorporated in volume 1 to make it more user friendly.
- ✓ Revision of a general chapter on maintenance, identification, preservation, and disposal of microorganisms to control the microbial quality of the entire medicinal range.
- ✓ For identification of an article, emphasis laid on more specific infrared, ultraviolet spectro-photometer and HPLC tests; general chemical tests and thin layer chromatography (TLC) almost eliminated.

❖ **National Formulary of India (NFI).**

NFI is a manual containing clinically oriented information on drugs and their formulations based on a broad consensus of skilled judgement of medical practitioners, nurses, pharmacists and drug manufacturers. NFI is not a regulatory document; it serves as a guidance document to healthcare professionals and other stakeholders and aims to promote rational and economic prescribing.

Criteria for inclusion of drugs in NFI:

- ◆ Drug related factors like relative advantages and disadvantages compared to other drugs, availability, affordability and extent of use in clinical practice.
- ◆ Drugs listed in IP and National List of Essential Medicines (NLEM).
- ◆ Drugs used in National Health Programmes.
- ◆ Drugs not covered but recommended by panel of experts.
- ◆ Any drug (s) considered appropriate by the IPC.

The latest edition of NFI, 5th edition (NFI 2016) was released by IPC in 2015; previous editions were published in 1960, 1966, 1979 and 2011.

DEPARTMENT OF BIOTECHNOLOGY (DBT)

The DBT was established in 1986 with an aim to evolve long term perspective for biotechnology, a newly emerging discipline in India. The department is actively engaged in promoting biotechnology research and improving capacity building across the country. DBT announced the first National biotechnology Development Strategy in September 2007which provided an insight into the enormous opportunities in this field. In 2015, the second strategy "National biotechnology Development Strategy 2015-2020" (also known as "Strategy –II") was announced which aims to establish India as a world class bio-manufacturing hub. Major objectives of the National biotechnology Development Strategy 2015-2020 are:

- ◆ Generating products, procedures and techniques in biotechnology to improve efficiency and profitability in the fields of agriculture, food and nutrition
- ◆ Providing cost-effective health care
- ◆ Steps to ensure environmental safety
- ◆ Promote clean energy, bio-fuel, bio-manufacturing etc.

Few schemes and programmes launched by the department to attain new heights in biotechnology research are:

- ❖ Research and development in the area of medical biotechnology e.g. stem cells and regenerative medicine, biomedical engineering and bio-design (devices, diagnostics and implants), human genetics and genome analysis, bioinformatics, genome engineering technologies (GET), basic research in modern biology, infectious and chronic diseases, vaccines, public health and nutrition etc.

❖ *North-East Region (NER) Biotechnology Programme* to strengthen biotechnology research and activities in north-east region of the country which is identified as a treasure house of bio-diversity with abundant mineral and forest resources.

❖ Translational and industrial development programmes to translate research into products and provide required facilities e.g. establishment of biotechnology parks/ incubators across the country; and flagship programs like "*Make-in India*" and "*Start-up India*".

❖ Mission programmes: *Innovate in India (i3) Program*-empowering biotech entrepreneurs and accelerating inclusive innovation; *Biotech KISAN Programme*; a farmer-centric scheme to stimulate innovation and entrepreneurship among farmers.

❖ *SAHAJ (Scientific Infrastructure Access for Harnessing Academia University Research Joint Collaboration)*; a portal launched by DBT to promote the availability of research resources and facilities across the country.

❖ *Biosafety Research programme*. Under this, emphasis is given to implement biosafety procedures, rules and guidelines under Environment Protection Act to ensure safety from the use of genetically modified organisms (GMOs) and products in research and clinical use. A three-tier system (Figure 4.4) has been established to grant permission for conducting research and development activities on recombinant DNA products.

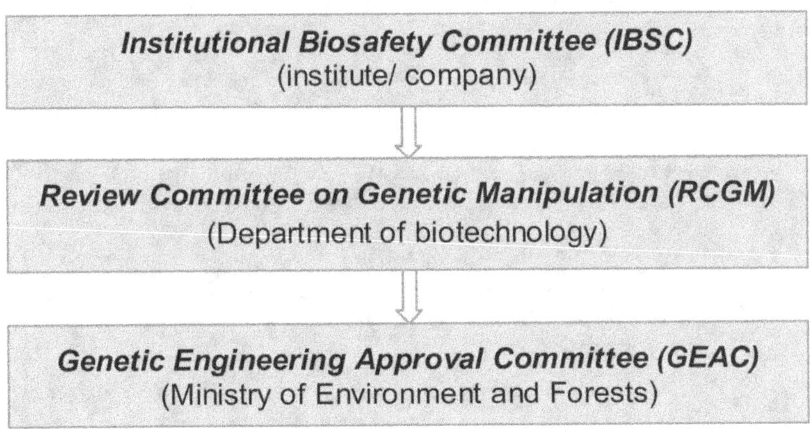

Figure 4.4 Three- tier system to regulate research on recombinant DNA products.

MINISTRY OF AYUSH

The Ministry of AYUSH (Ayurveda, Yoga & Naturopathy, Unani, Siddha and Homoeopathy) was established in 2014; it was formerly known as department of Indian System of Medicine and Homeopathy (ISM & H) and later renamed as department of AYUSH in 2003. The objectives of the Ministry are:

- To foster education and research in AYUSH systems of medicine,
- To formulate schemes to promote, cultivate and regenerate medicinal plants used in these systems,
- To establish Pharmacopoeial standards for AYUSH systems.

NATIONAL PHARMACEUTICAL PRICING AUTHORITY (NPPA)

NPPA is an establishment under the Ministry of Chemicals and Fertilisers aiming to implement the costs and accessibility of pharmaceutical products in the country under Drugs Prices Control Order (DPCO).

FUNCTIONS OF NPPA (FIGURE 4.5)

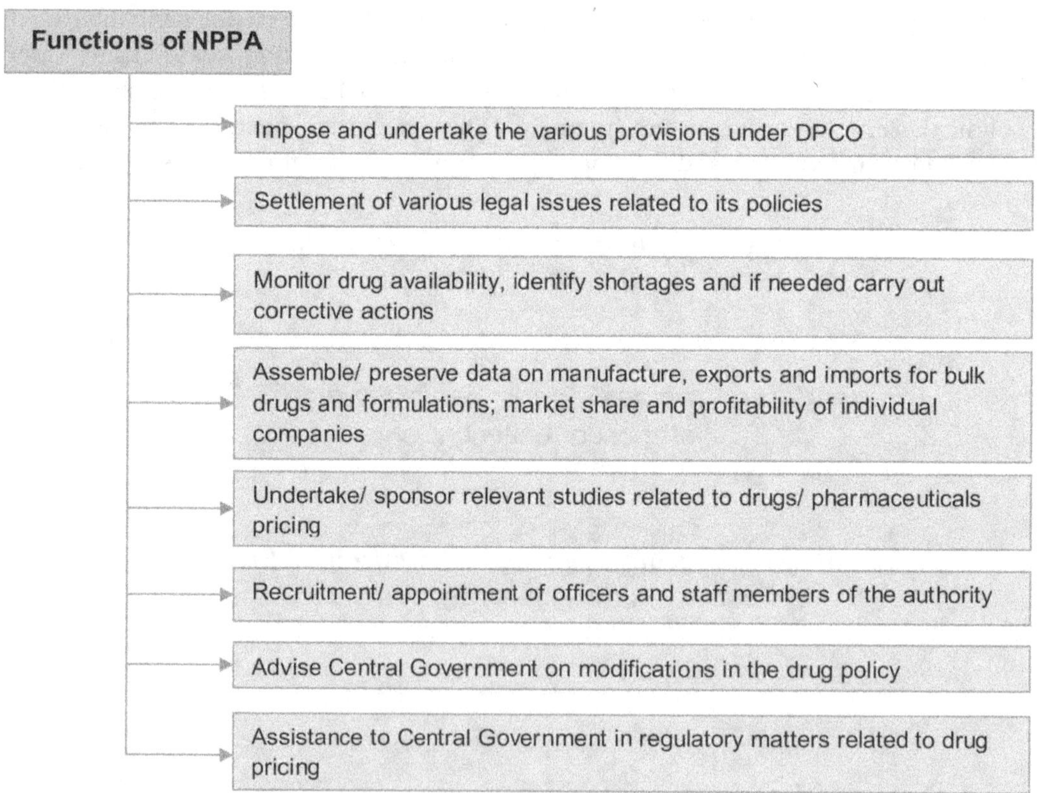

Figure 4.5 Functions of National Pharmaceutical Pricing Authority (NPPA).

DRUG PRICING MECHANISMS IN INDIA

An outline of how the drug pricing mechanisms evolved in India is given in Box 4.3.

Box 4.3 Drug Pricing Mechanisms In India.

Before 1970

Defense of India Act, 1915: Legal jurisdiction on costs of drugs and pharmaceuticals

Essential Commodities Act, 1955: Exercise control over manufacture, storage, delivery, and business related to certain commodities declared essential by Central Government.

Drug Prices (Display and Control) Order, 1966: Mandatory approval from Government prior to implementing price hike of any formulation.

Drug Price Control Order (DPCO), 1970

DPCO: an order released by the Government under the Essential Commodities Act, 1955 (Section 3) authorizing it to control the prices of essential bulk drugs and their formulations.

Features of DPCO, 1970:

✓ Direct control on profitability in pharmaceutical business (if company's per-tax profit exceeded 15% of pharma sales, the surplus had to be deposited with Government).

✓ No approval from Government for individual product prices.

Drug Price Control Order (DPCO), 1979

Based on recommendations of *Hathi Committee report, 1975.*

Controlled categories of bulk drugs and their formulations: *Ceiling prices* fixed by Government; *Retail prices* calculated using MAPE (Maximum Allowable Post manufacturing Expenses).

347 drugs under price control divided into 3 categories as Category I (Life saving drugs): MAPE 40%; Category II (Essential drugs): MAPE 55%; Category III (Less essential): MAPE 100%

Drawback: Steep fall in profitability margins urged the multinational pharmaceutical companies to discontinue a number of products, particularly life saving drugs in Category I.

Drug Price Control Order (DPCO), 1987

Based on the recommendations of *Kelkar Committee report, 1984* and *Drug Policy, 1986 entitled* "Measures for Rationalisation, Quality Control and Growth of Drugs & Pharmaceuticals industry in India"

Box 4.3 Contd...

Recommendations of the Kelkar Committee report:

- Proposal of keeping some drugs out of price control.
- Criteria for inclusion and exclusion suggested.
- Need to liberalise the strict profitability curbs.

Features of DPCO, 1987:

- ✓ The count of bulk drugs falling under price control reduced from 347 to 142 (20 and 122 drugs from Category I and II, respectively excluded from price control).
- ✓ Two categories of drugs under price control with higher MAPE viz. Category I (Drugs required for National Health Programmes): MAPE 75%; Category II (Others): MAPE 100%.

Drug Policy, 1994

Modifications of the basis for including bulk drugs or formulations under price control (data upto 31st March, 1990 to form the basis for applying these criteria):

- ✓ A single list of drugs and formulations included under price control having MAPE of 100%.
- ✓ Drugs with an yearly revenue of at least Rs 400 lakhs.
- ✓ Popularly used drugs in monopoly situation (only one manufacturer possessing 90% or greater market share in retail business) having annual turnover of Rs 100 lakhs
- ✓ If, for drugs outside price control, there is an unreasonable price hike then the Government may take measures like reclamping of price control.
- ✓ Genetically engineered drugs and targeted therapies i.e. drug formulations having specific cell/tissue targets will be outside price control for a period of 5 years from the date of manufacture in India.

Drug Price Control Order (DPCO), 1995

The count of drugs under price control reduced further to **74.**

Prices of controlled bulk drugs to be fixed from time to time by NPPA.

Cost based pricing (CBP) method for price control based on various components like

- cost of active pharmaceutical ingredient (API), excipients, packaging material, labour, overheads;
- application of MAPE;
- duties applicable and
- margins/ profits

Box 4.3 *Contd...*

Issues in DPCO, 1995:

- Based on outdated data i.e. 1990 turnover sales
- High span of control (60-65% of indigenous pharmaceutical industry)
- Poor stability on criteria deciding the inclusion or exclusion of any drug or formulation resulting in drastic changes in prices.
- No control over prices of input materials.
- Artificial disallowances in cases the Government does not recognize the actual input costs.
- Delays in announcing prices.

National Pharmaceutical Pricing Policy (NPPP), 2012

Objective:

Establishing a regulatory set up for drug pricing in such a way so as to assure accessibility of "essential medicines" at affordable costs and provide opportunity for competition and innovation to support industrial growth.

Features:

Price regulation of drugs is based on:

o Regulating the prices of formulations only.

o Drugs considered as 'essential' on the basis of NLEM-2011.

o Market Based Pricing (MBP) strategy to fix maximum costs of formulations.

Drug Price Control Order (DPCO), 2013

This is the latest and current regime followed for drug pricing in India.

Key features of DPCO, 2013:

✓ Market based pricing (MBP) approach used to implement price capping. For bulk drugs under price control, ceiling price i.e. a single maximum selling price applicable throughout the country is fixed.

✓ *Ceiling price* for a controlled drug is calculated as: average price to retailer (mean of costs of brands having greater than 1% market share) + 16% margin to retailer on the price to retailer.

✓ *Maximum retail price (MRP)* to be fixed by manufacturers as: ceiling price (notified by Government) + local taxes, as applicable. MRP of new drugs: Retail price (determined by Government) + local taxes, as applicable

Box 4.3 Contd...

> ✓ MRPs of the controlled formulations may be increased by the manufacturers once in a year (month of April) on the basis of wholesale price index (WPI). For drugs outside the price control, up to 10% annual price hike is allowed.
>
> ✓ Revision of ceiling prices by Government based on moving annual turnover (MAT) to be carried out as and when the NLEM is revised or five years from the date of fixing the maximum cost (ceiling price), whichever is earlier.
>
> At present, around 850 nationally essential drugs (as per NLEM) including various models of coronary stents, knee implants etc. are under price control.
>
> **2019: Amendment to DPCO 2013**
>
> Following amendments have been made in DPCO 2013 as per an order released by the Ministry of Chemicals and Fertilizers (Department of Pharmaceuticals) in 2019:
>
> **New Drug Exemption.** w.e.f. January 3, 2019 the Indian Government has exempted manufacturers, importers and marketers ("**Manufacturers**") of patented new drugs in India from price control for a period of five years.
>
> **Orphan drug exemption.** Drugs for the treatment of diseases qualifying as orphan diseases will be exempt from price control.

INTELLECTUAL PROPERTY RIGHTS

Intellectual property rights (IPR) aim to prevent the stealing or copying of a novel idea, process, product, invention or design. They are present in many different forms, the most common being *patents* (for discoveries and medicines etc.), *copyright* (for literature, books, images) and *registered trademarks* (for company logos, slogans and brand names).

Patents

A patent is a property right offered by the government to the discoverer of a ***new***, ***nonobvious*** and ***utility*** invention. The patent holder has the right to disallow others from manufacturing, applying, presenting for sale, or selling his or her invention for a period of 20 years from the date of filing the patent application. The process of determining whether the requirements of novelty, nonobviousness and usefulness have been fulfilled is carried out by weighing up the representations made by the patent applicant versus the existing literature in the relevant field, including the patents granted previously; this whole process is known as **examination**. The *market exclusivity* and *greater costs* provided by the patent rights serve as a reward to the persons involved in undertaking and financing the research and developing new technologies.

Patent rights are *territorial* in nature and apply only in the regional administrations in which the patentee has applied for and been granted the rights.

The application of patents varies in different industries. In the pharmaceutical industry, the patent normally refers to the product as it is often simpler to replicate the manufacturing process with a fraction of the finances needed during discovery and development process.

In India, the Office of CGPDTM acts as an advisory body to the Government on various issues related to IPRs. The Office of CGPDTM functions through patent offices (Delhi, Kolkata, Mumbai and Chennai) which carry out their statutory functions according to Indian Patents Act, 1970 (as amended).

Box 4.4 highlights the key developments in the field of Intellectual Property Rights in India.

Box 4.4 Intellectual Property Rights (IPR) in India.

Scenario before 1970

♦ *Product Patent regime* was followed (Patent given over a period of 12 years).

♦ Indian drug industry was virtually non-existent and India was dependent on foreign multinational companies for drugs.

♦ Drugs reached Indian market after a long gap of their introduction in the world markets (e.g. Penicillin became available in India in 1963 after a gap of 22 years; introduced in world in 1941).

1970: The Indian Patents Act

The Indian Patents Act was passed in 1970 (based on the recommendations of Justice N Rajagopala Ayyengar). This Act introduced many changes in the existing laws.

- *Process patent* for chemical substances (pharmaceuticals, food products and agrochemicals) instead of Product patents. Product patent for nonchemical substances.

- Generic drugs could be produced using *"Reverse engineering"*.

- Duration of patent: 7 years (or five years from the period of sealing the patent, whichever is lesser).

- It gave a *boost to growth of India's generic pharmaceutical industry* as firms in India could now manufacture the same drugs using different process and sell it at a lower price than the originator company.

- Resulted in *drop in drug prices* (e.g. drop in the prices of antiretroviral drugs by as much as 98% due to Indian generics production).

- *Sooner availability of drugs* in Indian markets.

- India became one of the *leading supplier of generic medicines to developing countries* which accounted for 66.7% of its exports (many African countries dependent on India for supply of generic anti-HIV drugs).

- Drawbacks:
  New drug development suffered although manufacturing processes were strengthened.

  Many *unsafe drugs reached Indian market* due to their sooner availability and lack of adequate surveillance systems in India.

Box 4.4 *Contd...*

General Agreement on Tariffs and Trade (GATT) - Trade Related Aspects of Intellectual Property Rights (TRIPS)

TRIPS was an alliance by the World Trade Organization (WTO) to assure the respect of intellectual property rights within the international trade. Under TRIPS agreement,

- the duration of patent protection was extended for at least a period of 20 years from the date of filing patent application.

- "Product patent" to be followed i.e. drugs could no longer be manufactured using "reverse engineering".

TRIPS came into force on 1ˢᵗ January 1995, however developing and least developed nations were given a longer grace period to bring their existing national patent system in accordance with the TRIPS Agreement.

India had a deadline of January 1, 2005 to follow the prerequisites in TRIPS which means for drugs discovered after January 1, 2005 generic versions would not be permitted for the life of the patent. For medicines that were patent protected outside of India since 1995 till 2005, a "mailbox" was established where patent applications during this period were filed. The mailbox was opened after January 1, 2005 and requests for patents considered by the Indian Patent Office.

Doha Declaration. In the *WTO Doha ministerial conference in 2001*, it was agreed that under certain conditions (e.g. when patent holder fails to provide their product or provide it at a very high unaffordable cost) Government can issue a license to enable both the production and import of patented drugs (***compulsory licensing***); here the Government can simply announce the general use of the patent by public without discussing with patent holder; the patent holder, however, receives adequate remuneration. Another strategy can be negotiated price discounts or ***voluntary licensing*** (the patent holder provides a voluntary license for the manufacture of generic version of the drug).

1999: Patents (Amendment) Act (came into force retrospectively from 1ˢᵗ January, 1995):

Provision for applying product patents in the areas of drugs, pharmaceuticals and agro-chemicals; however, such applications were to be examined after 31ˢᵗ December 2004. Meanwhile, Exclusive Marketing Rights (EMR) were granted to applicants under certain conditions.

2005: Indian Patent (Amendment) Act, 2005: w.e.f. 1ˢᵗ January 2005,

- ***Product patent regime*** was implemented in India for drugs, medicines, food and chemical processes.

- Provisions related to Exclusive Marketing Rights (EMR) were removed.

Box 4.4 *Contd...*

- Provision of **compulsory licensing** was made.
- Provision to appeal to Intellectual Property Appellate Board (IPAB) from the order of decision of the patent office.

2016: Patents (Amendment) Rules 2016

Key features:

Remote hearings can be carried out through video-conferencing or other communication means and relevant documents with written submission have to be submitted within 15 days of the hearing.

Refund of official fees if the applicant withdraws request for examination.

2016: National IPR Policy released with the aim to create awareness about the importance, creation, commercialization and enforcement of IPRs. The objectives of the policy are:

- To generate awareness among public regarding the social, cultural and economic aspects of IPRs.
- To encourage development of IPRs.
- To enforce effectual IPR laws maintaining harmony between owners of patent rights and public at large.
- To strengthen and modernize the administration process of IPRs.
- To value IPRs through commercialization.
- To combat IPR infringements by enforcing adjudicatory mechanisms.
- To expand human resources, capacities and skill building in IPRs.

STATE LICENSING AUTHORITIES (SLA)

All state Governments have their own SLA which work in coordination and under the guidance of Central Government. SLA is responsible for:

- Granting license to drug manufacturing and sales establishments.
- Granting license to establishment of drug testing laboratories.
- Granting license for manufacture and marketing of different drug formulations in India.
- Enforcement of laws as regards to quality and safety of medicines.
- Conducting pre- and post-license inspections.
- Recalling/withdrawing sub-standard drugs.
- Monitoring the quality of drugs and cosmetics.

IMPORTANT LINKS

1. Central Drugs Standard Control Organization; official website: https://cdscoonline.gov.in/CDSCO/homepage

2. Central Drugs Laboratory, Kolkata; https://cdsco.gov.in/opencms/opencms/en/Departments/Lab/CDL-Kolkata/

3. Indian Council of Medical Research: official website: https://www.icmr.nic.in/

4. *Indian Pharmacopoeia Commission;* official website: https://www.ipc.gov.in/

5. Department of Biotechnology; official website: www.dbtindia.nic.in/

6. National Pharmaceutical Pricing Authority; official website: http://www.nppaindia.nic.in/en/

CHAPTER 5

Drug Approval Process in India

OVERVIEW

Introduction

Investigational New Drug (IND)

New Drug Application (NDA)

NDA process in India

Regulatory requirements for permission to conduct clinical trial of a new drug or investigational new drug

Documents required for IND application in India

Abbreviated new drug application (ANDA)

Global clinical trial

Procedure for approval of clinical trials in India by regulatory authority

Application fee for various licenses as per the New Drugs and Clinical Trials Rules, 2019

INTRODUCTION

An overview of the various stages involved from the discovery of a drug molecule to its approval as a new drug is depicted in Figure 5.1.

INVESTIGATIONAL NEW DRUG (IND)

As per rule 122-DA of D & C Rules, IND means "a new chemical entity (NCE) or a product having therapeutic indication but which has never been tested on human beings earlier". Various steps involved in the regulatory approval of IND in India are depicted in Figure 5.2.

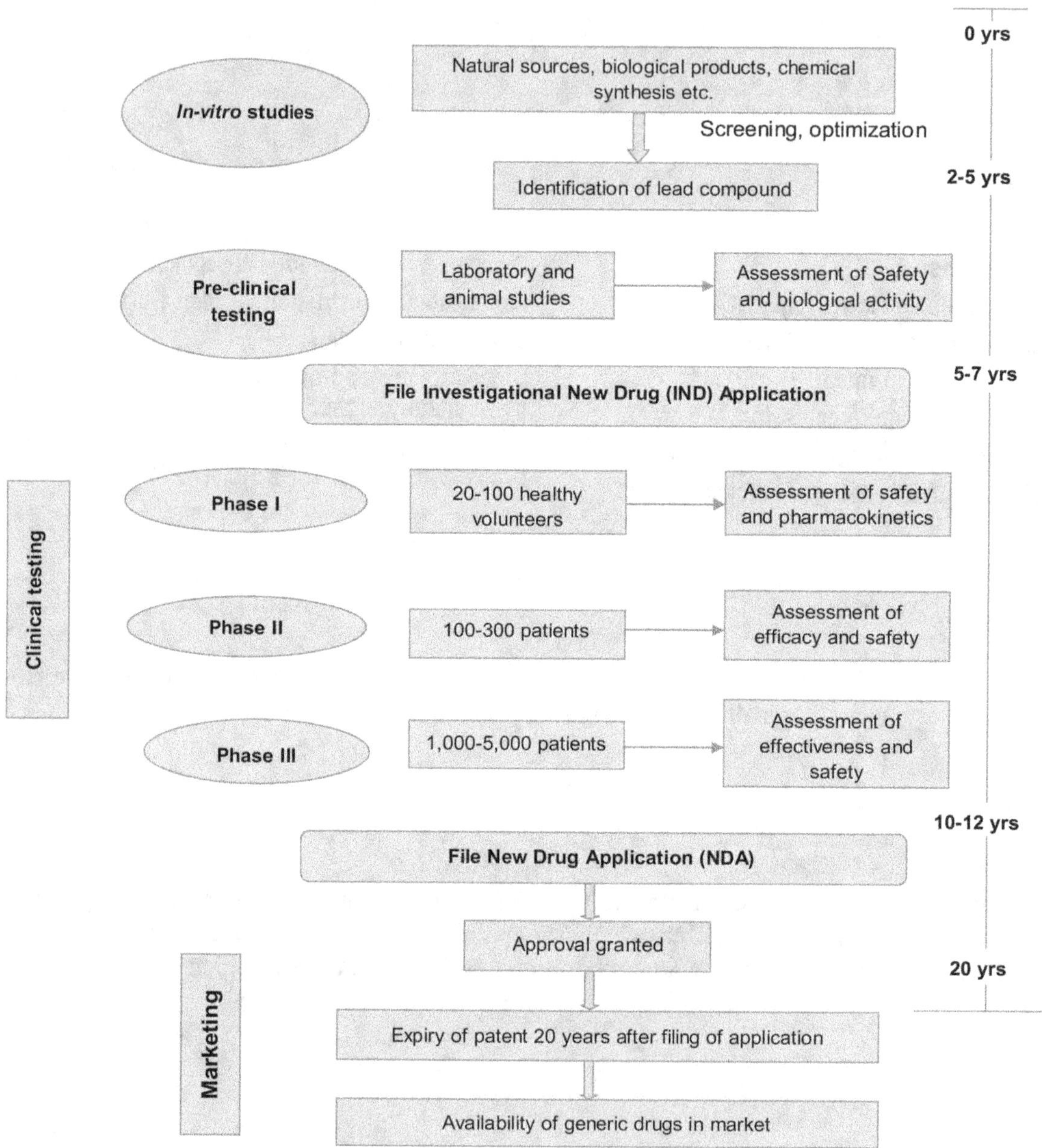

Figure 5.1 An overview of drug approval process.

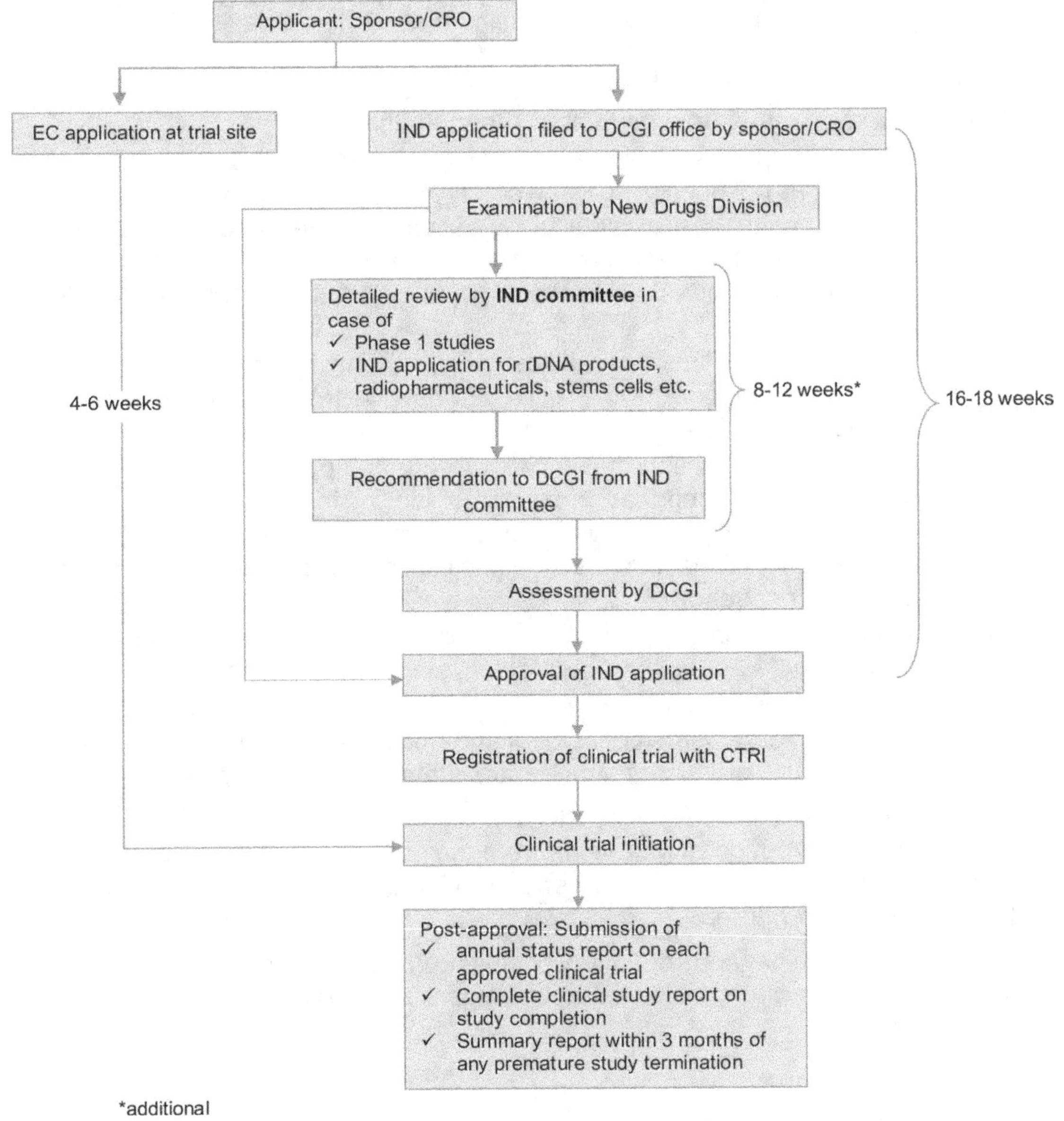

Figure 5.2 Regulatory approval process of IND in India.

NEW DRUG APPLICATION (NDA)

This refers to an application submitted to the regulatory authority to seek permission to import/manufacture and market a new drug in India (Box 5.1).

> **Box 5.1** The New Drugs and Clinical Trials Rules, 2019, India.
>
> ***Modification of the definition of "new drug".***
>
> As per the new rules, a **new drug** shall mean and include
>
> (i) "a drug, including active pharmaceutical ingredient or phyto-pharmaceutical drug, which has not been used in the country to any significant extent, except in accordance with the provisions of the Act and the rules made there under, as per conditions specified in the labeling thereof and has not been approved as safe and efficacious by the Central Licensing Authority with respect to its claims"; or
>
> (ii) "a drug approved by the Central Licensing Authority for certain claims and proposed to be marketed with modified or new claims including indication, route of administration, dosage and dosage form"; or
>
> (iii) "a fixed dose combination of two or more drugs, approved separately for certain claims and proposed to be combined for the first time in a fixed ratio, or where the ratio of ingredients in an approved combination is proposed to be changed with certain claims including indication, route of administration, dosage and dosage form"; or
>
> (iv) "a modified or sustained release form of a drug or novel drug delivery system of any drug approved by the Central Licensing Authority"; or
>
> (v) "a vaccine, recombinant Deoxyribonucleic Acid (r-DNA) derived product, living modified organism, monoclonal anti-body, stem cell derived product, gene therapeutic product or xenografts, intended to be used as drug";
>
> For drugs referred to in clauses (i) to (iii) a drug shall continue to be considered as new drug for a period of four years from the date of permission granted by Central Licensing Authority; drugs referred to in clauses (iv) and (v) shall always be deemed as new drugs.
>
> *Note:* According to previous definition of new drug, modified/ sustained release formulations were not considered new drugs after 4 years from the time of initial approval.

NDA PROCESS IN INDIA

The regulatory approval process of NDA may vary depending on whether the new drug is discovered and/or approved within or outside India (Figure 5.3). The average approval time period for NDA ranges from 12-20 months depending on whether the local data from clinical trials is requested by the regulatory authority. However, depending on the benefits offered by the new drug "expedited approval" may be granted on an individual case basis.

Till now, there was no provision of *fast tracking* or *orphan drug status* in Indian regulations unlike in some key countries worldwide. However, in the New Drugs and Clinical Trials Rules, 2019, special situations for approval of NDA have been incorporated (Box 5.2).

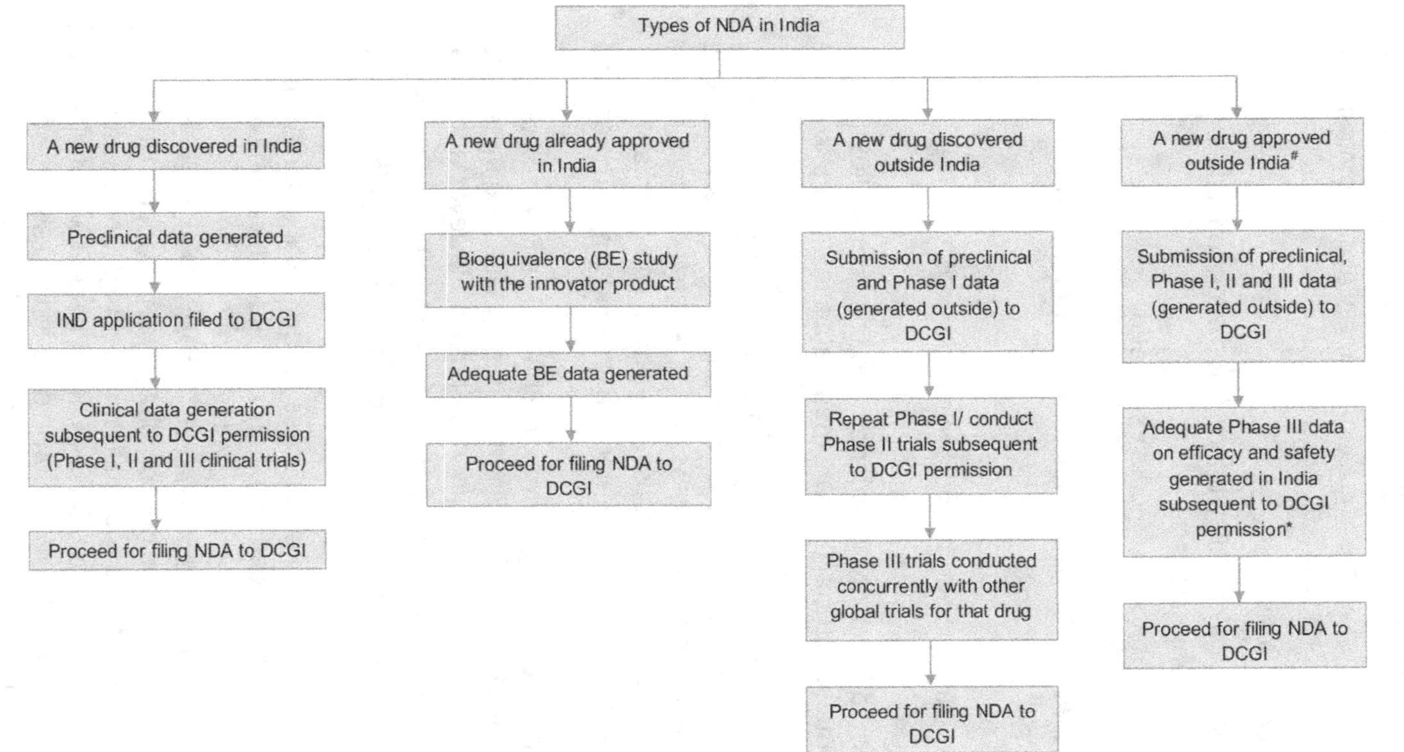

Figure 5.3 Types of New Drug Applications (NDAs) in India.

Box 5.2 The New Drugs and Clinical Trials Rules, 2019.

Special situations for a new drug where relaxation, abbreviations, omission or deferment of data may be considered.

❖ *Accelerated approval process*.

Accelerated approval process may be allowed for drugs intended to be used in:
- serious/ life threatening / rare diseases,
- diseases with particular importance in Indian scenario,
- unmet clinical need,
- haemostatic and rapid wound healing in disaster and defence purpose
- improving oxygen carrying capacity,
- radiation safety,
- drugs to combat chemical, nuclear, biological infliction etc.

Procedure for accelerated approval process:
- Approval may be granted for above mentioned conditions provided there is evidence that the product affords significant therapeutic advantage over the available treatment.
- Approval may be given based on data generated in a clinical trial using surrogate end-point/s which should be measurable earlier than standard outcomes (e.g. survival, disease progression, irreversible morbidity or mortality (IMM)) and are fairly likely to anticipate clinical end-point/s.
- Mandatory post-marketing studies will be needed for validating the predicted clinical benefit.
- Marketing approval may be granted based on Phase II clinical trial data of INDs for unmet medical needs, serious/life threatening diseases if the drug shows remarkable efficacy with a defined dose in Phase II. However, additional post-licensure studies will be required to generate data on larger population.

❖ *Quick or Expedited review process* for approval of a new drug after clinical development.

An application for expedited/ quick review process for approval of a new drug can be made by the sponsor to the licensing authority under the conditions as mentioned below:
- New drug with established evidence of clinical efficacy and safety even if the clinical trial phases for the drug have not completed yet provided (i) the drug is indicated for the treatment of a serious/life threatening/ rare disease, (ii) on approval, the drug is expected to offer significant benefit with respect to efficacy and safety, (iii) a substantial reduction in drug-limiting adverse events and improvement in patient compliance is assumed with the drug.

Box 5.2 *Contd...*

- New drugs developed for disaster or defence use like war time, accidental or incidental radiation exposure, situations where conduct of clinical trial in real life situation might not be feasible etc. provided certain criteria are fulfilled such as (i) claimed efficacy from preclinical data, (ii) lack of availability of established therapeutic/ management strategy, (iii) conditions where it is not possible to have strict protocol adherence, adoption of eligibility criteria for each subject and obtaining informed consent, (iv) such approval can be used only once and subsequent approval may be granted upon generation of detailed efficacy report of the intervention.
- New drug is an orphan drug.

After the marketing authorization for new drugs is obtained from CDSCO, an application is made to the state FDA to receive permission to manufacture the drug which then grants a license for drug manufacture.

In the New Drugs and Clinical trials Rules, 2019, few provisions pertaining to drug approval have been embodied (Box 5.3). Also, a new provision for import or manufacture of unapproved new drug for use in Government hospital or medical institution has been added (Box 5.4).

Box 5.3 The New Drugs and Clinical Trials Rules, 2019.

❖ Provision of formal **pre-submission and post-submission meetings** with the Central Licensing Authority by a person filing an application for grant of license or permission for import or manufacture of new drugs or to conduct clinical trial.

❖ **Debarment of applicant**
- If an applicant or any other person on his behalf is found to be guilty of submitting misleading or fake or fabricated documents may after giving an opportunity of being heard be debarred by CLA for a period as considered appropriate.
- In such a case the applicant, if aggrieved by an order of CLA, may make appeal to the Government within 30 days of the receipt of order.

Box 5.4 The New Drugs and Clinical Trials Rules, 2019.

Introduction of a new provision

Import or manufacture of unapproved new drug (but under clinical trial) for treatment of patients (with life threatening disease) in Government hospital and Government Medical Institution

❖ The application for permission to import/manufacture an unapproved drug for treatment of patients has to be made by the concerned (medical officer) to the Central Licensing authority in Form CT-24 and Form CT-26, respectively.

*Box 5.4 **Contd...***

❖ The license granted would be viable for a period of 1 year from the date of issue; a half-yearly report about the status of unapproved imported/ manufactured drug (e.g. amount utilized/ destroyed etc.) would be deposited to the Central licensing authority by medical officer/ manufacturer as the case may be.

❖ Use of the unapproved drug shall strictly be restricted for the treatment of patient/s and no part of the drug shall be used for selling or supplying purposes.

❖ The amount of any single new drug imported/ manufactured would not be above one hundred average doses per patient; however under special situations larger quantities can be imported/ manufactured after obtaining due permission from regulatory authority.

❖ If there is report of any serious adverse event, the Central licensing authority has to be informed by the permission holder about such event and the action taken thereafter.

REGULATORY REQUIRMENTS FOR PERMISSION TO CONDUCT CLINICAL TRIAL OF A NEW DRUG OR INVESTIGATIONAL NEW DRUG

As per rule 122 DAC, Drugs and Cosmetics Rules, 1945 [Drugs and Cosmetics (second amendment) Rules *(G.S.R. 63 (E), dated February 1, 2013)]*

❖ The application for permission to conduct clinical trial of a new drug or IND is to be submitted to the Central licensing authority in Form 44; permission is granted as approval letter, not in any specific format.

❖ The approval timeline is 120 days (as per DCGI office order dated 30 May 2014).

❖ The Licensing authority issues permission to conduct clinical trial provided below mentioned criteria are fulfilled:

- The data furnished with the application for proposed clinical trial is complete in all aspects,

- The clinical trial would be conducted in accordance with approved protocol, GCP guidelines and requirements as per Schedule Y,

- Ethics Committee approval is obtained prior to study initiation,

- Trial is registered with CTRI before the enrolment of first patient,

- Annual status report of each trial would be submitted to the Licensing authority,

- SAE reporting to concerned authorities would be done within stipulated timelines,

- In case of any clinical trial related injury or death, compensation and medical management would be provided according to applicable guidelines,

- Officers authorized by CDSCO would conduct inspection of the premises of sponsor and clinical trial sites,
- The Sponsor would permit the designated personnel to inspect the premises and data, and provide appropriate comments to the queries of the personnel.

❖ The Licensing authority may, if deemed necessary, direct additional conditions for issue of permission to conduct clinical trial.

❖ In case of non-compliance with any of the required conditions, the Licensing authority can:
  - ✓ issue warning letter,
  - ✓ recommend the study rejection/ discontinuation,
  - ✓ suspend or withhold the permission to conduct CT,
  - ✓ disqualify the Sponsor, Investigator and the involved staff from conducting any CT in future.

The Sponsor can make a plea to the central government within 90 days of the receipt of the order from Licensing authority.

The regulatory requirements for conduct of clinical trials of IND or new drug in accordance with the New Drugs and Clinical Trials Rules, 2019 are detailed in Box 5.5.

Box 5.5 The New Drugs and Clinical Trials Rules, 2019.

Permission to conduct clinical trials

- An application to obtain permission for conducting clinical trial of a new drug or IND can be submitted to the central licensing authority (CLA) in form CT-04.
- The licensing authority, after scrutiny of the information and documents submitted, shall give its decision within 90 working days.; approval is granted in Form CT-06.
- If the application is rejected, the applicant may put requisition to the CLA, for reconsidering the application within 60 working days from the date of rejection after submitting fees and documents as applicable.
- In case the applicant is aggrieved by the judgement of the CLA, he/she may appeal to the Central Government within 45 days of receiving such decision and the Government, may after conducting enquiry and hearing to the appellant, discard or retain the appeal, as the case may be, within 60 working days.
- ***Permission to conduct clinical trial of a new drug or investigational new drug as part of discovery, research and manufacture in India*** *(no such differentiation as per previous regulations)*: Such application shall be processed or approved or rejected, as the case may be, by the CLA within 30 working days of receiving the application.

Box 5.5 Contd...

- ***Provision of deemed approval***: If the applicant does not receive any communication from the CLA within 30 working days, the application is deemed to be approved. In such a case, the applicant can submit Form-CT-4A to CLA as legal record which is considered as automatic approval of CLA. *(There was no provision of deemed approval in previous regulations).*
- The permission to conduct such clinical trial granted by the CLA in form CT-06 or CT-4A holds validity till 2 years after the issue date, unless extended by the CLA. *(Validity/ expiry of permission granted was not defined previously).*

Conditions of permission for conduct of clinical trial

- Before initiation of a clinical trial, prior approval needs to be obtained from Ethics committee of the respective site.
- In cases of non-existence of EC at a clinical trial site, prior approval can be obtained from EC of another trial site or an independent EC. In such a case, the EC granting approval holds responsibility for trial conduct at the site. Further, the approving EC and the clinical trial site or BABE study centre needs to be situated within same city or within a radius of 50 kilometers.
- In case the study protocol is rejected by an EC of a clinical trial site, detailed information on the same needs to be submitted to CLA before seeking permission of another EC to conduct clinical trial at same site.
- Information about EC approval of the protocol should be submitted to CLA within 15 working days of grant of approval.
- Prior to enrolment of first subject in the trial, the clinical trial needs to be registered with the CTRI maintained by ICMR.
- CLA should be informed about the status of subject enrolment in clinical trial on quarterly basis or as appropriate depending on trial duration as mentioned in the approved protocol, whichever is earlier.
- Electronic submission of the trial status report (ongoing/ completed/ terminated) should be made to CLA in SUGAM portal at six monthly intervals.
- Under situation of premature termination of clinical trial, report on the same including reasons for termination in details should be submitted to CLA within 30 working days of trial termination.

DOCUMENTS REQUIRED FOR IND APPLICATION IN INDIA

- Cover letter with summary of the investigational product (IP).
- Form CT-04; Fees as per the clinical trial phase.
- Data to be submitted depending on various conditions as mentioned in Second Schedule of the New Drugs and Clinical Trials Rules, 2019*.
- Final version of the protocol.

- Final version of the Informed Consent Document.
- Case report form.
- Investigator's brochure; accompanied by an affidavit stating that the information included is factual.
- Curriculum vitae, medical registration certificates of all the participating investigators.
- Undertaking by all the investigators.
- IEC approvals.

*"*Data to be submitted along with the application to conduct clinical trials or import or manufacture of new drugs for sale in the country"*.

*"*Data required to be submitted by an applicant for grant of permission to import or manufacture a new drug already approved in the country"*.

*"*Data required to be submitted by an applicant for conduct of clinical trial of an approved new drug with new claims, namely, new indication or new dosage form or new route of administration or new strength or to import or manufacture such new drug for sale or distribution"*.

*"*Data to be submitted along with application to conduct clinical trial or import or manufacture of a phytopharmaceutical drug in the country"*.

ABBREVIATED NEW DRUG APPLICATION (ANDA)

For generic drugs, an abbreviated new drug application (ANDA) is filed by the applicant for marketing authorization. An ANDA is different from NDA in that it requires lesser data for approval; generally there is no need to repeat the entire drug development process (pre-clinical, phase 1-3), however the following data should be submitted:

- *in-vitro* tests (dissolution profile etc.); and
- *in-vivo* tests (bioequivalence study or a clinical equivalence study with the reference product)

GLOBAL CLINICAL TRIAL

The New Drugs and Clinical Trials rules, 2019 have included the definition of global clinical trial as mentioned in the box below (Box 5.6).

> **Box 5.6** The New Drugs and Clinical Trials rules, 2019.
>
> **Global clinical trial:** "a clinical trial conducted as part of the clinical development of a drug in more than one country".

Data required to be submitted for global clinical trial

For a global clinical trial application, some additional information is needed to be submitted as:

- Names of the countries participating in the trial;
- Number of subjects planned for enrolment globally;
- Number of subjects to be enrolled in India;
- Number of centres participating in India;
- Regulatory/ IEC approvals from all the participating countries;
- Status of the trial in other countries e.g. data on number of patients enrolled/ completed/ discontinued;
- Data on any reported SUSARs (Suspected Unexpected Serious Adverse Reactions) from other participating countries;
- Affidavit from the sponsor/ MAH (marketing authorization holder) regarding study discontinuation in any participating center along with the reasons and that any future discontinuation would be communicated to DCGI.

PROCEDURE FOR APPROVAL OF CLINICAL TRIALS IN INDIA BY REGULATORY AUTHORITY

PROCEDURE FOR **APPROVAL OF CLINICAL TRIALS IN INDIA BY REGULATORY AUTHORITY**

Till 2010 — **Single tier approval process**- review at CDSCO office only. Approval timelines: 8-12 weeks.

2010 — DCGI constituted 12 **New Drug Advisory Committees (NDAC)** comprising of experts from eminent institutions to review all submitted protocols.

Increase in CT approval timelines upto 18 months
Drop in CT approval rate

2013 — NDAC replaced by **Subject Expert Committees (SEC)**. (Since 2014, there exist 25 panels of SECs across various therapeutic domains)

Three tiered regulatory approval process

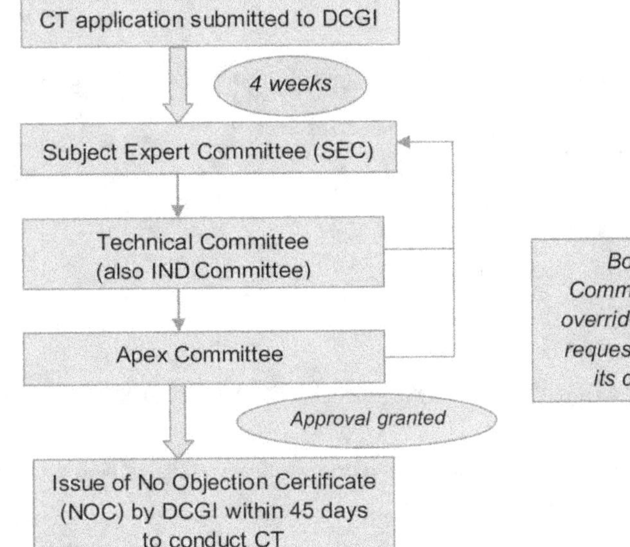

- Simultaneous review by IEC/IRB
- Resulted in delay in approval timelines due to infrequent meetings of the 3 review committees.

2017 **Proposals to simplify the 3 tier review process.**

✓ ***Review of Global Clinical Trials (GCTs) by SEC only.*** Proposals relating to global clinical trials should be placed before the SEC only; and regardless of their approval or rejection by the SEC, no further review by the Technical or Apex Committee is needed.

✓ ***Simplification of the IND approval process.*** 'IND clinical trial applications are to be submitted to the IND Committee and its report will be final. In rare situations, if deemed necessary by the IND Committee, the Apex Committee can be consulted for guidance. (IND Committee is now independent of Technical Committee and has final decision making authority).

✓ ***Role of Technical Committee in case of disapproval from SEC.*** In case of rejection from SEC and discontentment of applicant on the decision, the case can be submitted to the Technical Committee for review. Should the Technical Committee disagree with the SEC decision, it can overrule and its decision will be final.

✓ ***Role of Technical Committee in case of conflict between DCGI and SEC.*** In situations where there is disagreement between DCGI and SEC's decision on a clinical trial application, the issue may be brought to the notice of the Technical Committee within 1 month of SEC decision, whose decision would then be considered as final.

Table 5.1 gives a list of application fee for various licenses as per the New Drugs and Clinical Trials Rules, 2019.

Table 5.1 Application fee for various licenses as per the New Drugs and Clinical Trials Rules, 2019.

Type of application	Fees
Clinical trial – Phase I	3,00,000 INR
Clinical trial – Phase II,III	2,00,000 INR
Clinical trial – Phase IV	2,00,000 INR
Reconsideration of clinical trial application	50,000 INR
BABE study	2,00,000 INR
Registration of BA BE centre	5,00,000 INR
Permission to manufacture new drugs or investigational new drugs for clinical trial or BE BE Study	5000 INR per product
Import of new drugs or investigational new drugs for clinical trial or bioavailability or bioequivalence study or for examination, test and analysis	5000 INR per product
Permission to import new drug (Finished Formulation or API) for marketing	5,00,000 INR
Permission to import new Drug (Finished Formulation or API) already approved in the country for marketing	2,00,000 INR
Application for permission to import approved new drug for new claims, new indication or new dosage form or new route of administration or new strength for marketing	3,00,000 INR
Application for permission to import fixed dose combination having one or more of the ingredients as unapproved new molecules for Marketing	5,00,000 INR
Application for permission to import fixed Dose combination having approved ingredients for marketing	4,00,000 INR
Application for permission to import fixed dose combination already approved for Marketing	2,00,000 INR
Application for permission to import fixed dose combination for new claims, new indication or new dosage form or new route of administration or new strength for marketing	3,00,000 INR
Application for permission to manufacture new drug (Finished Formulation or Active Pharmaceutical Ingredient) for sale or Distribution	5,00,000 INR
Application for permission to manufacture new drug (Finished formulation or Active Pharmaceutical Ingredient) already approved in the country for sale or distribution	2,00,000 INR
Application for permission to manufacture approved new drug for new claims, new indication or new dosage form or new route of administration or new strength for sale or distribution	3,00,000 INR
Application for permission to manufacture fixed dose combination having one or more of the ingredients as unapproved new molecules for sale or distribution	5,00,000 INR

Table 5.1 *Contd...*

Application for permission to manufacture fixed dose combination having approved ingredients for sale or distribution	3,00,000 INR
Application for permission to manufacture fixed dose combination already approved for sale or distribution	2,00,000 INR
Application for permission to manufacture fixed dose combination for new claims, new indication or new dosage form or new route of administration or new strength for sale or distribution	3,00,000 INR
Application for Import of unapproved new drug by Government hospital and medical institution	10,000 INR
Application for permission to manufacture unapproved new drug but under clinical trial, for treatment of patient of life threatening disease	5,000 INR
Pre-submission meeting	5,00,000 INR
Post-submission meeting	50,000 INR
Any other application	50,000 INR

CONTENTS

Clinical Research on Biologics

INTRODUCTION

Biologicals are defined as "Structurally complex compounds such as a virus, therapeutic serum, toxin, antitoxin, vaccine, blood, blood component or derivatives, allergen product or analogous product applicable to the prevention, treatment or cure of a disease or condition of human beings" *(as per Public Health Services (PHS) Act, section 351)*.

The biological medicinal products or therapeutic biological products are referred to as "**Biopharmaceuticals**"; which are defined as "a protein or nucleic acid based pharmaceutical substance used for therapeutic or in vivo diagnostic purposes, which is produced by means other than direct extraction from a native (non-engineered) biological source". Key properties of biopharmaceuticals are their inherent biological nature and use of biotechnology in their manufacturing process.

Biosimilar: A biological therapeutic product similar in terms of quality, safety and efficacy to an already licensed reference biological therapeutic product. These are also referred to as:

Follow on biologics (as per US-FDA) defined as "highly similar to an existing FDA-approved reference product without clinically meaningful differences in safety, purity and potency".

Similar biologics (as per Indian guidelines) defined as "a biological product/drug produced by genetic engineering techniques and claimed to be "similar" in terms of safety, efficacy and quality to a reference biologics authorized for safe use in India by Drug Controller General of India (DCGI)" (Box 6.1).

> **Box 6.1** The New Drugs and Clinical Trials Rules, 2019.
>
> **Similar biologic:** "a biological product which is similar in terms of quality, safety and efficacy to reference biological product licenced or approved in India or any innovator product approved in International Council of Harmonisation (ICH) member countries".

Interchangeable biologics: It is a biosimilar product which may substitute the reference biological product without prescription. It should meet additional requirements based on further evaluation and testing as:

- it is assumed to yield the clinical effect comparable to the reference product in a particular patient.
- switching between interchangeable and reference biological does not alter the effectiveness or risk in a given patient.

SPECIAL CONCERNS WITH BIOLOGICS

Immunogenicity

Biologicals are inherently immunogenic. The intrinsic immunogenicity is expected to increase along the range from fully human analog to non-human mammalian source to non-mammalian source. The neutralizing antibodies to the biologicals commonly result in reduction of efficacy. For biologics having structural relationship with endogenous proteins, the antibodies generated may also bind to endogenous proteins. Hence, studies evaluating the immunogenicity of biological products hold great significance in the development of new biological drugs or biosimilars.

Pharmacokinetic issues

The substantially different physicochemical properties of biologics affect not only their pharmacokinetics, but the whole preclinical and clinical testing strategy. Traditional absorption, distribution, metabolism and excretion studies carried out during the preclinical phases of development of small drug molecules do not apply to biologics.

- Oral route of administration for delivering biologicals has limitations like enzymatic and pH-determined inactivation in the gastrointestinal tract, limited permeation through epithelial barriers, and formulation instability. Oral delivery is, hence, not an option for commercial use despite efforts made to increase the bioavailability of small proteins to around 10 percent. Biologics are mostly administered parentally. The extent of absorption is influenced by molecular weight, hydrophobicity, hydrophilicity, stability etc. and also by other associated factors e.g. blood flow and temperature at injection site, depth of injection, concomitant administration of albumin, physical activity etc.

- The biologics are generally confined to plasma and/or extracellular fluids.
- Biologics are degraded to small peptides and amino acids through processes similar to endogenous compounds; the resulting metabolites (amino acids) enter the endogenous amino acid pool and are used for the *de novo* synthesis of structural or functional body proteins. Mass balance (excretion) studies are not applicable as biologics are usually not eliminated in unchanged forms in urine and feces.
- Metabolism studies are also of limited value and generally focus on those compounds for which metabolism is likely to differ from normal protein catabolism. As biologics are cleared by non-cytochrome P450 enzymatic systems, there is very limited role of *in-vitro* metabolism based interaction studies in their case.

Bioanalytics

Appropriate bioanalytical methods form the cornerstone for obtaining valid pharmacokinetic/toxicokinetic and immunogenicity data during preclinical and clinical phases of development of biologics. Small molecule drugs usually require one pharmacokinetic assay for quantitative assessment of the parent molecule and its (major) metabolite(s). In contrast, biologics need multiple assays for the quantitative analyses of protein, its biological action and the identification and characterization of antibodies. This whole process is more time and capacity demanding.

USFDA REGULATIONS GOVERNING BIOLOGICS

Biologics Control Act, 1902. This was the first ever law to regulate biologics in United States. It was enacted in response to death of 22 children developing tetanus after being injected with contaminated biologicals [13 children injected with diphtheria anti-toxin at St. Louis, Missouri (contaminated vaccine produced from the blood of a horse, Jim, infected with tetanus); and 9 children received contaminated small-pox vaccines in Camden, New Jersey]. The Act regulated the manufacture and sale of biologics and licensure of facilities/ laboratories producing them.

In USA, FDA's *Center for Biologics Evaluation and Research (CBER)* and *Center for Drug Evaluation and Research (CDER)* are involved in the process of regulating biological products, including premarketing review and oversight. These are regulated under the provisions of Food, Drugs and Cosmetics (FDC) Act and Section 351 of the Public Health Service (PHS) Act; accordingly the applications for approval are made as New Drug Application (NDA) and Biologics License Application (BLA), respectively (Figure 6.1).

Biosimilars and interchangeable biologics are approved by an abbreviated licensure pathway under the Biologics Price Competition and Innovation Act (BPCI Act), 2009.

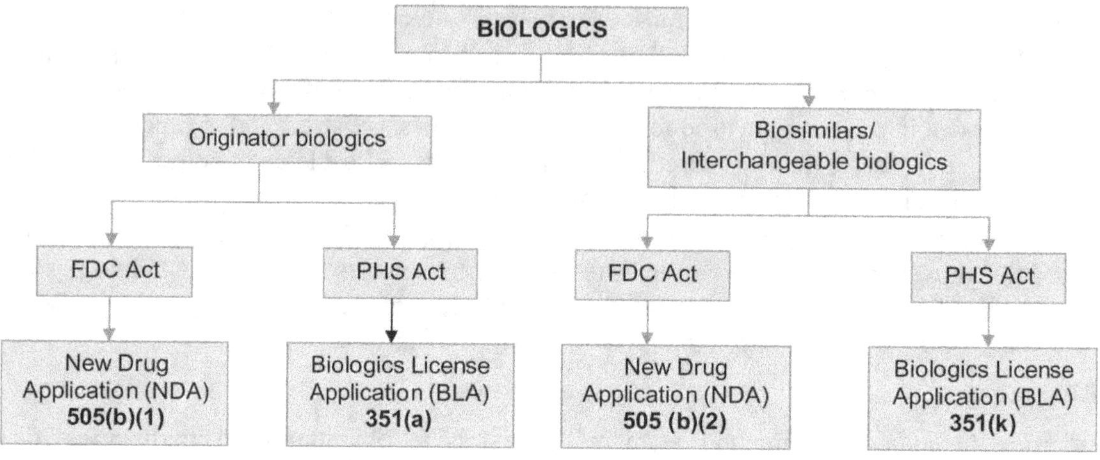

Figure 6.1 US-FDA approval pathways for biologics.

REGULATORY REQUIREMENTS FOR APPROVAL

❖ **Traditional 351 (a) pathway for biologics (Figure 6.2)**
  ♦ Need to develop the entire preclinical and clinical profile demonstrating the compounds safety and effectiveness, including the clinical trials in proposed indication/s.
  ♦ Drug development starts with preclinical research moving to Phase 1, 2 and 3 trials to show efficacy and safety.

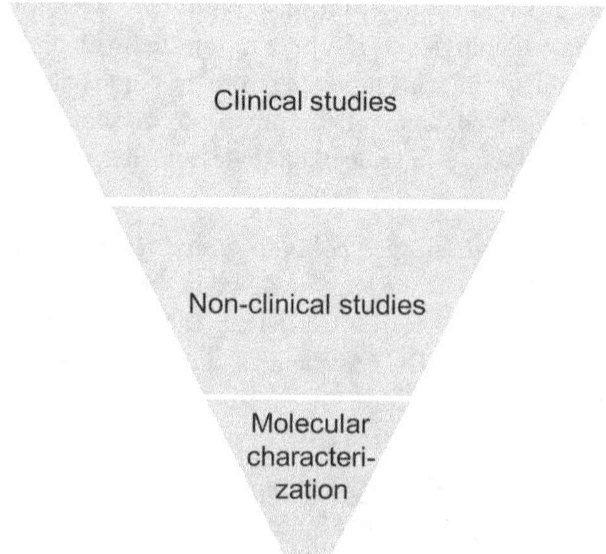

Figure 6.2 351 (a) approval pathway requirements.

❖ **Abbreviated licensure 351(k) pathway for biosimilars (Figure 6.3)**
- ♦ No need to generate the entire preclinical and clinical profile as the reference biologic.
- ♦ Need to exhibit *biosimilarity* and *absence of clinically significant dissimilarities in safety, purity and potency* between the proposed and FDA-approved reference product; generate the comparative data in a step-wise fashion with evaluation of residual uncertainty at each step.
- • Detailed analytical (physico-chemical and biological) characterization.
- • Preclinical studies including toxicity evaluation.
- • A clinical study or studies (including evaluation of immunogenicity, pharmacokinetics and/or pharmacodynamics) to demonstrate safety, purity and potency in 1 or more indications approved for the reference biologic.
- ♦ The type and purview of clinical studies depends on the amount of *residual uncertainty* after carrying out detailed analytical characterization and where relevant, animal studies.

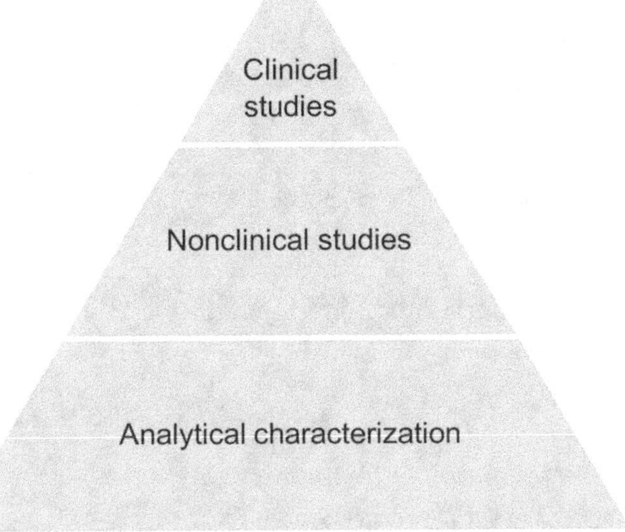

Figure 6.3 351 (k) approval pathway requirements.

US FDA maintains a "**Purple book**", which contains the lists of biological products and any biosimilar or interchangeable biologic approved by FDA.

REGULATORY SYSTEM FOR BIOLOGICS IN INDIA

In India, biologicals are regulated as per the Drugs and Cosmetics Act (1940) and Rules (1945) and Rules for the manufacture, use, import, export and storage of hazardous microorganisms/ genetically engineered organisms or cells, 1989 (Rules, 1989) notified under the Environment Protection Act, 1986. The regulatory authorities involved in the control of biologicals are Drug Controller General of India (DCGI) and Department of Biotechnology (DBT). All the biological products are considered as "new drugs" as per the Indian "Drugs and Cosmetics Act".

APPROVAL PROCESS FOR INDIGENOUSLY DEVELOPED BIOLOGICAL PRODUCTS

- Recombinant biological products that are indigenously developed are subject to regulation from the stage of cell line or clone development.
- Cell line development protocols should be reviewed and approved by the Institutional Bio-Safety Committee (IBSC) at the institute/company; and further notified to Review Committee on Genetic Manipulation (RCGM), department of biotechnology.
- The data on consistency of manufacturing, product characterization and proposed preclinical study protocols are submitted by the manufacturers to RCGM for review and approval before initiating the preclinical studies.

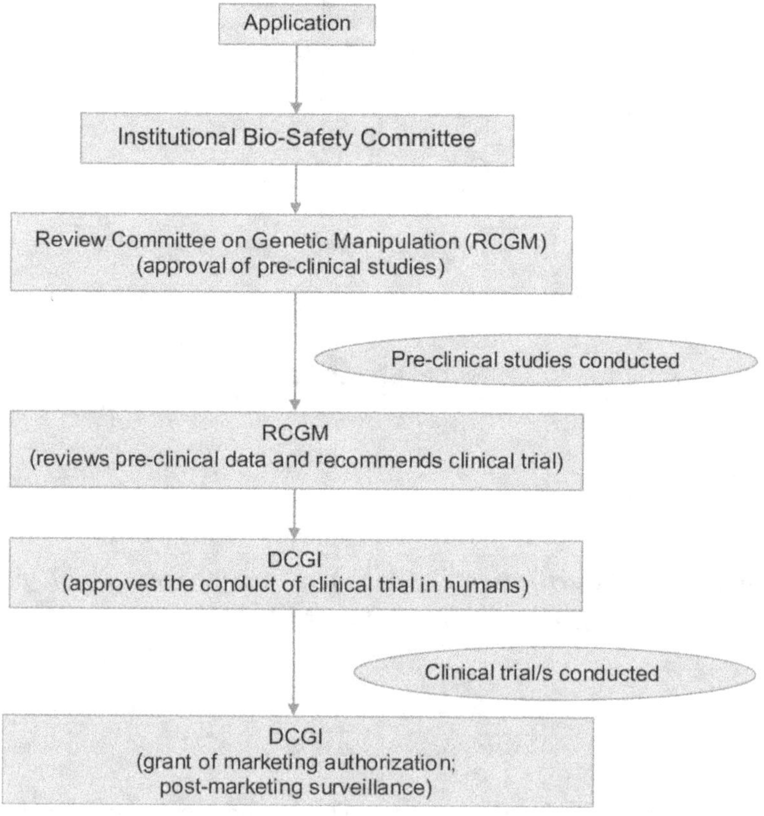

Figure 6.4 Approval process for indigenously developed biological products in India.

- On completion, the preclinical studies are then reviewed by RCGM; recommendation from RCGM about the safety of product is required for all clinical studies for biological products developed in India.
- In cases where the final product contains genetically modified organisms/ living modified organisms, applications need to be reviewed and approved by GEAC (Genetic Engineering Appraisal Committee), a statutory body under the Ministry of Environment and Forests (MoEF).
- The DCGI may direct the companies to conduct additional clinical studies in India for biological products that are intended for import and marketing.

Figure 6.4 illustrates various steps associated with the approval of indigenously developed biological in India.

NEW DRUG APPLICATION (NDA) FOR BIOLOGICALS

In 2008, CDSCO released a guidance document for industry regarding NDA for biologicals. The format of the document conforms with the international submission requirements and is in line with ICH- Common Technical Document (CTD). The scope of this document is applicable to all biologicals to be registered for human use, regardless of whether they are manufactured or licensed in the country of origin.

Suggested format of NDA for biologicals as per the guidance document:

Module I: Administrative and legal information

Module II: Summaries

Module III: Quality information (Chemical, Pharmaceutical and Biological)

Module IV: Non-clinical information

Module V: Clinical information

REGULATORY REQUIREMENTS FOR BIOSIMILARS OR SIMILAR BIOLOGICS

Biosimilars are relatively large and complex proteins; their characterization using simple analytical methods is a tedious process. Hence, the techniques available for generic non-biological molecules are not applicable to the development, evaluation and licensing of biosimilars.

The extent of data needed to evaluate efficacy and toxicity of biosimilars is quite variable and depends on the molecule evaluated; data required to be submitted is decided on an individual basis by the regulatory authority. One of the most important requirements for a biosimilar product is comparability to the innovator product and includes evaluation of physico-chemical properties, biological, preclinical, clinical and quality comparability.

Biosimilars or similar biologics had so far been getting approvals by CDSCO (DCGI) and RCGM using abbreviated version of the process applicable to new drugs as the case may be. However, need to establish a robust and clear regulatory pathway for similar biologics was felt and by the combined efforts of experts from CDSCO and DBT, a guidance document (Guidelines on similar biologics: regulatory requirements for marketing authorization in India) was released in 2012 which was revised in 2016. The objectives of the guidance document are:

- ✓ to provide information on the requirements to ensure comparability of similar biologic to reference biologic in terms of efficacy, safety and quality;
- ✓ to assist the applicants in understanding and complying with the regulatory requirements for marketing authorization of similar biologics in India.

Box 6.2 gives a summary of the key features of the DBT-CDSCO guidance document on similar biologicals.

Box 6.2 Guidelines on similar biologics: regulatory requirements for marketing authorization in India, 2016.

- ❖ The guidelines are applicable to similar biologics containing well-characterized proteins as active substance, synthesized by modern technology like recombinant DNA technology.

- ❖ Similar biologics can be developed only against the reference biologic that is approved in India or in an ICH country.

- ❖ There are less stringent requirements for preclinical and clinical evaluation of the similar biologics as compared to reference biologic, however, sufficient testing should be done to ensure comparability of similar biologic to reference biologic in terms of safety, efficacy and quality to safeguard public health.

- ❖ In general, data requirements are abbreviated for preclinical and clinical data but not for the quality components to demonstrate comparability to reference biologic.

- ❖ Similar biologics should be manufactured using a process which is validated, having high consistency and robustness. The same host line as used for manufacturing reference biologic should be used, if disclosed. Details on molecular biology viz. host cell cultures, vectors, gene sequences etc. should be provided. For clinical trial application, compliance of manufacturing process and facilities with the applicable GMP guidelines should be ensured.

- ❖ The characterization of similar biologics should include quality; structural, physico-chemical and immunological properties; biological activity; functional assays; purity; strength; content and stability.

Box 6.2 *Contd...*

❖ Data requirements for pre-clinical studies:
- proof of congruity of the process and product, product characterization and specifications as per RCGM requirements;
- general information about the reference biologic (drug, route of administration, therapeutic index, pharmacokinetics, bioequivalence, available toxicity data, tissue specific localization etc.) and similar biologic (indication, target population, dosage, route of administration, formulation, adjuvants, diluents, presentation etc.);
- preclinical studies (pharmacodynamic, toxicology, immune responses in animals).

❖ Data requirements for clinical trials
- pharmacokinetic studies;
- pharmacodynamic studies;
- confirmatory safety and efficacy study;
- safety and immunogenicity data.

CHAPTER 7

Clinical Research on Traditional Medicine

OVERVIEW

Introduction
General Regulatory Considerations
Good Clinical Practice Guidelines for
Clinical Trials in Ayurveda,
Siddha and Unani Medicine (GCP-ASU)

Phytopharmaceuticals
Research and Development (R & D) in the Sphere
of Translational Medicine in India
WHO Traditional Medicine Strategy 2014-2023

INTRODUCTION

WHO defines **traditional medicine (TM)** as "the knowledge, skills and practices based on the theories, beliefs and experiences indigenous to different cultures, used in the maintenance of health and in the prevention, diagnosis, improvement or treatment of physical and mental illness". **Complementary medicine (CM) or alternative medicine** refers to a "wide range of health care practices which are not considered to be part of conventional or traditional medicine and are not entirely included in the predominant health-care system". They are used as substitute to conventional medicine in some countries. **Traditional and complementary medicine (T&CM)** merges the terms TM and CM, encompassing products, practices and practitioners.

The recognized traditional systems of medicine in India are Ayurveda, Siddha and Unani (ASU), Yoga, Naturopathy and Homeopathy. In 2012, *Sowa Rigpa* (amchi or Tibetan medicine) was also included under the list.

GENERAL REGULATORY CONSIDERATIONS

- These systems are regulated in India by the Ministry of AYUSH (Ayurveda, Yoga & Naturopathy, Unani, Siddha and Homeopathy). Under AYUSH, drugs/formulations are classified in two categories:

o ***Classical preparations/formulations:*** those which are to be examined clinically for the same condition in which they are already in use or as have been mentioned in classical scholarly literature. Such traditional or classical drugs are synthesized and given nomenclature as per the formulations mentioned in scholarly literature.

o ***Patent or proprietary products:*** formulations comprising of only those ingredients as described in the formulae given in the authoritative books (of Ayurveda, Yoga, Naturopathy, Unani, Siddha, Homoeopathy, SOWA–RIGPA systems, as the case may be), medicine mentioned under the first schedule, but different from the classical medicine in terms of being combination/s, or use of invention, innovation or intellectual mediation to manufacture products. However, this group does not include products to be administered by parenteral route.

- The general principles of clinical trials are also applicable to herbal remedies. However, when there is a need to conduct clinical trials involving herbal remedies and products used in the traditional Indian systems of medicine in allopathic settings, it is desirable to associate physicians from the concerned system of medicine as collaborators/ co-investigators/ study team members for planning and executing the study. In situations where comparators are from more than one traditional system of medicine, investigators from the concerned systems should be involved as co-investigators.

- For the ethical review of research proposals involving any traditional system of medicine, the ECs must co-opt an expert from the respective system.

- When a folklore medicine / ethno-medicine is developed for commercialization after demonstrating its effectiveness on scientific grounds, the legitimate rights/ dues of the tribe or community which imparted the knowledge should be duly considered when applying for intellectual property rights for the product.

- The plants and herbal remedies being used already or described in authoritative texts of traditional system of medicine should be manufactured in strict accordance with the described text and as per the GMP standards.

- Clinical trials with herbal products must be conducted after their appropriate standardization and identification of suitable markers for their evaluation.

- Good manufacturing Practices (GMP) standards for the formulations to be tested are generally not required for Phase I and II trials. For Phase III trials, however, GMP standards need to be maintained due to involvement of larger number of subjects followed by applying for marketing approvals.

- All formulations containing herbal ingredients must fulfill criteria as described by WHO document "Operational Guidance: Information needed to support clinical trials of herbal products (2005)":

❖ **For Phase I/II studies**

Herbal Substance:
- description of the plant: genus, species (cultivar when applicable); region(s) and country(ies) of origin, time of harvest, parts to be harvested;
- plant processing: drying, mechanical disruption, solvent extraction (aqueous or organic solvents, others);
- analytical methodologies;
- specification;
- storage conditions/shelf life.

Herbal Product:
- amount of active ingredient
- list of excipients
- type of product (tablet, capsule, etc.) and its method of manufacture
- analysis of putative active ingredient(s) via chemical or biological parameters
- analysis of a sizeable chemical constituent (analytical marker compound)
- analysis via chemical fingerprint (analytical markers)
- analysis for lack of contamination by pesticides, herbicides, heavy metals, synthetic drug adulterants, microbials, toxins, etc.
- dissolution studies
- storage conditions and stability during the duration of the trial
- specification against which a certificate of analysis can be assessed before the release of clinical trial material.

❖ **For Phase III studies**: Generally the same procedures are followed as for Phase I/II trials, but in a more extensive and stringent manner.

Herbal Substance:
- as mentioned under Phase I/II trials.
- Additionally, a statement that the cultivation of plant was done as per the Good Agricultural Practices or harvesting done as per the Good Wildcrafting Practices.
- reference batch in addition.

Herbal Product:
- as mentioned under Phase I/II trials.
- Additionally, environmental impact statement.

GOOD CLINICAL PRACTICE GUIDELINES FOR CLINICAL TRIALS IN AYURVEDA, SIDDHA AND UNANI MEDICINE (GCP-ASU)

In 2010, the Drugs and Cosmetics Rules 158(B) released guidelines for issuing license to patent or proprietary ASU medicines based on demonstration of proof of effectiveness. This was followed by release of GCP-ASU guidelines by Department of AYUSH, MoHFW, Government of India in 2013 aiming to guide the researchers conducting such trials. The main objectives of the guidelines were to:

- encourage the culture of conducting ASU-intervention based clinical trials according to applicable ethical and scientific standards and
- assure safety and safeguard of the rights of study subjects.

The guidelines, in general, adopt the basic principles outlined in CDSCO document of GCP guidelines (2001) with deemed changes as applicable to ASU principles and treatment methodologies.

As per the GCP-ASU guidelines:

- The Phase 1 studies should include healthy volunteers an exception being studies on ASU drug/patent or proprietary medicine with possible toxicity (e.g. medicines containing Schedule E-1 ingredients) where patients should be studied.
- For ASU drug / patent or proprietary medicines supposed to be administered for long duration, trials including expanded exposure to the medicine are usually undertaken during Phase III, although they may be started in Phase II. Such studies conducted in Phase III aim to gather comprehensive information required to support prescribing information for the medicine/ drug.

PHYTOPHARMACEUTICALS

Phytopharmaceuticals, a separate class of drugs, was defined in Drugs and Cosmetics Rules, 2015 as "purified and standardised fraction with defined minimum four bio-active or phyto-chemical compounds (qualitatively and quantitatively assessed) of an extract of a medicinal plant or its part, for internal or external use in human beings or animals for diagnosis, treatment, mitigation or prevention of any disease or disorder but does not include administration by parenteral route".

The regulatory requirements for phyto-pharmaceuticals are within the scope of CDSCO (Box 7.1).

Being the newest category of drugs in India, the standards and guidance documents for pharmaceuticals are still getting evolved. As per current regulations, every herbal formulation seeking approval under phytopharmaceutical category shall be considered as new drug for 5 years and hence, it is mandatory for phytopharmaceutical drug to undergo clinical trials and submit non-clinical as well as clinical data to obtain license for marketing. This is in contrast to a herbal drug under the categorization of AYUSH which needs demonstration of *in vitro* bioequivalence with the reference standards mentioned in the respective monographs.

> **Box 7.1** The New Drugs and Clinical Trials Rules, 2019.
>
> ***Regulatory requirements to conduct clinical trials, import or manufacture a phytopharmaceutical drug in the country***
>
> Data to be submitted:
>
> - Summary of phytopharmaceutical drug with information on botanical name of the plant, formulation and route of administration, dosages, proposed indication/s, etc.
> - Supportive information from published scientific literature on plant or product or phytopharmaceutical drug, as a traditional medicine or as an ethno medicine, including efficacy, safety, human and clinical pharmacology for the pharmaceutical drug/ product intended to be marketed.
> - Data generated on:
>   - ✓ identification, authentication, and source of the plant used for extraction and fractionation (toxonomical identity of plant; morphological and anatomical description; natural habitat and geographical distribution; season or time of collection; harvest location and time; stage of plant growth at harvest; collection, washing, drying and storage conditions; quality specifications etc.);
>   - ✓ procedure for extraction, fractionation and purification;
>   - ✓ formulation details of phytopharmaceutical drug;
>   - ✓ manufacturing process of formulation;
>   - ✓ stability data;
>   - ✓ efficacy and safety; human and clinical pharmacology.
> - Regulatory and marketing status.
> - Post marketing surveillance (PMS) by means of PSURs.
> - Any other relevant information.
>
> Once NDA approval is obtained from CDSCO, the phyto-pharmaceutical drug would be granted marketing status as that of a new chemical entity- based drug.

RESEARCH AND DEVELOPMENT (R & D) IN THE SPHERE OF TRANSLATIONAL MEDICINE IN INDIA

The Department of Biotechnology has taken various initiatives to promote research and development in this area across the country using a multi-disciplinary approach. Some of these initiatives are:

- ◆ With an aim to develop a herbal drug line, provisions have been laid for supporting translational research to convert research leads from medicinal plants into potential drug products.

- Launch of *"Phytopharmaceuticals Mission Programme in North East Region"* with a goal to develop worldwide acceptable phytopharmaceuticals from medicinal plants of North East Region.
- Identification of centre of excellence for *"National Centre for Microbial Resource (NCMR)"*, National centre for cell science, Pune in 2017 previously known as Microbial Culture Collection (MCC). DBT has notified NCMR to function as "Bio-repository for resistant microbes/infective agents (Bacteria and Fungi)" to conduct collection, storage, maintenance, preservation and characterization of these microbes across the country.
- Launch of *"Indian Bioresource Information Network (IBIN)"* as a gateway to access bi-resource database available in the country. Currently, IBIN is the largest database with information on 73,276 species of plants, animals, marine organisms and microbes including the spatial database.
- Establishment of *"Virtual Centre of Excellence for Marine Biodiversity and Biotechnological Interventions"* for exploring ocean resources with an aim to escalate research in modern marine biology and biotechnology.

WHO TRADITIONAL MEDICINE STRATEGY 2014-2023

This strategy was launched with an aim to support the member states to strengthen the field of traditional medicine and prioritize health services and systems including traditional and complementary medicine products, practices and practitioners. For this, three strategic sectors have been identified as:

- Active management by means of national policies recognizing the role and potential of T & CM.

Clinical Research on Medical Devices

INTRODUCTION

Medical device: An instrument, equipment, implant, appliance, or other similar articles, whether used alone or in combination, including any component, part, or accessory which does not attain its primary intended purpose through pharmacological, immunological or metabolic methods but may be aided in its proposed action by such methods. It may be intended to be used for one or more specific purposes like:

- ✓ diagnosis of ailments or disorders or in the cure, alleviation, therapy, or prevention of illness in human beings or other animals;
- ✓ to introduce any structural or functional modifications in the body of humans or other animals;
- ✓ as replacement or for modification or support of congenital deformity;
- ✓ control of conception;
- ✓ supporting or sustaining life.

Medicated devices: These are devices containing pharmacologically active substances and act like drugs.

CLASSIFICATION OF MEDICAL DEVICES

❖ **As per Indian GCP:**
- *Non critical devices:* An investigational device not posing significant risk to the subjects e.g. thermometer, B.P. apparatus.

- *Critical devices:* A device presenting a potential risk to the health and safety of subjects e.g. implants, pacemakers, internal catheters etc.

❖ Depending upon the risks involved (for medical devices apart from *in-vitro* diagnostic devices)
  - *Class A*: Low level of risk e.g. thermometers, bandages, tongue depressors.
  - *Class B*: Low to intermediate level of risk e.g. hypodermic needles, suction equipment.
  - *Class C*: Intermediate to high level of risk e.g. lung ventilator, bone fixation plate.
  - *Class D*: High level of risk e.g. heart valves, implantable defibrillator.

❖ Diagnostic devices can be classified as:
  - *Notified devices*. These are *in-vitro* diagnostic devices for testing HIV, HBsAg, HCV and blood grouping.
  - *Non-notified devices*. These are devices for testing malaria, TB, dengue, chikungunya, typhoid, syphilis, cancer markers, etc.

❖ **As per 21 CFR 860:**

Class I (Low risk devices)

- Routine control measures are enough to offer reasonable affirmation of safety and efficacy.
- Simple in design.
- Subject to least regulatory control- require Premarket Notification (510k application) if they are not exempt.
- e.g. elastic bandages, hand-held surgical instruments, wound dressings etc.

Class II (Moderate risk devices)

- Routine and special control measures (e.g. performance standards, surveillance) required to assure safety and effectiveness.
- Subject to more regulatory control than class I including special labeling requirements, post market surveillance, mandatory performance standards, design controls, tracking requirements etc.
- e.g. electronic wheelchairs, infusion pumps, surgical drapes, sutures, ECGs, urology catheters.

Class III (Moderate and high risk devices)

- Routine and special control measures required to reasonably ensure the efficacy and safety of such devices.
- Most stringent regulatory requirements- clinical data and pre- market approval required
- Such devices are life sustaining or life supporting, hold crucial role to prevent deterioration of human health, important in preventing impairment.
- e.g. pacemakers, defibrillators, silicone gel filled breast implants, vascular grafts, angioplasty catheters, cardiac stents.

USFDA REGULATIONS GOVERNING MEDICAL DEVICES

Regulatory clearance processes of medical devices

Premarket Notification 510(k)

Used for devices that are substantially equivalent (SE) to a predicate (legally marketed) device. The manufacturer must notify FDA 90 days before proposing to market a device.

Premarket Approval Application (PMA)

PMA process is used for class III devices, new types of devices and devices identified to be not substantially equivalent to predicate devices. May require pre-clinical and clinical data obtained from an investigational device exemption (IDE).

Investigational device exemption (IDE)

An IDE permits the use of an investigational device in a clinical study aiming to gather data on its safety and efficacy, which is needed to support a Premarket Approval (PMA) application or a Premarket Notification [510(k)] submission to FDA.

An approved IDE grants permission for lawful shipment of the device with the purpose to conduct investigations on it without the need to comply with other requirements of the Food, Drug, and Cosmetic Act, which are otherwise applicable to devices used commercially. Sponsors are not required to submit a PMA or Premarket Notification 510(k), register their organization, or enlist the device while it is under investigation. Sponsors of IDE's are also not liable to quality system regulation except the design control requirements.

Humanitarian Device Exemption (HDE)

- ✓ The purpose of HDE pathway is to foster development of medical devices which will be of use to patients having rare disorders (i.e. <4000 patients per year). The process of applying for HDE is identical to that for a PMA, except that there is no need to prove effectiveness. The use of these devices is permissible under IRB approval.
- ✓ There should be no profit margin for these devices i.e. price cannot exceed the costs accrued during their research, development, manufacturing and distribution.
- ✓ There is less regulatory burden on manufacturers for HDEs due to less stringent data requirements with respect to effectiveness of these devices. Hence, the process for approval is less time consuming.
- ✓ E.g. the vertical expandable prosthetic titanium rib was given an HDE. This device was developed to treat thoracic insufficiency syndrome, including fused ribs and scoliosis in infants and small children. It is now a Humanitarian use device (HUD).

De novo classification pathway

The FDA "de novo" classification pathway comprises of a streamlined reclassification procedure for low risk devices having no substantially equivalent predicate (i.e. do not have any identical device which has already received 510(k) clearance). Hence, these low-risk devices, due to their novelty, are automatically given a Class III status (conventionally for high-risk devices and require a very demanding application process). By virtue of the de novo pathway, novel low-risk devices can be re-categorized under Class I or II, aiding manufacturers to bypass the highly resource and time demanding process of Premarket Approval (PMA).

REGULATIONS GOVERNING MEDICAL DEVICES IN INDIA

In India, the clinical research on medical devices and their import, manufacture, sale and distribution are regulated under the Medical Device Rules, 2017.

Medical Device Rules, 2017

The Medical Device Rules were released by MoHFW, Government of India in 2017 (GSR 78E) (Box 8.1). The guidelines to conduct clinical investigation of medical devices and assessment of clinical functioning of new *in-vitro* diagnostic medical devices are included in Chapter VII of the Medical Device Rules, 2017. The guidelines, in general, focus on the basic principles of clinical research as described in Indian GCP guidelines developed by CDSCO in 2001 with necessary modifications as applicable to medical devices (Box 8.2).

Box 8.1 Important definitions included in the Medical Device Rules, 2017.

Active diagnostic medical device: "any active medical device whether used independently or along with other medical devices to impart information for identifying, diagnosing or monitoring, or to provide support in the treatment of any physiological condition, state of health, illness or congenital deformity".

Active medical device: "a medical device, the functioning of which is dependent on a source of electrical energy or any other source of energy other than the energy generated by human or animal body or gravity".

Active therapeutic medical device: "any active medical device used independently or along with other medical devices to assist, alter, replace or restore biological functions or structures with an aim to treat or alleviate any disease, physical damage or handicap".

Predicate device: "a device, first time and first of its kind, approved for manufacture for sale or for import by the central licensing authority and has the similar intended use, material of construction, and design characteristics as the device which is proposed for license in India".

Medical devices claiming substantial equivalence to predicate device but requiring clinical investigation shall not be marketed without prior approval by central licensing authority.

Registration of the clinical investigation is mandatory with the clinical trial registry prior to enrolment of first patient.

The sponsor, investigator, clinical research organization or any other organization conducting a clinical investigation are required to maintain data, records, and other relevant documents for seven years after the investigation is completed.

> **Box 8.2** Application to conduct clinical investigation on medical devices.
>
> Application in Form MD-22 along with following data:
> - Design analysis data;
> - Biocompatability and animal performance study data;
> - Investigator's brochure, clinical investigation plan, case report form, informed consent form, adverse event form, undertaking by investigator, ethics committee approval;
> - Regulatory status in other countries;
> - Proposed instructions for use or directions for use and labels;
> - Report of clinical investigation, certified by Principal Investigator.
>
> (Permission to conduct investigation is granted in Form MD-23 by the licensing authority within a period of 90 days from the date of application).
>
> ***Investigational medical device developed in India:*** Pilot clinical investigation or first in human study is required and data generated needs to be submitted.
>
> ***Investigational medical device developed and studied in country other than India:*** Data from pilot clinical investigation or relevant clinical study to be submitted along with application. Central licensing authority may grant permission to repeat pilot study or conduct pivotal clinical investigation. Pivotal clinical investigation should be carried out in India prior to marketing authorization application for medical device in India except for investigational medical devices classified under class A.
>
> The number of study subjects and trial sites required depends on the nature and objective of clinical investigation.

BIOMEDICAL ENGINEERING AND BIO-DESIGN

There is an increasing demand for medical devices in India which are affordable, simple, reliable and flexible. In this direction, the department of biotechnology has taken many initiatives to develop indigenous affordable medical technologies (Box 8.3).

> **Box 8.3** Biomedical engineering and Bio-design.
>
> - ***"Bio-medical engineering"***, a multi-disciplinary field of research involving application of engineering techniques for basic understanding and invention of novel technologies for improvement of quality of life.

Box 8.3 Contd...

- ◆ Implementation of ***"med-tech innovation bio-design programmes"*** whose objectives are:
  - promoting multi-disciplinary approach in innovation by collaboration of medical and engineering institutes;
  - providing hands-on training to medical technology innovators in bio-design process;
  - creating easily accessible processes and facilities to support the entire innovation process;
  - establish an effective network of biologists, engineers, clinicians, and medical technology personnel for design process;
  - promote industry participation for scale-up of technology transfer and commercialization;
  - take steps to establish national and international partnerships.

IMPORTANT LINKS

1. Medical device Rules; GSR 78E:
   https://mohfw.gov.in/sites/default/files/Medical%20Device%20Rules%2C%202017.pdf

CHAPTER 9

Clinical Research on Stem Cells

OVERVIEW

Introduction
Specific Principles Applicable to
Stem Cell Research
Categories of Research on Stem Cells

Responsibilities for Conduct of Stem Cell
Research (Investigator, Institution and Sponsor)
Procedure for Review and Regulatory
Surveillance of Stem Cell Research

INTRODUCTION

"Guidelines for Stem Cell Research and Therapy" were released jointly by the Indian Council of Medical Research and the Department of Biotechnology in 2007. These were further revised in 2013 and 2017 as "National Guidelines for Stem Cell Research". The guidelines have been constituted to assure that research involving human stem cells is carried out ethically and responsibly and in compliance with all regulatory guidelines applicable to biomedical research in general and stem cell research in particular (Box 9.1).

Box 9.1 Stem Cell Research - Points to consider.

- The guidelines are applicable to only stem cell research, both experimental and clinical, and not their therapeutic applications.

- The guidelines are applicable to research conducted on any kind of human stem cells and their derivatives; these are not applicable to research involving non-human stem cells and their derivatives.

- Using stem cells for any condition in patients besides that for hematopoietic stem cell reconstitution for approved indications (hematological, immunological and metabolic disorders), is investigational at present.

- Any application/s of stem cells for research in patients should only be conducted within the purview of an approved clinical trial with an objective to enhance medical and scientific knowledge, and not proposing it for treatment. Any use of stem cells in patients outside the purview of an approved clinical trial shall be taken as malpractice.

- Protein rich plasma (PRP) and autologous chondrocyte/osteocytes implantation are categorised as other cell based applications and not stem cell transplantation; hence these do not fall within the range of these guidelines.

The guidelines describe specialized provisions of stem cells, due to their potential for unlimited proliferation, differentiation to cells of the germ layers, regeneration of tissues, and their involvement in pre-implantation stages of human development. The guidelines therefore include:

- Procurement of gametes, embryos and somatic cells for derivation and propagation of pluripotent and multipotent stem cell lines, their banking and distribution.
- Regulated differentiation into desired progenitor cells and their characterization.
- Use of human stem cells and other progenitors derived from them, or their products for basic and clinical research.

SPECIFIC PRINCIPLES APPLICABLE TO STEM CELL RESEARCH

The general principles pertaining to all biomedical research conducted in human subjects also apply to stem cell research. However, stem cells are distinctive due to their potential for self-renewal and multi lineage differentiation; they might also lead to tumors such as teratomas. Hence, there are few major issues with regard to their collection, processing, storage and use, especially the human embryonic stem (ES) cells for translational research.

Health and Safety of Donors

Before procuring stem cells for research, it is essential to acquire informed consent from the donor.

- The donor should be imparted information regarding the need to screen transmissible diseases (about which he/she may or may not be aware of) and potential risks associated with donation especially during major invasive procedures like ovum or bone marrow donation, under local or general anaesthesia.
- The donor must also be briefed that cell lines might be produced from donated material which can further be banked and shared with other scientific groups. The cell lines might also be genetically manipulated and commercialized , however, the Intellectual Property Rights (IPR) will not be conferred on the donor.
- The donor should be informed that he/she may be approached in future for particular requirements.
- The donation of gametes and embryos are associated with distinct ethical and moral issues. It is required to assure the donors that they are not exploited and commoditized.

Manufacture and Quality Assurance of Stem Cell Product

Adequate quality control and assurances need to be in place during processing, enrichment, preparation and administration of stem cells. Therapeutic cell products should be manufactured in accordance with the applicable guidelines and other laboratory conditions as per the purpose of each use. Rigorous characterization of the product with regard to its identity, purity safety, genomic stability, tumorigenicity and potency is required prior to being released for use in humans.

CATEGORIES OF RESEARCH ON STEM CELLS (FIGURE 9.1)

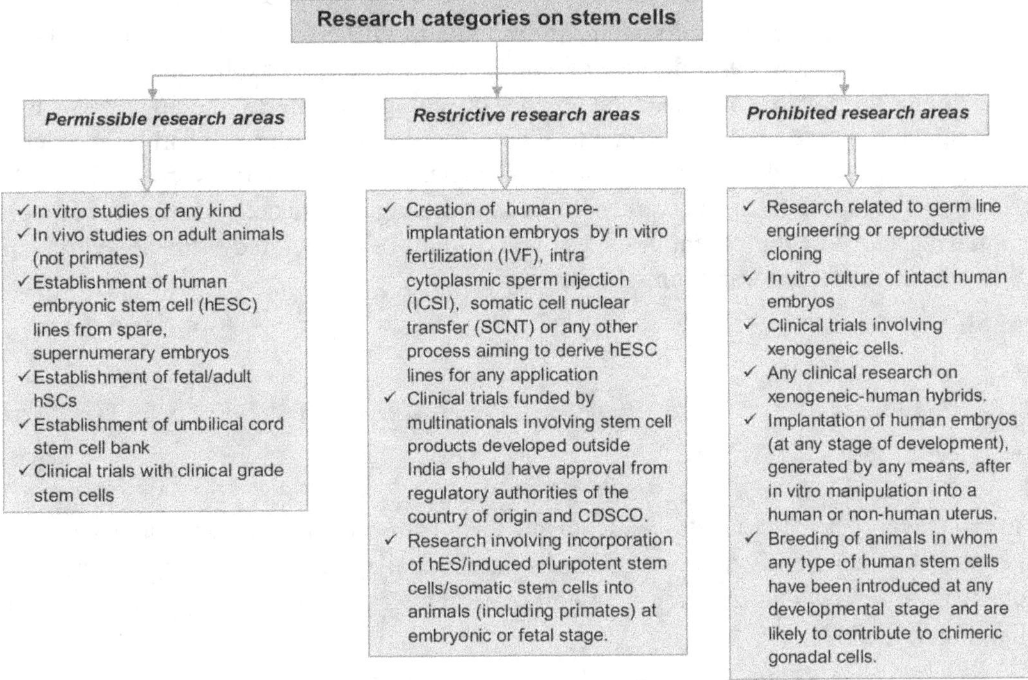

Figure 9.1 Categories of research on stem cells.

RESPONSIBILITIES FOR CONDUCT OF STEM CELL RESEARCH (INVESTIGATOR, INSTITUTION AND SPONSOR)

- The investigators and institutions carrying out stem cell research are ultimately responsible for ensuring that research activities are in compliance with the national regulations and guidelines. Sponsors are also responsible and liable under various statutes, regulations and guidelines governing research and development in this area in the country. Members of the regulatory committee should be updated on any advances in this field.
- The study participants and their family members should be informed adequately about the trial protocol, its constraints and possible harmful effects. They must also be given information regarding the indication for treatment.
- Every institution should maintain a record of its investigators involved in stem cell research and ensure that all registered users hold updated knowledge on existing guidelines and regulations regarding stem cells. The institution should also ensure the application of most current standards in this field.

- Every institution shall establish an Institutional committee for Stem Cell Research (IC-SCR) as per national stem cell guidelines and lend proper support for its performance. All records related to clinical adult stem cell research should be archived for a minimum period of 5 years and those for ES/iPS cell research for atleast 10 years.

- The basic scientists involved in human stem cell research should be vigilant for safeguarding rights and dignity of human donors and aborted foetuses from whom samples for research have been obtained. The biological material should be given utmost respect and care in all experiments. The use of human embryos shall be restricted to minimum required, and under situations when no other alternatives are available. Also, utmost precautions need be taken while introducing human cells in animals, especially during early developmental stages, which may be associated with development of chimeras or incorporation into brain/gonads.

PROCEDURE FOR REVIEW AND REGULATORY SURVEILLANCE OF STEM CELL RESEARCH

Stem cell research has unique ethical, legal and social concerns that needs an added oversight and expertise to efficiently conduct scientific and ethical evaluation. Hence, an independent mechanism to review and monitor stem cell research is essential both at the institutional as well as the national level.

National level: **National Apex Committee for Stem Cell Research and Therapy (NAC-SCRT)** *Institutional level:* ***Institutional Committee for Stem Cell Research (IC-SCR).*** This is a multidisciplinary body at the institutional level. The committee should have at least 7 members and comprise of representatives from public and persons having expertise in clinical medicine, developmental biology, stem cell research, molecular biology, assisted reproduction technology, and ethical and legal issues in stem cell research. It should have adequate resources for coordinating reviews of various protocols.

- The major role of these oversight committees is to ensure that review, approval and monitoring of all research projects in the area of stem cell research is carried out in an efficient and stringent manner according to the national guidelines.

- All organizations and investigators whether public or private, conducting research on human stem cells need to be registered with the NAC-SCRT through IC-SCR.

- It is mandatory for Institutional Committee for Stem Cell Research (ICSCR) to get registered with National Apex Committee for Stem Cell Research and Therapy (NAC-SCRT).

- Stem cell research should be conducted only at institutions having registered IC-SCR, IEC, and Good Manufacturing Practice (GMP) and Good Laboratory Practice (GLP) certified facilities.

- Research on stem cells should be undertaken only by medical professionals registered with the Medical Council of India (MCI) and possessing MCI approved post graduate qualification in the key area of the concerned trial.

- Stem cell research should be conducted after getting prior approval of IC-SCR for permitted research and of the NAC-SCRT for restricted research areas. All new human pluripotent stem cell lines, regardless of the source and methodology used, can be developed after obtaining approval of IC-SCR. However, the use of human embryonic and iPS cells in clinical trials shall be done after prior approval from NAC-SCRT. Permission for procurement of human embryonic stem cell lines from abroad or from laboratories/banks in India needs to be obtained from IC-SCR.

- All clinical trials with SSCs, apart from those with genetic modifications, need to have prior approval of IC-SCR and Institutional Ethics Committee (IEC). Clinical trials involving genetically modified SSCs, and ES or iPS cells or derivatives should have prior approval from the NAC-SCRT after obtaining clearance from IC-SCR and IEC.

- Approval of the Drug Controller General of India (DCGI) is obligatory for stem cell based IND products and application for new indications (stem cells for therapies are considered as drugs) with prior clearance from IC-SCR and IEC. All clinical trials using stem cells that have undergone more than minimal manipulation need to be approved by IC-SCR, IEC and DCGI.

- In order to obtain marketing authorization of stem cell derived products, all clinical trials approved by the DCGI need to be registered with the clinical trials registry of India (CTRI) established by ICMR.

CHAPTER 10

Clinical Research in Special Populations

OVERVIEW

INTRODUCTION

Depending on the proposed therapeutic profile of a new drug and its presumed use in population, specific information supporting its use in special subgroups (pediatric, geriatrics, pregnant and lactating women etc.) needs to be submitted to regulatory bodies. It is important to study these subgroups of population as they are usually not involved during the developmental phases of new drugs and hence there is paucity of data supporting the efficacy and safety of new drugs in these subgroups. Different regulatory authorities worldwide have laid down recommendations on conducting clinical research in special populations and data required to be submitted before considering a drug as suitable for their use.

CLINICAL RESEARCH IN PEDIATRICS

Children are unique biologically and in their interphase with environment. The observations in adults cannot be automatically assumed to be true in children. Adequately designed and conducted clinical trials involving children are necessary to promote the health of children and future adults. There should be justified and reasonable involvement of children in clinical research; subgroups of children should neither be unduly burdened as participants nor unnecessarily excluded from taking part in research.

AGE CLASSIFICATION IN PEDIATRICS

Age classification of pediatric population is dubious to some extent with a lack of consensus among various authorities.

US FDA guidance (E11: Clinical investigation of medicinal products in the pediatric population) provides one possible categorization for guiding study design in pediatric research as:

- Preterm newborn infants
- Term newborn infants (0 to 27 days)
- Infants and toddlers (28 days to 23 months)
- Children (2 to 11 years)
- Adolescents (12 to 16-18 years (depending on region))

WHO pediatric age categories as basis for Model Essential Medicines List for children:
- Premature newborns (< 38 weeks gestational age)
- Term newborns (>38 weeks gestational age)
- Neonates (0 to 30 days of age)
- Infant (1 month to 2 years)
- Young child (2 to 6 years)
- Child (6 to 12 years)
- Adolescent (12 to 18 years)

Nevertheless, there is some degree of overlap in developmental issues (e.g. physiological, psychological, social, cognitive etc.) across various age categories.

NEED FOR BIOMEDICAL RESEARCH IN CHILDREN

The conduct of biomedical research in children becomes imperative in today's era of evidence based medicine due to a number of reasons:
- To advance knowledge in the area of diseases affecting only children with no adult counterparts e.g. hyaline membrane disease, neonatal hyperbilirubinemia, infantile spasms etc.
- For diseases affecting both children and adults e.g. nephrotic syndrome, rheumatoid arthritis etc. there may be pathophysiological differences in disease processes and response to treatment between children and adults. Hence, the drugs approved in adults cannot be simply extrapolated for use in children.
- Age-dependent variations in the pharmacokinetics of many drugs e.g. metabolism; rapid metabolism of many drugs in children compared to adults may necessitate the administration of a higher dosage (per kilogram body weight) of the drugs in children.
- Age-related differences in the adverse effect profile of some drugs e.g. Reye's syndrome in children associated with aspirin use, grey baby syndrome with chloramphenicol.

- Need for age-appropriate drug delivery approaches like syrups to ensure accurate, palatable and safe drug administration in children.
- Limited information regarding pediatric drug usage in drug product labeling.

CHALLENGES IN CONDUCTING BIOMEDICAL RESEARCH IN CHILDREN

- Practical issues in enrolling sufficient number of pediatric subjects in trials particularly if the disease under study is rare which may adversely affect the statistical power of the clinical trial.
- Special study design considerations in pediatric research e.g. incorporation of developmentally appropriate end-points, long duration follow up studies to assess long term outcomes, preference for non-invasive procedures etc.
- Ethical concerns revolving around pediatric research such as diminished autonomy, inherent vulnerability etc.
- Need to take into consideration familial and societal concerns due to the involvement of parents, guardians and families in research involving children.
- Relatively lesser inclination of pharmaceutical companies towards developing drugs for pediatric use due to smaller market compared to adults and lack of funding sources.

REGULATIONS GOVERNING PEDIATRIC BIOMEDICAL RESEARCH

The first regulations specifically governing research involving children were published by the U.S. Department of Health and Human Services (DHHS) in 1983 as Subpart D of 45 CFR 46. Under this, there were four categories under which pediatric research may be approved:

- ❖ Research exposing the children to not more than minimal risk.
- ❖ Research involving more than minimal risk but the risk is reasonably explained by the expected benefit to subjects and benefit-risk profile is favorable and comparable to available treatment options.
- ❖ Research involving more than minimal risk and no anticipated direct benefit to participants but (a) very small increase in risk over the minimal risk, (b) the research is expected to enhance existing knowledge about the pediatric disease or illness.
- ❖ Research not otherwise permissible but considered as essential by IRB and the Secretary of DHHS to understand, prevent or treat some serious illness affecting children provided research is carried out in compliance with sound ethical principles.

U.S. laws governing drug development in pediatrics

- ❖ *Pediatric Research Equity Act (PREA).* PREA was signed into law in 2003 as an amendment to the Federal Food, Drug and Cosmetic Act. PREA was an attempt to handle the inadequacy of information on pediatric use in drug product labeling. PREA requires the pharmaceutical companies to conduct pediatric assessment of new drugs/ biologics which encompasses:

♦ assessment of effectiveness and safety for the proposed indication in relevant pediatric population.

♦ data supporting dosage and administration in pediatric population.

Specifically, the Act requires NDAs and BLAs for a new active ingredient, new dosage form, new dosage regimen, new indication or new route of administration to include data on pediatric evaluation unless a waiver or deferral has been obtained by the applicant.

❖ *Best Pharmaceuticals for children Act (BPCA).* Under this Act, provisions are laid down to provide financial incentives to companies for voluntarily conducting pediatric studies. It also authorizes FDA to request pediatric studies for approved and /or unapproved indications.

The New Drugs and Clinical Trials Rules, 2019 recommendations on pediatric clinical research

❖ **The appropriate time to conduct pediatric studies** during the clinical development program of a new drug depends on the drug being evaluated, the type of disorder being treated, safety concerns, and the benefit-risk profile of existing therapies (Figure 10.1).

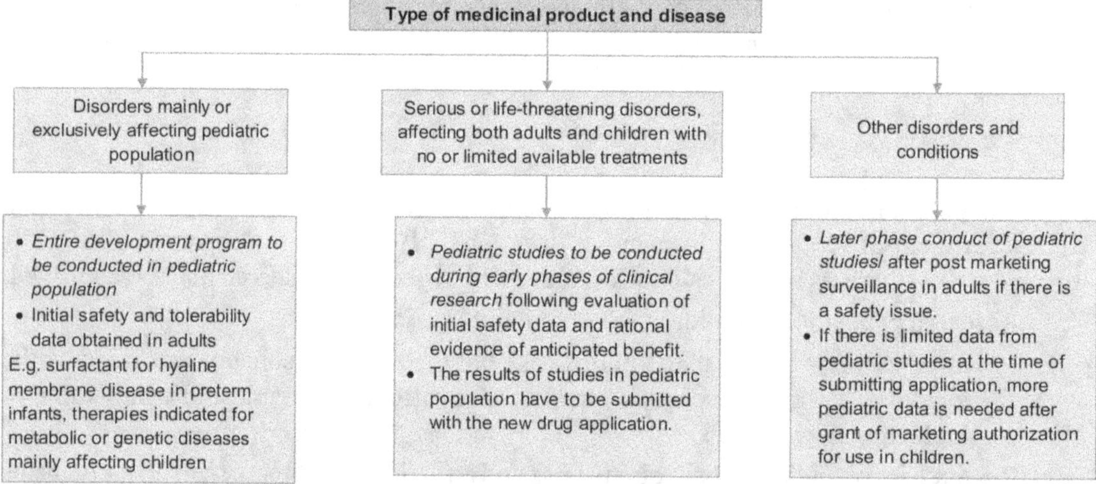

Note: In cases where the clinical development program of new drug involves children, it is preferable to take older children during initial period with subsequent involvement of younger children and then infants during later phases.

Figure 10.1. Time frame of pediatric clinical studies on the basis of type of medicinal product and disease to be treated.

❖ *Types of pediatric studies*
- clinical trials,
- studies involving comparison of relative bioequivalence of the pediatric formulations with the adult formulations carried out in adults, and
- pharmacokinetic dose ranging studies for selecting dose across the wide age ranges of pediatric patients; performed in pediatric patients with the disease under study.

BIOMEDICAL RESEARCH IN PEDIATRICS UNDER SPECIAL SITUATIONS

♦ *Research involving children in emergency situations*

This should be conducted only when justified on scientific grounds and if research cannot be conducted in any other setting. Here an important ethical issue is obtaining informed consent. Under such emergency and critical care situations, when immediate informed consent is not possible, it is suggested to have *deferred consent*. In deferred consent, initially minimum information is given verbally, later full information is given and formal consent taken. The time frame within which formal consent should be taken would be reviewed and approved by EC.

♦ *Research involving neonates*
- ✓ There is need to focus on special aspects relevant to neonates e.g. delayed or long term consequences of interventions comprising developmental effects.
- ✓ The inclusion of critically ill neonates in research should be adequately justified.
- ✓ Important considerations regarding informed consent should be taken into account as:
  - In case of research exposing the neonates to no or minimal risk and having potential to benefit participants, the consent of one parent is necessary.
  - In studies having high risk and no anticipated benefit to participants, the consent of both parents should be taken except in cases where one parent is deceased, incompetent, not known, not available for reasonable reasons and one parent is legally responsible for custody of neonate.

♦ *Research involving adolescents i.e. children in the age group of 12- 18 years*

The researcher conducting research involving this group of pediatric population should be adequately familiar with peculiar aspects relevant to social, psychological, behavioral and physical development of adolescents. In community based studies, the youth advisory committees can be involved during planning and implementation of research.

CLINICAL RESEARCH IN GERIATRICS

The classification of elderly population is so far arbitrary with age > 65 years considered as elderly by most authorities while > 75 years considered by some. Gerontologists usually categorize elderly population into sub-groups as:
- Young-old: 65-74 years,
- Middle-old: 75-84 years and
- Very old: > 85 years

NEED FOR BIOMEDICAL RESEARCH IN GERIATRICS

Adequate representation of geriatric population in clinical trials is required to assess the benefit/ risk balance of drugs with potential indications in geriatrics. The need to conduct research in geriatrics arises due to a number of reasons such as:

- Globally, recent era has witnessed an increase in the proportion of elderly population. By 2050, elderly population worldwide is expected to rise to more than 2 billion. With a rapid rise in geriatric population, the importance of generating safety/ efficacy data in elderly during drug development program has increased.
- Differential response to drug therapy in geriatric patients as compared to younger patients due to:
  - ✓ age - related physiological changes affecting the drug pharmacokinetics which may demand dosage adjustments; and pharmacodynamics which can have a bearing on drug response and dose response relationship.
  - ✓ increased susceptibility of elderly patients to adverse effects of drugs due to comorbidities and concomitantly administered drugs. Also, the pattern of adverse effects in geriatrics can vary from non-geriatrics in terms of severity, tolerability or consequences etc.
- Insufficient information on geriatric usage in drug product labeling as a result of under representation of elderly population during drug development program due to reasons like:
  - ✓ protocol restrictions with respect to age for inclusion
  - ✓ challenges with informed consent process in special cases like "frail" geriatric patients i.e. vulnerable elderly at high risk of adverse outcomes
  - ✓ issues of compliance with study procedures
  - ✓ need to have age-relevant formulations and packaging in some cases
  - ✓ co-morbidities influencing outcome assessment
  - ✓ high incidence of polypharmacy leading to drug interactions with investigational drug.

REGULATIONS GOVERNING GERIATRIC BIOMEDICAL RESEARCH

US FDA guidance on geriatric research (E7: Studies in support of special populations: Geriatrics)

- For diseases not specific to but present in elderly, it is recommended to include more than 100 geriatric patients in phase 2 and 3 clinical trials and patients should represent the entire spectrum of geriatric population. When the disorder under investigation is primarily confined to elderly population e.g. Alzheimer's disease, geriatric patients should constitute the major portion of clinical database.
- Data across various age categories of geriatric population should be presented for marketing application to assess consistency in treatment effect and safety profile in geriatric compared to non geriatric populations.

- Both geriatric and non- geriatric populations should preferably be included in same study to facilitate assessment of age related differences.
- Certain specific age- related efficacy end points and safety parameters should be actively included in studies on geriatric population e.g. effects on cognition, urinary incontinence or retention, balance and falls etc. which in turn may require specific testing.
- Pharmacokinetic evaluation should be conducted across the entire spectrum of geriatric patients to identify age-related differences not explained by other factors like impaired renal/hepatic function.
- As a general principle, for drugs having narrow therapeutic range and high likelihood of concomitant therapy, the need to conduct specific drug-drug interaction studies should be determined on a case-to-case basis.

The New Drugs and Clinical Trials Rules, 2019 recommendations on geriatric research

Geriatric patients should be enrolled in Phase III clinical trials (and in Phase II trials, if desired by manufacturer) in significant proportions, if

- the disorder under investigation characteristically affects elderly population e.g. Alzheimer's disease;
- the population for which investigational drug is indicated comprises substantial numbers of elderly patients; or
- when the response to new drug is expected to differ in geriatric as compared to non-geriatric population;
- when the disorders/ conditions prevalent in elderly are expected to be encountered during the clinical use of investigational drug.

CLINICAL RESEARCH IN PREGNANT OR NURSING WOMEN

Many women need to take drugs during pregnancy and/or lactation to treat a chronic health condition e.g. asthma, epilepsy etc. or to treat a new condition associated with pregnancy or getting worsened because of pregnancy. However, since most approved drugs have not been studied in pregnant and lactating women, there is limited knowledge regarding their safe and effective use in this subgroup.

NEED FOR BIOMEDICAL RESEARCH IN PREGNANT AND NURSING WOMEN

- Drug labeling information for pregnant and nursing women is generally based on preclinical studies with limited human safety data. Such lack of information leads to reluctance on part of prescribers and patients to prescribe drugs in pregnant and nursing women; in some cases this may lead to more harm to women or fetus than if she had received treatment.

- Physiological changes during pregnancy may be associated with alterations in pharmacokinetics (demanding dose/ dosage regimen adjustments) and pharmacodynamics (leading to differences in drug response). Hence, knowledge needs to be gained regarding the safe and effective dose in this subgroup.

- Inclusion of pregnant and nursing women in clinical trials may sometimes offer direct therapeutic benefit to women and /or fetus which is not available outside the clinical research setting.

- Most of the information pertaining to drug usage in pregnancy and lactation is gathered during post marketing phase through surveillance methods and observational studies like pregnancy exposure registries. However, certain situations may demand data collection in this subgroup in a clinical setting e.g. non availability of any approved treatment options, based on clinical need etc.

REGULATIONS GOVERNING CLINICAL RESEARCH IN PREGNANT AND NURSING WOMEN

US FDA regulations governing research in pregnant and lactating women

✓ As per US FDA recommendations, it is ethically justifiable to conduct clinical trials on pregnant women with the disease being studied under the following conditions:

For FDA approved drugs i.e. postmarketing phase

- Completed non-clinical studies including studies on pregnant animals.
- Completed clinical studies including studies in non-pregnant women with proven safety.
- Existence of preliminary safety data regarding drug usage in pregnancy in literature or other medical sources.
- Efficacy and /or safety cannot be evaluated by other methods.

For investigational drugs i.e. premarketing phase:

- Completed non-clinical studies including studies on pregnant animals.
- Trial holds promise to directly benefit pregnant women and/or fetus.
- In the absence of any assumed benefit, fetus is not exposed to a greater than minimal risk.
- Trial imparts benefit to pregnant women and /or fetus which is otherwise not available outside the research setting.
- Circumstances like no available treatment options, absence of response to existing approved therapies.

✓ Adequate data from reproductive and developmental toxicology studies in preclinical models should be available before including pregnant women in clinical trials.

✓ Conventionally, results from phase 1 and 2 studies involving non-pregnant women including females of reproductive potential should be available before studying pregnant women in later phase clinical trials.

✓ Due consideration needs to be given to the gestational timing of exposure to the investigational treatment in relation to fetal development.

✓ Need to consider the conduct of pharmacokinetic (PK) trials under situations such as:
  - Drug is generally prescribed in pregnant women, particularly during second and third trimesters.
  - New drug or indication with anticipated use in pregnancy
  - Used rarely in pregnancy, but may lead to detrimental consequences in improper dosages e.g. narrow therapeutic index drugs.
  - Pharmacokinetics of drug is likely to be significantly altered in pregnant women e.g. renally excreted drug.
✓ It is preferable to include an ethicist during planning of clinical research in pregnant women.
✓ Minimum safety data collected should comprise:
  - gestational age at the time of enrolment.
  - gestational time and duration of drug exposure.
  - pregnancy outcomes comprising maternal, fetal and neonatal events.
  - follow-up safety data in infants.
✓ USFDA recommends conduct of clinical studies in lactating or nursing women under following circumstances:
  - investigational drug is expected to be used by women of reproductive age.
  - once approved, drug is anticipated to be used by nursing women as per literature reports.
  - new indication for an approved drug and evidence of its anticipated use in nursing women.
  - approved medications used commonly by women of reproductive age e.g. anti-hypertensives, anti-infectives etc.

Since 2015, USFDA has implemented the Pregnancy Lactation Labeling Rule (PLLR), the highlights of which are mentioned in Box 10.1.

Box 10.1 The Pregnancy Lactation Labeling Rule (PLLR).

✓ PLLR, implemented by US FDA since 2015, is an amendment to the Physician labeling rule and replaces the pregnancy letter categories (A, B, C, D, X) printed on drug labels with a summary of drug information.
✓ PLLR provides a framework regarding the information to be included in drug product labeling about benefits and risks of prescription drugs and biologics during pregnancy and lactation.
✓ The rule aims to provide updated information to clinicians regarding the benefit-risk profile of drugs in pregnant and lactating women including the fetus/newborn.
✓ In accordance with the rule, the prescribing information has been updated in three labeling subsections viz. Pregnancy, Lactation, and Females and males of reproductive potential.

The New Drugs and Clinical Trials Rules, 2019 recommendations

- ♦ Pregnant or lactating women should be enrolled in clinical trials only under circumstances like:
    - ✓ the study drug is expected to be used by pregnant/nursing women or fetuses/nursing infants
    - ✓ when data from non-pregnant or non-lactating women is not suitable.
- ♦ When investigational drug is intended to be used by pregnant women, follow-up data (relevant to a period adequate for study drug) regarding outcomes of drug on pregnancy, fetus and child needs to be submitted. Where applicable, the excretion of drug or its metabolites into human milk should be assessed and infants should be closely monitored for anticipated pharmacological effects.
- ♦ The inclusion of these women in clinical trials should be justifiable on certain grounds e.g. if the trial provides direct benefit to women /fetus/infant and objectives of the trial cannot be achieved otherwise. Examples of such trials include testing the efficacy and safety of a drug to reduce perinatal transmission of HIV infection from mother to fetus, trials to detect fetal abnormalities and for conditions related to or exaggerated by pregnancy etc.
- ♦ Women should not be encouraged to discontinue nursing in order to participate in research and in case she decides to do so, consequences of cessation of breast feeding to the nursing child should be properly assessed except in situations where breast feeding is harmful to the infant.
- ♦ *Research related to termination of pregnancy*: Pregnant women who wish to undergo Medical Termination of Pregnancy (MTP) can be included in such research as per The Medical Termination of Pregnancy Act, GOI, 1971.
- ♦ *Research related to pre-natal diagnostic techniques*: In pregnant women this type of research should only be conducted for detection of fetal abnormalities or genetic disorders in accordance with the Prenatal Diagnostic Techniques Act (Regulation and Prevention of Misuse), GOI, 1994 and not for sex determination of the fetus.

Bioavailability and Bioequivalence Studies

INTRODUCTION

Bioavailability (BA) and bioequivalence (BE) focus on the liberation of an active drug from its dosage form followed by its absorption in systemic circulation or site of action. The bioavailability of an active drug from a pharmaceutical product and bioequivalence of various products marketed by various manufacturing companies and containing same active ingredients are very important parameters from clinical as well as regulatory aspects.

Bioavailability is usually estimated by the exposure profile of an active drug and /or metabolite systemically; BA determined during early phases of clinical drug development serves as a benchmark for further BE studies. BE studies are conducted to determine the clinical/ therapeutic equivalence and interchangeability of two drug products having same active pharmaceutical ingredient/s. According to The New Drugs and Clinical Trials Rules, 2019. BA/BE data needs to be furnished with applications for new drug products based on the type of application.

The documentation of BE is required for comparing the bioavailability of:
- generic medicinal products with the brand name product.
- drug formulations used during early and late phases of clinical trials.
- clinical trial formulations and products launched in market.
- formulations utilized in clinical trials and stability tests, if not identical.

IMPORTANT DEFINITIONS (BOX 11.1 AND 11.2)

Box 11.1 Important definitions.

Bioavailability: defined as the rate and extent of absorption of the active pharmaceutical ingredient from its dosage form and its availability at the site of action.

Bioequivalence: is comparable bioavailability of pharmaceutical equivalent or pharmaceutical alternative products when studied under similar experimental conditions.

Reference product: defined as a pharmaceutical product containing the same active ingredient(s) as the new drug and has been identified as "designated reference product" by the licensing authority. This is generally the brand name drug having a full NDA.

Generic name: the established non-proprietary or common name of the active drug in a drug product (e.g. acetaminophen).

Brand name: is the trade name of a drug; the name privately owned by the manufacturer and distinguishes the specific drug product from existing competitor products (e.g. paracetamol).

Generic substitution: the process of dispensing some other brand or an unbranded medicinal product instead of the prescribed medicinal product.

Pharmaceutical equivalents: medicinal products which are in similar dosage forms containing the same active ingredient(s) i.e. same salt or ester, are having similar strength or concentration and use the similar route of administration. However, they may be different in terms of some features e.g. shape, mode of release, packaging, excipients, and up to specific limits labeling.

Pharmaceutical alternatives: medicinal products comprising of the same active therapeutic ingredient but as some other salts, esters or complexes. e.g. tetracycline hydrochloride or tetracycline phosphate equivalent to 250 mg tetracycline base are deemed as pharmaceutical alternatives.

Pharmaceutical substitution: the process of dispensing a pharmaceutical alternative for the prescribed drug product. This needs physician's approval.

Therapeutic alternatives: medicinal products comprising of different active ingredients (from the same pharmacological class) which are indicated for same therapeutic objective e.g. ibuprofen and diclofenac, omeprazole and pantoprazole.

Therapeutic equivalents: medicinal products which are pharmaceutical equivalents and their efficacy and safety profile is assumed to be similar on administration in patients under specified conditions.

Therapeutic substitution: the process of dispensing a therapeutic alternative instead of the prescribed drug product.

Box 11.2 The New Drugs and Clinical Trials Rules, 2019..

Definitions

- **Bioavailability (BA) study**: "a study to assess the rate and extent to which a drug is absorbed from a pharmaceutical formulation and becomes available in the systemic circulation or availability of the drug at the site of action".

- **Bioequivalence (BE study)**: "a study to establish the absence of a statistically significant difference in the rate and extent of absorption of an active ingredient from a pharmaceutical formulation in comparison to the reference formulation having the same active ingredient when administered in the same molar dose under similar conditions".

- **BA/BE study centre**: "a centre created or established to undertake bioavailability study or bioequivalence study of a drug for either clinical part or for both clinical and analytical part of such study".

ORANGE BOOK (BOX 11.3)

Box 11.3 Orange book.

US FDA maintains an "Orange Book" which is comprised of therapeutic equivalence assessments for approved drug products manufactured by various companies. The evaluations, however, do not apply to unapproved, off-label indications.

Link: https://www.fda.gov/drugs/drug-approvals-and-databases/approved-drug-products-therapeutic-equivalence-evaluations-orange-book

---

METHODS FOR ASSESSING BA AND BE

❖ **IN-VIVO STUDIES**

1. Pharmacokinetic (PK) methods

(i) Plasma drug concentration

- C_{max} (peak plasma/blood concentration)
- T_{max} (time for peak plasma/blood concentration)
- AUC (area under the plasma drug concentration-time curve)

(ii) Urinary drug excretion

- D_u (cumulative amount of drug excreted in urine)
- dD_u/dt (rate of drug excretion in urine)
- t (time for maximum urinary excretion)

2. Pharmacodynamic (PD) methods

- Acute pharmacodynamic effect
- E_{max} (maximum pharmacodynamic effect)
- Time for maximum pharmacodynamic effect
- Area under the pharmacodynamic effect- time curve
- Onset time for pharmacodynamic effect

3. Clinical methods

Well controlled clinical trials

❖ **IN – VITRO STUDIES**

Drug dissolution studies

CIRCUMSTANCES FOR THE REQUIREMENT OF BE STUDIES

Tables 11.1 and 11.2 give a list of conditions where BA/BE studies are required and where they can be waived off.

Table 11.1 Conditions where BE studies are required.

In-vivo studies required:

1. Orally administered immediate release dosage forms having systemic action with at least one of the below mentioned criteria:
   - indicated in serious disorders;
   - narrow therapeutic index;
   - complex pharmacokinetics: incomplete/ variable absorption, non-linear kinetics, high first pass metabolism;
   - unacceptable physico-chemical characteristics like instability, low solubility etc.;
   - low ratio of active ingredient to excipients;
2. Systemically acting non-oral, non-parenteral preparations e.g. transdermal patches, suppositories;
3. Systemically acting modified or sustained release preparations;
4. Fixed dose combination drug products acting systemically;
5. Non- solution, non-systemic formulations (oral, nasal, ocular, dermal, vaginal, rectal etc.) – need to conduct comparative clinical or pharmacodynamic studies.

In-vitro studies required:

- ❖ Drugs for which data substantiates all of the below mentioned criteria:
  - solubility of maximum dose strength in 250 ml aqueous media at pH range of 1-7.5 at 37° C.

Table 11.1 *Contd...*

- absorption of at least 90% of orally administered dose on mass balance estimation or compared to intravenous reference dose
- speed of dissolution as >80 % dissolution within 15 minutes at 37° C using IP apparatus 1, at 50 rpm or IP apparatus 2, at 100 rpm in 900 ml or less of each of three media- 0.1 N HCl or artificial gastric juice (without enzymes), a pH 4.5 buffer and a pH 6.8 buffer or artificial intestinal juice (without enzymes)

❖ Different strengths of drug manufactured by same manufacturer when:
- different strengths have same qualitative composition, same ratio of active pharmaceutical ingredients and excipients
- similar method of manufacture
- linear PK demonstrated over therapeutic dose range
- an equivalence study has been performed on atleast one strength, usually the highest.

Table 11.2 Conditions where BE studies are not required (Waivers for BE studies).

❖ When the new drug/s consists of the same active ingredient(s) and excipients in similar concentration and is/are:
- parenterally administered drugs (e.g. intravenous, intramuscular, subcutaneous) as aqueous solutions or
- orally administered solutions or
- otic or ophthalmic or topical product as aqueous solution or
- inhalational product or nasal spray or
- powder for reconstitution as a solution.

❖ When the new drug is a gas .

Considerations related to seeking permission to conduct BA/BE study from regulatory authority as given in the New Drugs and Clinical Trials Rules, 2019 (box 11.4).

Box 11.4 The New Drugs and Clinical Trials Rules, 2019.

Permission to conduct BA/BE study

General considerations related to conduct of BA/BE study are similar to other clinical trials. Few peculiar aspects include:
- An application for permission to conduct a BA/BE study can be filed to the central licensing authority in form CT-05.
- The licensing authority, after scrutiny of the information and documents submitted, shall give its decision within 90 working days.

Box 11.4 *Contd...*

- The permission to conduct the BA/BE study shall be granted by the central licensing authority in form CT-07 which holds validity for a period of one year from the issue date. In exceptional circumstances, on written request by the applicant, CLA if satisfied, may extend the permission further by one year.
- The BA/BE study shall begin by enrolling the first subject within a period of one year from the date of grant of permission, failing which prior permission from the Central Licencing Authority should be obtained.
- The central licencing authority shall be informed about EC approval within 15 working days of the grant of such approval.
- In situations where the study protocol is rejected by the EC of a BA/BE study centre, the details of the same shall be submitted to the CLA before applying for approval of another ethics committee to conduct BA/BE study at the same site.

DESIGN AND CONDUCT OF BA/BE STUDIES

STUDY DESIGN

Cross-over design

For comparing two medicinal formulations, the design of choice is 2-period, 2-sequence cross-over design with adequate wash out period (equal to or greater than 5 half-lives of the moieties to be measured) between two periods of treatment. (As per US FDA guidelines, wash out period should be equal to about 10 elimination half-lives).

The order of administering the drug treatments should be modified in order to avoid any bias due to residual effect from previously administered treatment.

Other designs

In some situations, other designs can be used e.g.

- *Parallel design* in case the substances have very long half- lives,
- *Replicate cross-over design* in case the substances have highly variable disposition. (Generally, a 4- period, 2-sequence, 2-formulation design is recommended by US FDA)

STUDY SUBJECTS

Healthy adult volunteers are preferred in order to minimize variability. For drugs with high risks of side-effects/ toxicity, patients with the concerned disease in stable state may be included. For drugs mainly indicated in elderly population, attempt should be made to include subjects in the age group of 60 years or more.

Both males or females may be used; the selection of gender should be in accordance with expected use and safety aspects. If the indications of medicinal product extend to both sexes, males and females should be involved in identical proportions.

STUDY TYPES

For solid oral dosage forms, three different studies may be required:

Fasting study.

This is usually conducted as a single dose, 2-period, 2-sequence, 2-treatment, open label, randomized cross-over design evaluating equal doses of the test and reference products in fasting, adult, healthy participants. This study is needed to be conducted for all immediate release and modified release orally administered dosage forms. (Fasting: overnight fast of minimum 10 hours before drug administration followed by 4 hours fasting after drug administration).

No other medication is generally given to the subjects for at least 1 week before conducting the study.

Fed-state/ Food intervention/ Food effect study.

Fed-state studies are required:

- for all modified- release dosage forms.
- for immediate release dosage forms if it is known that food may affect bioavailability of active drug ingredient.
- when evaluation of C_{max} and T_{max} is tedious in fasting studies.

Concomitant administration of food with an oral drug product may affect the bioavailability of drug, hence these studies are generally carried out under meal conditions which are assumed to highly affect GI physiology and thus maximally affect the systemic drug availability. The test meal is given as breakfast with high fat content before dosing (high calorie content of 950-1000 calories, with minimum of 50% calories from fat, 15-20% from proteins and remaining from carbohydrates). Due to diverse ethnicity and cultural backgrounds, no specific recommendations for test meal are included in Indian guidelines. The meal should be consumed approximately 15 minutes prior to dosing.

(US FDA guidelines: Subjects (after an overnight fast of 10 hours) are given the recommended meal 30 minutes prior to dosing, meal is consumed over 30 minutes and medicinal product is administered immediately after meal. The drug product is given with 240 mL water. Food intake is not permitted for a minimum of 4 hours after dose administration).

Multiple-dose/ steady state study.

These may be preferred in certain cases:

- drugs having very long elimination half-lives;
- poor assay sensitivity to follow terminal elimination phase for desired period of time;
- modified release forms demanding evaluation of fluctuations in plasma concentration over a dosage interval;
- drugs with non-linear (dose or time dependent) pharmacokinetics;
- drugs with large intra-individual variability.
- drugs having tendency to accumulate in body

In such studies, the dosing schedule should be as per the clinically recommended dosing regimen.

Generally, a multiple-dose, steady state, randomized, 2-treatment, 2-sequence cross-over study comparing equal doses of the test and reference products may be conducted in adult, healthy individuals.

SAMPLING POINTS/ SCHEDULES

For immediate release products in single dose trials, blood sampling should be carried over a minimum duration of 3 elimination half-lives. Blood sampling should be continued for a duration sufficient enough to ensure that the area extrapolated from time of measurement of last concentration to infinite time is less than 20% of total AUC. The number of sampling points should be

- minimum of 3 during absorption phase,
- 3-4 at projected T_{max},
- 4 during elimination phase.

For urinary excretion data, urine should be collected for seven or more half-lives.

DATA EVALUATION

Analytical method

The bio-analytical method used for determining the drug/ metabolites in biological fluids must be validated for

- Accuracy (extent to which the 'true' value of drug concentration is determined by assay);
- Precision (degree of reproducibility of individual assays);
- Specificity/ selectivity (free from interference by endogenous compounds, degradation products, other drugs/ metabolites etc.);
- Sensitivity (capacity to record small variations in concentration);
- Recovery (documentation of extraction recovery at high, medium and low concentrations).

Pharmacokinetic evaluation of data

For single dose studies. PK parameters evaluated are:

- Area under the curve (AUC) to the last quantifiable concentration i.e. AUC_{0-t} and infinity i.e. $AUC_{0-\infty}$;
- T_{max};
- C_{max};
- elimination rate constant, k;
- elimination half-life ($t_{1/2}$).

For multiple dose studies. Pk parameters evaluated are:

- Steady state area under the curve AUC_{0-t};
- T_{max};

- C_{max};
- C_{min};
- Percent fluctuation $[(C_{max} - C_{min})/C_{min} \times 100]$.

CRITERIA FOR ESTABLISHING BIOEQUIVALENCE

To document bioequivalence, the acceptable range for the calculated 90% confidence interval for AUC and Cmax is 80-125%. However, narrow limits for bioequivalence range may be required for drugs having:

- narrow therapeutic index;
- dose related serious toxicity;
- steep dose-response curve;
- non-linear pharmacokinetics.

BA/BE STUDY REPORT

The BA/BE study report should comprise an entire documentation of the study plan, execution and assessment (Table 11.3).

Table 11.3 BA/BE study report.

- ✓ Table of contents.
- ✓ Title of the study.
- ✓ Names and credentials of study investigators along with their signatures.
- ✓ Site where study conducted and facilities employed.
- ✓ Time periods over which clinical and analytical procedures were performed.
- ✓ Names and batch numbers of the products compared, a signed declaration that the products used were similar to proposed marketed products.
- ✓ Results of assays and other pharmaceutical tests carried out on batches.
- ✓ Complete protocol of study including a copy of ICF.
- ✓ Protocol deviations/ violations, if any.
- ✓ Evidence of IEC approval and compliance with GCP/GLP guidelines.
- ✓ Subjects: demographic details, names and addresses.
- ✓ Details of study withdrawals and drop outs.
- ✓ Details of analytical procedures utilized, quality control data, criteria used for assay results.
- ✓ Representative chromatograms over the whole concentration range for all samples analyzed.
- ✓ Sampling schedules and deviations, if any.
- ✓ Details of pk parameters calculations.
- ✓ Details of all statistical analyses performed.

GUIDELINES FOR CONDUCT OF BA/BE STUDY OF NEW DRUGS OR INVESTIGATIONAL NEW DRUGS (BOX 11.5)

Box 11.5 The New Drugs and Clinical Trials Rules, 2019, India.

Introduction of guidelines on BA/BE studies (not explicitly defined in previous regulations)

Fourth Schedule : **Requirements and guidelines for conduct of BA/BE study of new drugs or investigational new drugs.**

These include clearly defined processes for:
- General principles.
- BA/BE study centre.
- Maintenance of records.
- Retention of samples.

Table 1: Document required for registration of BA/BE centre.

Table 2: Data and information required for grant of permission to BA/BE study of a new drug or investigational new drug.

Table 3: Data and information required for grant of permission to conduct BA/BE study of a new drug already approved in the country.

General principles
- BA/BE focus on the liberation of an active drug component from its dosage form followed by its absorption into the systemic circulation. BA/BE study holds significance for ensuring efficacy and safety of pharmaceutical product.
- BA is generally determined by a systemic exposure profile attained by measuring the concentrations of drug or metabolites in the systemic circulation over time.
- The aim of BE study is to ensure therapeutic equivalence between pharmaceutically equivalent test product and a reference product.
- The aim of BA/BE study is to ensure therapeutic equivalence between an approved new drug formulation and reference product.
- BA/BE study is also carried out to ensure therapeutic equivalence during any clinical trial phase of a new chemical entity to establish bioequivalence between two products of the chemical entity, which is essential for any changes in manufacturing process or pharmaceutical formulation occurring during different stages of drug development.
- In cases where the drugs are approved in other nations and undergo systemic absorption, bioequivalence with the reference formulation should be demonstrated as the case may be. Such studies should be carried out in accordance with the labeled conditions of administration. For formulations not designed for systemic absorption, data on the degree of systemic absorption might be needed.

- For solid oral dosage forms, data regarding food effects on absorption and dissolution studies should be submitted.
- Dissolution and bioavailability data accompanying the NDA must provide information assuring bioequivalence or bioavailability and demonstrating dosage correlations between the formulations used in clinical trials and those to be marketed.
- All BA/BE studies should be conducted as per the Guidelines for Bioavailability and Bioequivalence studies issued by Central Drugs Standard Control Organisation, Ministry of Health and Family Welfare.
- All BA/BE studies should be carried out in a registered BA/BE study centre after approval from the Central Licensing authority.

BIOAVAILABILITY AND BIOEQUIVALENCE (BA/BE) STUDY CENTRE

The New Drugs and Clinical Trials Rules, 2019 have clearly defined the BA/BE centre, facilities required at such a centre and guidelines for its registration (Box 11.6 and 11.7).

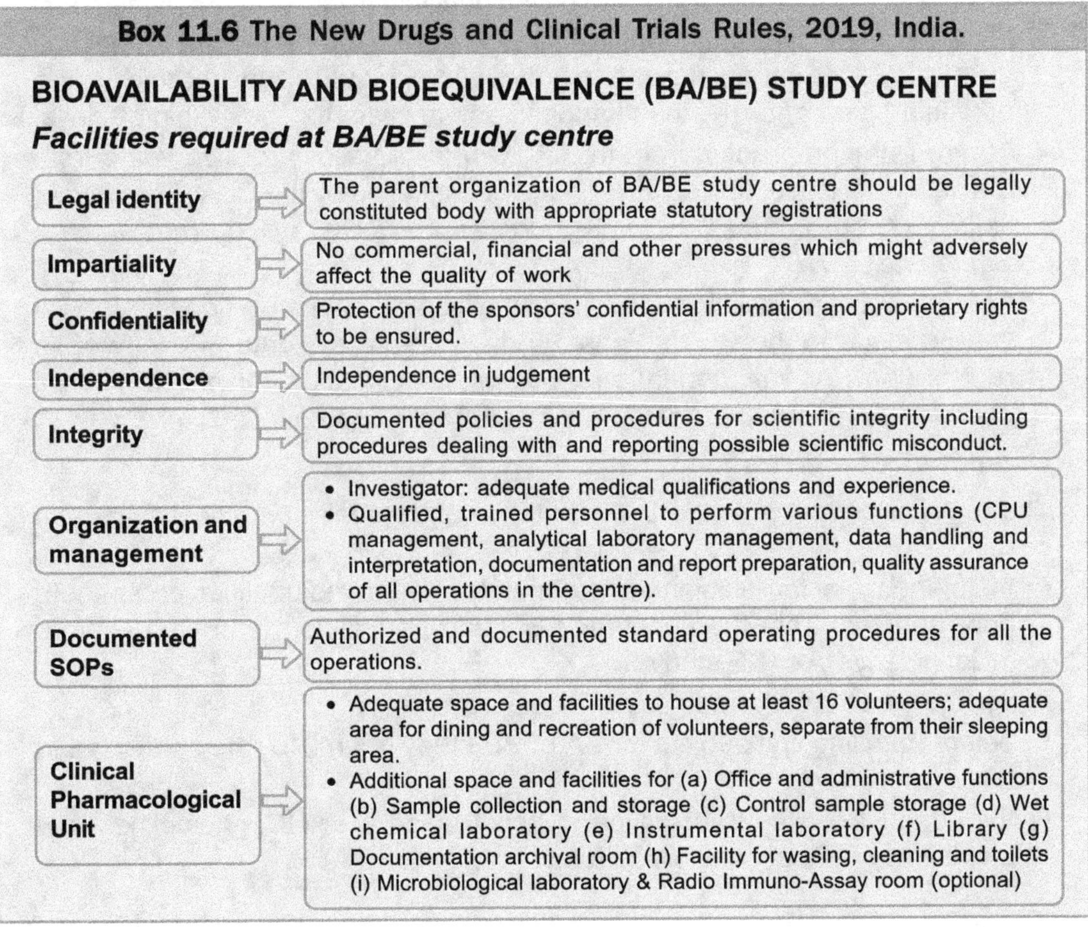

Box 11.6 The New Drugs and Clinical Trials Rules, 2019, India.

BIOAVAILABILITY AND BIOEQUIVALENCE (BA/BE) STUDY CENTRE

Facilities required at BA/BE study centre

Legal identity	The parent organization of BA/BE study centre should be legally constituted body with appropriate statutory registrations
Impartiality	No commercial, financial and other pressures which might adversely affect the quality of work
Confidentiality	Protection of the sponsors' confidential information and proprietary rights to be ensured.
Independence	Independence in judgement
Integrity	Documented policies and procedures for scientific integrity including procedures dealing with and reporting possible scientific misconduct.
Organization and management	• Investigator: adequate medical qualifications and experience. • Qualified, trained personnel to perform various functions (CPU management, analytical laboratory management, data handling and interpretation, documentation and report preparation, quality assurance of all operations in the centre).
Documented SOPs	Authorized and documented standard operating procedures for all the operations.
Clinical Pharmacological Unit	• Adequate space and facilities to house at least 16 volunteers; adequate area for dining and recreation of volunteers, separate from their sleeping area. • Additional space and facilities for (a) Office and administrative functions (b) Sample collection and storage (c) Control sample storage (d) Wet chemical laboratory (e) Instrumental laboratory (f) Library (g) Documentation archival room (h) Facility for wasing, cleaning and toilets (i) Microbiological laboratory & Radio Immuno-Assay room (optional)

Box 11.7 The New Drugs and Clinical Trials Rules, 2019.

Registration of BA/BE study centre

- No BA/BE study centre can conduct any BA or BE study of a new drug or IND without being registered with the Central Licensing Authority (CLA).
- An application for registration of BA/BE study center shall be filed to the CLA in Form CT-08.
- Following receipt of application, an officer authorized by CLA accompanied by officers authorized by State Licensing Authority (SLA) may conduct inspection of the BA/BE study centre to verify its capacity and facilities.
- If satisfied as per the requirements laid down, registration may be granted by CLA to the applicant in Form CT-09 within 90 working days from the date of receipt of application.
- If the application is rejected, applicant may request the CLA to reconsider the application within 60 working days from the date of rejection of application.
- In case the applicant is aggrieved by the decision of CLA he/she may appeal to the Central Government within 45 days from the date of receipt of rejection and the Government may after conducting enquiry and hearing to the appellant, discard or retain the appeal, as the case may be, within 60 days.
- The registration granted in Form CT-09 retains validity for five years from the date of its issue, unless suspended or cancelled by the CLA. *(Previously, validity of registration was for 3 years, as per DCGI office order dated 5 September, 2016)*
- For renewal of registration of BA/BE study centre, an application for renewal can be made to the CLA at least 90 days before the date of expiry of its registration. *(As per previous regulations, application for renewal to be submitted 4 months before the expiry of present approval).*

Conditions of registration

The registration granted to a BA/BE study centre shall be subject to certain conditions as:

- maintenance of facilities and appropriately trained and qualified personnel; prior approval from the concerned EC and permission from CLA before initiating any BA or BE study;
- the CLA shall be informed about EC approval;
- before enrolling first subject for BA or BE study of an IND, the study should be registered with CTRI;
- the conduct of study should be in accordance with GCP guidelines and provisions of the act and these rules;

Box 11.7 *Contd...*

- in case of premature termination of a study, the reasons for termination in details should be communicated to CLA;
- SAE reporting to the concerned authorities should be done within stipulated timelines;
- in case of any clinical trial related injury or death, compensation and medical management would be provided according to applicable guidelines;
- in case of any change in ownership or constitution of BA/BE study center, the information shall be intimated to CLA in writing within 30 days of change;
- maintenance of data, records and other documents related to the conduct of BA or BE study for a period of 5 years after study completion or for at least 2 years after the expiry date of the batch of new drug or IND studied, whichever is later;
- the BA/BE study centre would permit the designated personnel by CLA and SLA (state licensing authority) to inspect the premises and data, and provide appropriate comments to the queries of the personnel;
- the CLA may if deemed necessary, inflict supplementary condition, in writing with justification, with regard to a specific BA/BE study pertaining to study objective, design, conduct, eligibility or assessment as the case may be.

RECORD MAINTENANCE

All data from BA/BE studies including in-vitro and in-vivo tests performed on any batch of a new medicinal product should be archived by the sponsor for a minimum duration of 5 years after study completion or for at least 2 years after expiry date of the batch of new drug product whichever is later. *(As per previous regulations, records shall be maintained for at least 2 years after expiry date of the batch).*

RETENTION OF SAMPLES

- ✓ All the test and reference drug samples used in BA/BE study have to be retained for 5 years after study conduct or 1 year after expiry date of drug, whichever is later.
- ✓ The batches of test and reference drug products should be provided to the testing centre by study sponsor or drug manufacturer.
- ✓ The samples should be preserved in their original holders sufficient to carry out twice all the in-vitro and in- vivo tests required during BA/BE study.
- ✓ The storage of reserve samples should be in accordance with product labeling and in an area isolated from the testing area and with restricted access to authorized personnel.

THE BIOPHARMACEUTICS CLASSIFICATION SYSTEM (BCS)

(9th amendment to D& C Rules; G.S.R. 327 (E), dated 3 April 2017)

(Link: http://www.cdsco.nic.in/writereaddata/GSR%20327(E)%20Dated%2003_04_2017.pdf)

The BCS is a system to correlate *in-vitro* drug dissolution of immediate release solid oral drug products with *in-vivo* bioavailability. This system classifies drugs on the basis of their solubility (aqueous solubility) and permeability (through gastrointestinal tract) into 4 categories (Table 11.4).

Table 11.4 Bio-pharmaceutics Classification System (BCS).		
Category	**Solubility/ Permeability**	**Comments**
Category 1	High/ High	Drug undergoes rapid dissolution and good absorption. BA problem not predicted for immediate release drug products.
Category 2	Low/ High	Drug has limited dissolution and good absorption. BA is determined by dosage form and rate of release of drug substance.
Category 3	High/ Low	Drug has limited permeability. BA may not be complete if the drug's release and dissolution does not occur within absorption window.
Category 4	Low/ Low	Inconsistent BA of drug. Need to administer the drug through an alternate route.

Contents

CHAPTER 12

Evolution of Ethics in Research

OVERVIEW

Introduction
History of Medical Ethics
Evolution of International Research Ethics
Declaration of Helsinki

CIOMS International Ethical Guidelines
Evolution of Research Ethics in India
Few Unethical Trials in Past

INTRODUCTION

Ethics. Term for various means of apprehending and assessing the moral life.

Medical ethics or Bioethics. Application of moral issues in the domain of medical treatment and research.

HISTORY OF MEDICAL ETHICS

The origin of medical ethics dates back to traditional system of medicine when the code of conduct for physicians was formed.

***Charaka Samhita* (1600 B.C.):** included guidelines for:
- professionalism of physicians,
- rational approach to the causation and cure of diseases,
- objective methods of clinical examination.

***Hippocratic oath* (4ᵗʰ century B.C.):** moral of conduct to be used by physicians, respect for all human life.

EVOLUTION OF INTERNATIONAL RESEARCH ETHICS

Figure 12.1 depicts important historical landmarks in the evolution of research ethics internationally and the formulation of various ethical codes and guidelines.

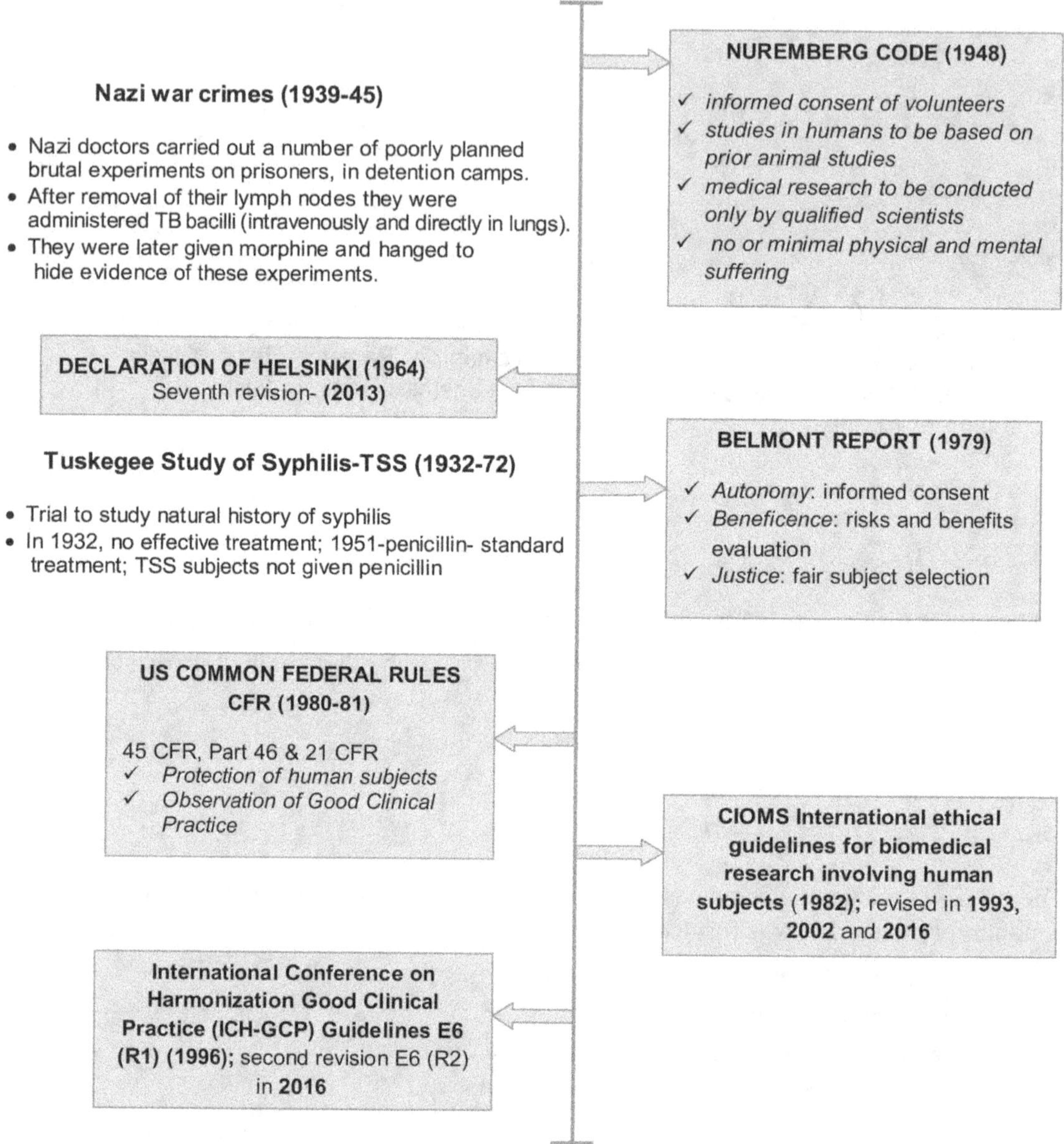

Figure 12.1 Evolution of International research ethics.

DECLARATION OF HELSINKI

The Declaration of Helsinki was laid down by the World Medical Association (WMA), as a framework of ethical guidelines for the medical fraternity pertaining to experimentation in humans, and is broadly considered as the fundamental report of human research ethics. The Declaration was originally endorsed in June 1964 in Helsinki, Finland, and has gone through seven revisions and two clarifications since then (the most recent in October 2013).

CIOMS INTERNATIONAL ETHICAL GUIDELINES

Council for International Organizations of Medical Sciences (CIOMS) in collaboration with WHO prepared the ethical guidelines for the first time in 1982 which were entitled *"Proposed International Ethical Guidelines for Biomedical Research Involving Human Subjects"*. The main aim of these guidelines was to provide internationally acceptable ethical principles and their application in clinical research with particular focus on research in low-resource settings. The guidelines were revised in 1993 as *"International Ethical Guidelines for Biomedical Research Involving Human Subjects"* and later in 2002. The fourth and the latest revision was made in 2016 which includes several developments like emphasis on translational research, community engagement in research, inclusion of vulnerable groups etc.

EVOLUTION OF RESEARCH ETHICS IN INDIA

Figure 12.2 depicts the timelines for the formulation of various ethical codes and guidelines in India.

Examples of few trials violating ethics conducted in recent past are given in Box 12.1.

Box 12.1 Few Unethical Trials in Past.

TGN 1412 trials in London in 2006. Phase 1 trial of anti-inflammatory drug, TGN 1412 in six healthy volunteers; initial administration of the compound resulted in potentially fatal multi-organ failure in the subjects. Later it was noticed that essential information on the assumed effects in humans in comparison to monkeys was not available at the time of regulatory approval of trial. *Ethical violation:* Essential data from preclinical evaluation was not included in the documentation for regulatory approval of trial; subjects were not appropriately informed.

Letrozole trials in India. Letrozole, an aromatase inhibitor, was tested by the pharmaceutical company to induce ovulation. More than 400 women were enrolled in 2003 in clinical trials conducted at multiple centres across India. *Ethical violation:* Participants were not informed regarding their involvement in a trial; informed consent process was not performed.

Ragaglitazar (antidiabetic) trials in 32 countries including India in 2002. Ethical concerns regarding the conduct of phase 3 clinical trials before completion of adequate preclinical studies were raised by Indian scientists. The trials were withheld by the company after there were reports of development of urinary bladder tumors in a mouse (and several rats) who were administered the drug. *Ethical violation:* It was questioned whether required preclinical testing/s were done; as per Indian Council of Medical Research (ICMR) regulations, the results of toxicity studies for drugs intended to be used in chronic diseases need to be submitted for regulatory approval of phase III clinical trials.

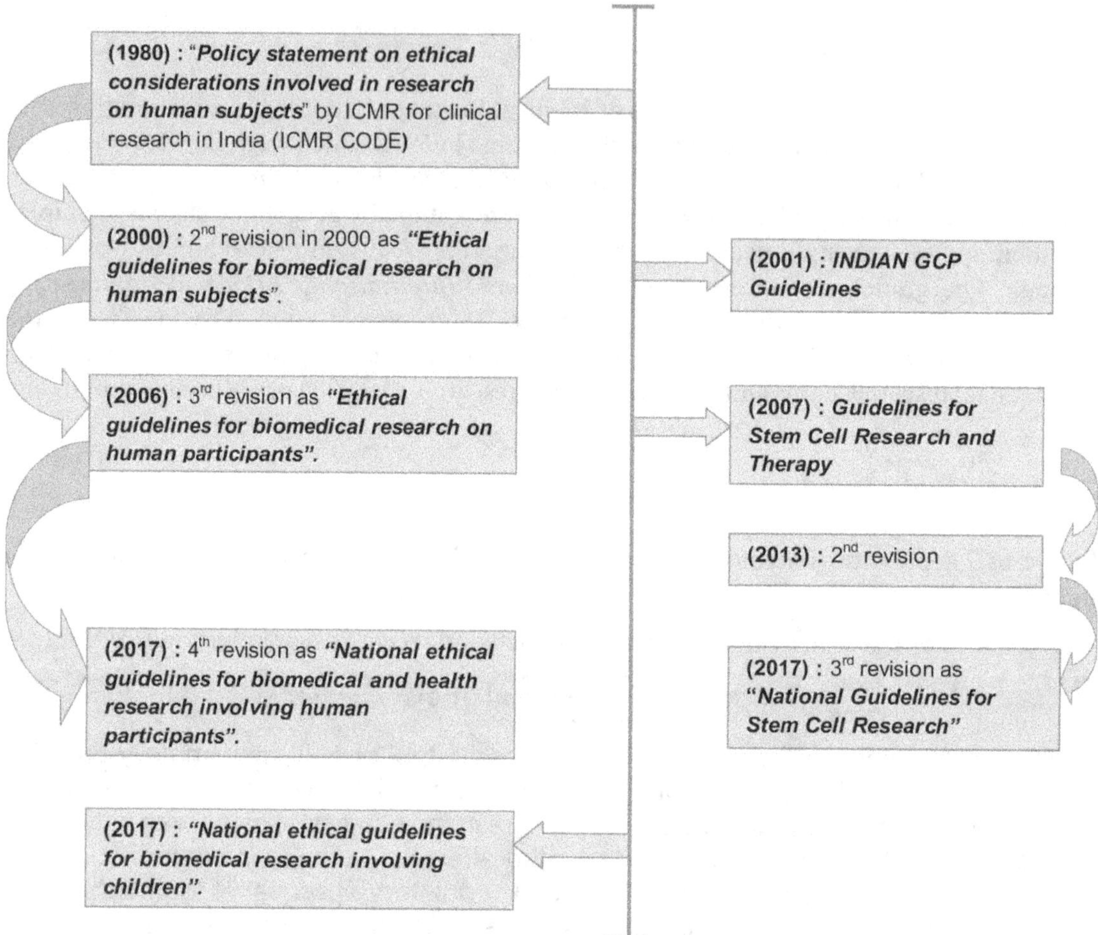

Figure 12.2 Evolution of research ethics in India.

IMPORTANT LINKS

1. Declaration of Helsinki. https://www.wma.net/what-we-do/medical-ethics/declaration-of-helsinki/
2. Code of Federal Regulations. https://www.accessdata.fda.gov/scripts/cdrh/cfdocs/cfcfr/cfrsearch.cfm

CHAPTER 13

Ethical Principles and Issues in Research

OVERVIEW

INTRODUCTION

The ethical justification for an RCT is generally described as ***"Principle of therapeutic or clinical equipoise"*** which is fulfilled in the absence of a conclusive evidence about the relative merits and/or demerits of interventions being compared in RCT e.g. intervention A has better efficacy or safety profile than intervention B. Equipoise depends on a therapeutic obligation of not allocating a treatment known as inferior or denying an effective and available treatment. The presence of uncertainty regarding superiority or inferiority of the interventions provides justification and ethical acceptability for randomizing subjects to different intervention groups. Biomedical ethics is comprised of four cardinal principles (Figure 13.1).

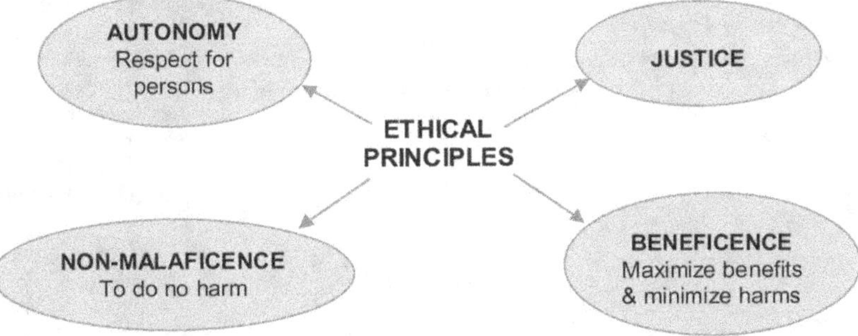

Figure 13.1 Cardinal Principles of biomedical ethics.

DECLARATION OF HELSINKI: GENERAL ETHICAL PRINCIPLES IN RESEARCH (BOX 13.1)

Box 13.1 Declaration of Helsinki (2013) on *"General ethical principles in research".*

- Encourage and protect the health, well-being and rights of subjects participating in biomedical research.
- Medical research should abide by the ethical principles aiming to assure respect and safeguard the health and rights of human subjects.
- Interests of subjects must always be given preference over societal and scientific interests.
- It is the responsibility of physicians or investigators undertaking biomedical research to safeguard the health, respect, morals, rights of human subjects involved in research and to maintain privacy and confidentiality of the subject's personal information.
- Biomedical research should be carried out in a manner which poses minimal risk to the environment.
- Research should be undertaken by personnel possessing adequate qualification, training and experience in ethical and scientific areas.
- Underrepresented groups to be given adequate access to research participation.
- Appropriate compensation and treatment for subjects harmed during research.

ETHICAL ISSUES DURING VARIOUS STAGES OF CLINICAL RESEARCH

Issues related to ethics play a crucial role during all stages of clinical research viz. planning, conduct and post completion (Figure 13.2).

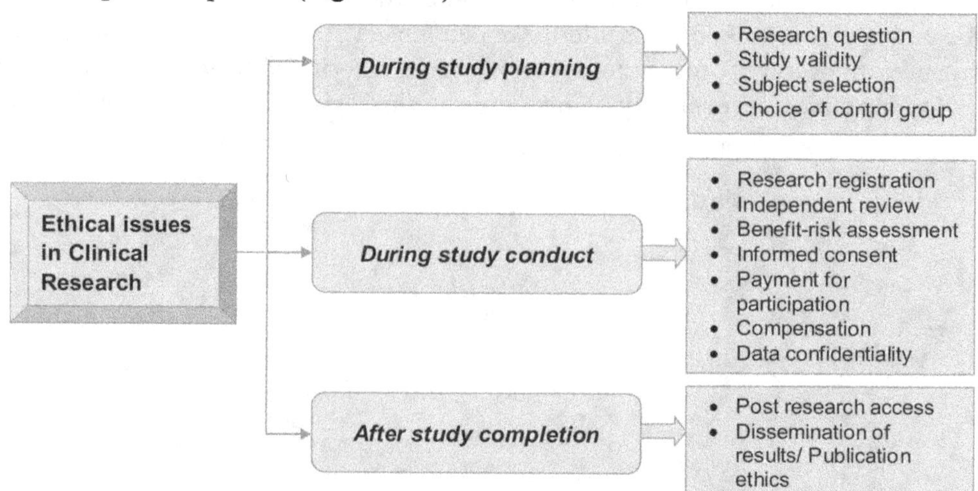

Figure 13.2 Important ethical issues of concern at various stages of clinical research.

ETHICAL ISSUES DURING STUDY PLANNING

1. ***Research question***: Research should aim to answer a question which is based on a scientific rationale, holds clinical relevance, is socially valuable and is expected to contribute knowledge in the field of health (Box 13.2).
2. ***Study validity***: Study possesses an adequate and feasible design, valid end points and stringent methods to ensure the acquirement of valid and interpretable data.

Box 13.2 Declaration of Helsinki (2013) on *"Scientific Requirements"*.

"Medical research carried out on human subjects should adhere to universally applicable scientific principles, be built around a meticulous knowledge of scientific literature, other appropriate origins of information, and relevant laboratory and animal experimentation".

---

3. ***Subject selection***: The process and outcomes of subject and site selection should be equitable and based on scientific principles, pose minimal risks and maximal benefits.

❖ *Healthy volunteers.* The inclusion of healthy humans in phase 1 studies, although is voluntary and done after obtaining safety information about new drug from preclinical studies, but still the ethical issue remains of administering a new drug to healthy persons who are not going to get any benefit.

❖ *Vulnerable groups.*

Vulnerable groups include:
- Socially, economically or politically disadvantaged e.g. sexual minorities, unemployed, orphans, ethnic minorities, tribals, refugees, migrants etc.
- Incapable of making voluntary informed decisions e.g. children under 18 years of age.
- Can give consent but have compromised autonomy e.g. mentally ill, unconscious, cognitively impaired.
- Diminished autonomy due to dependency e.g. students, prisoners, employees, defence personnel, institutionalized individuals etc.
- Terminally ill or having rare or stigmatizing diseases.

Principles of conducting research in vulnerable groups (Box 13.3)
- The selection of individuals or communities for participating in research should be made in a manner that the risk/s and advantage/s of biomedical research are uniformly distributed (distributive justice).
- Adequate rationale for the involvement of vulnerable groups in research needs to be provided.
- Appropriate safety measures should be adopted to protect the rights and welfare of the individuals and maintain privacy and confidentiality of the data obtained.
- Mandatory audio-visual recording of the informed consent process.

- Care should be taken to avoid any undue influence, force, coercion, threat or incentives to participate through the entire research period.
- Involvement of legally acceptable representative (LAR) where the participants lack the ability to give consent. Fresh or re-consent to be obtained in cases where participant gains mental competence or consciousness (from unconscious state) during the course of study.
- Permission to be taken from appropriate authorities where relevant e.g. tribal communities (tribal welfare commissioner, district collector), institutionalized individuals etc.
- Ethics committee should ensure the justification for inclusion of vulnerable groups, meticulously ascertain benefits and risks involved and risk-minimization strategies, additional protective measures e.g. more frequent reviews and monitoring, to have separate SOPs for handling proposals involving vulnerable groups. The initial and continuing reviews of the proposals involving vulnerable groups should be done by the full EC. Representatives from specific populations should be involved during meetings.

Box 13.3 Declaration of Helsinki (2013) on *"Vulnerable groups and individuals"*.

- Especially contemplated protection to be given to vulnerable individuals and populations.
- Medical research involving vulnerable group is reasonable only if the research aims to cater the healthcare needs or priorities of this group and research cannot otherwise be conducted in non-vulnerable group.

❖ *Special populations: Children, pregnant and nursing females, geriatric population etc.*

The recommendations and conditions for the inclusion of these special groups of populations as subjects in clinical research have been discussed in Chapter 10.

❖ *Community*

- Depending on the type of research, participants can be taken from a community.
- In cases where community engagement is there, a community advisory board/group acts as interface between the participating community, the researchers and the EC.
- The EC may include community representatives during proceedings of such proposals.
- Individual informed consent needs to be obtained.
- After study completion, the results may be communicated to the community representative for their dissemination to the entire community.

4. Choice of control group (Box 13.4)

Use of placebo. The use of placebo in placebo controlled studies is always a matter of ethical debate since the group receiving placebo is deprived of existing standard effective treatment.

> **Box 13.4** Guidelines on the use of placebo.
>
> ***Principles of Declaration of Helsinki (2013 revision)***
>
> - The advantages, harms, burdens and efficacy of a new intervention should be evaluated in comparison to the best proven intervention(s), except in the below mentioned situations:
>   - ✓ in the absence of a proven intervention, the use of placebo or no intervention is admissible; or
>   - ✓ when due to convincing and scientifically justified methodological issues, the use of any intervention/ treatment having less efficacy than the best proven one, the use of placebo, or no intervention is essential to evaluate the efficacy or safety of an intervention and the subjects receiving such an intervention are not exposed to undue risks of serious or irreversible harm due to being deprived of the best proven intervention.
> - Utmost caution should be exercised to prevent abuse of placebo.
>
> ***ICMR guidelines (2017)***
>
> A placebo may be used as control under following conditions:
>
> - No effective established therapy available.
> - Self-limiting disease
> - Participant is not exposed to serious harm on withholding the standard effective treatment, though there may be some short term uneasiness or delay in symptom alleviation.
> - Participants are not subjected to any added risk of irreversible or serious harm.

ETHICAL ISSUES DURING STUDY CONDUCT

1. **Research registration:** Clinical trial registration is the process of submitting and updating the trial information in a structured web-based registry that is accessible to public before starting patient enrolment. The registration of clinical trials in a public database is a major step towards increasing transparency, accessibility and accountability in clinical research; curtailing inadequate reporting of results and increasing awareness among public and regulatory bodies about ongoing trials (box 13.5).

> **Box 13.5** Declaration of Helsinki (2013) on *"CT Registration".*
>
> "Every research study involving human subjects must be registered in a publicly accessible database before recruitment of the first subject".

Steps in clinical trial registration

Figure 13.3 gives an outline of the major steps involved during the process of clinical trial registration and disclosure of results.

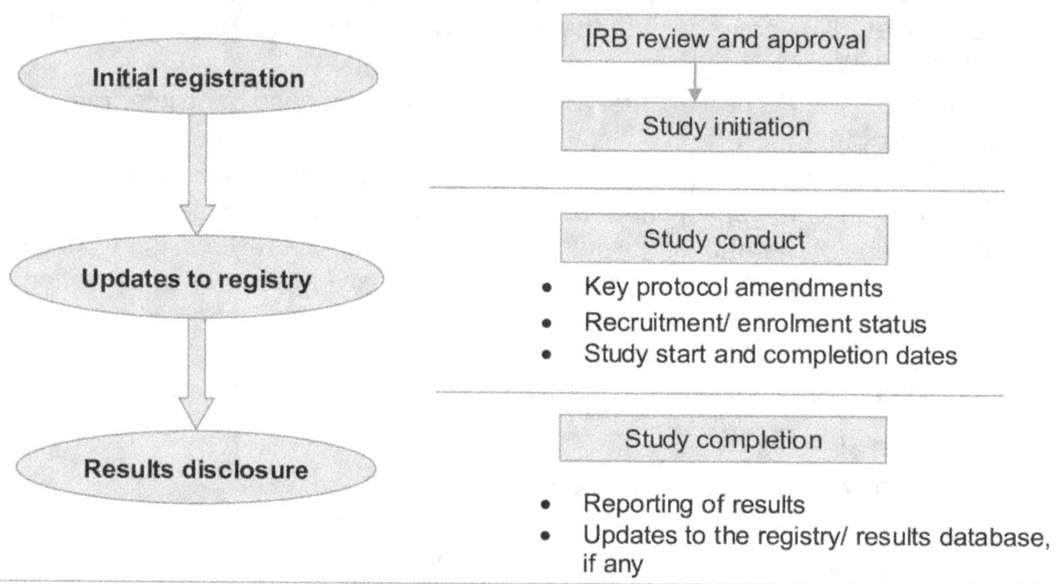

Figure 13.3 Steps in clinical trial registration.

In 2005, the International Committee of Medical Journal Editors (ICMJE) commenced a policy regarding registration of clinical trials for considering the trial results for publication. In 2007, the FDA passed the FDA Amendment Act mandating prospective registration and reporting of trial results in an online data bank viz. www.clinicaltrials.gov that was established in 1999.

In India, clinical trial registry of India (CTRI) was launched on 20th July 2007 by National Institute of Medical Statistics (NIMS), an arm of ICMR for registering the clinical trials. Additionally, the editors of major Indian biomedical journals have made a declaration that only the trials registered on a public database would be given consideration for publication in journals (Box 13.6).

In May 2017, under the aegis of WHO, ICMR signed a joint statement on public disclosure of results from all international trials.

Box 13.6 Research Registration with CTRI.

- Registration of any research conducted on human subjects involving any intervention such as drugs, surgical practices, preventive methods, lifestyle modifications, devices, educational or behavioral therapy, rehabilitation measures, as well as trials conducted under the purview of Department of AYUSH should be done with CTRI prior to enrolment of first patient.

Box 13.6 *Contd...*

- Submission of EC approval and DCGI approval (if applicable) is mandatory to get the trial registered with CTRI.
- The prospective registration of clinical trials in India was made compulsory by DCGI since 15th June, 2009.
- From 1st April 2018, only prospective trials i.e. those trials where the date of enrolment is a future date and the status is "Not yet recruiting" can be submitted with CTRI. Retrospective registration i.e. submission of any ongoing/ closed to recruitment/completed trials would no longer be feasible after this date.
- Multi-national trials with India as one of the centre already registered with an international registry should also be registered with CTRI wherein the details of Indian investigators, trial sites, Indian target sample size and date of enrolment are captured.
- After trial registration, information regarding trial status and other aspects should be regularly updated with CTRI.
- Trials registered with CTRI simultaneously get registered with WHO-International Clinical Trials Registry Platform (ICTRP); hence are freely searchable both from the WHO's search portal (http://www.who.int/ictrp/search/en/) as well as from CTRI (www.ctri.in).

2. ***Independent review by Ethics Committee.*** Independent assessment of conformance to ethical principles and guidelines in the planning, conduct and interpretation of research (Box 13.7).

Box 13.7 Declaration of Helsinki (2013) on *"Research Ethics Committees".*

- In biomedical research, before study initiation, the protocol should be presented to the concerned research ethics committee for due consideration, review and approval.
- After the study termination, a final report including a summary of the study's observations and inferences should be submitted by the researchers to the ethics committee.

3. **Benefit-risk assessment (Box 13.8)**
- The scientific rationale of research should be able to justify the underlying risks or harms associated with the research and whether the risks involved outweigh the expected benefits.
- Attempts should be made at the levels of researcher, sponsor and EC to optimize the benefits and minimize the risks incurred by the subjects.

Box 13.8 Declaration of Helsinki (2013) on *"Risks, burdens and benefits"*.

- Biomedical research in human participants may only be carried out if the significance of the objective overshadows the risks and harms to the research subjects.
- Measures to minimize the risks must be executed.
- When the risks/ harms are observed to overshadow the benefits, the need to continue, modify or terminate the study should be duly considered by the investigators.

---

4. Informed consent (Box 13.9)

Box 13.9 Declaration of Helsinki (2013) on *"Informed consent"*.

- In medical research, the participation by human subjects who are competent to give written informed consent should be entirely voluntary.
- Every prospective participant should be appropriately acquainted with the objectives, strategies, potential benefits and harms, source of funding, conflicts of interest, post trial access or provisions and any other pertinent aspects of the study.
- The prospective participants should be informed of the right to disagree to take part in the research or to withdraw consent for participation at any time without retaliation.
- For medical research involving recognizable human material or data e.g. material or data from bio-banks or similar repositories, investigators should obtain informed consent for its collection, storage and/or reuse. In unusual situations where it is not possible to get consent, research may be conducted only after review and approval of research ethics committee.

---

5. Payment for participation

Indian GCP and ICMR ethical guidelines

- Human participants may be paid for the *inconvenience* caused, *time* spent and *expenses* incurred, related to their participation in research. *Free medical services* may also be provided to them. However, payments and medical services should not be too large to induce prospective subjects to give their consent for participation in research against their better judgement (inducement).
- All payments, reimbursement and medical facilities to be delivered to research subjects must be approved by the IEC.
- Caution should be exercised:
  - ✓ when consent is obtained from a guardian in the interest of an incompetent person, in such a case remuneration should not be provided except a payment of out of pocket costs;

✓ if a subject is withdrawn from study due to research related medical reasons, he should be offered compensation equivalent to complete participation;

✓ in cases where a subject withdraws for any other reasons, he/she should be given compensation proportionate to the extent of his participation.

♦ Unjustifiable inducement through payment for individual subjects, families and populations must be disallowed. Undue compensation comprise of providing assistance for transporting body for cremation or burial, providing insurance for unrelated conditions, free transportation to and fro for examination for non routine visits, free of cost trip to town for rural participants, free meals, freedom for prisoners, free medication which is generally not available, academic credits and disproportionate compensation to researcher/team/institution.

6. **Compensation for research related harm** (For details, please refer to Chapter 16).

7. **Data confidentiality**

The research team has an obligation towards the participant to protect the information collected from unauthorized access, disclosure, use, modification, loss or theft. This holds true strictly in case of sensitive data like HIV status, genetic information, sexual orientation etc. where loss of confidentiality may be associated with discrimination or stigmatization.

At the time of publication of results, care should be taken to avoid publishing any data which may reveal the identity of participants.

Re-consent should be taken in case of possibility of identity revelation through data presentation or photographs (which should be camouflaged appropriately).

A useful strategy in this direction would be anonymization as it helps in delinking the data from personal identifiers.

ETHICAL ISSUES AFTER STUDY COMPLETION

1. **Post research access (Box 13.10 and 13.11).** An important issue faced by researchers and sponsors after completion of clinical trial is to provide post trial access of study intervention/s to the trial participants especially in cases where trial intervention is proven effective in life threatening conditions/ conditions where no effective established therapy is available. However in chronic conditions a debatable aspect would be the duration for which post trial access will be provided.

• The findings of the research study, wherever relevant, should be communicated to the study participants.

• The arrangements planned for post trial access should be described in study protocol for their due consideration by EC during its review.

• Regulatory approvals need to be taken *a priori* in order to provide study intervention to the participants after trial completion.

• In academic studies e.g. student projects, post trial access may not be feasible. However, the institution should make efforts to continue to provide support and care to the participants.

> **Box 13.10** Declaration of Helsinki (2013 revision) on *"Post-trial provisions"*.
>
> In medical research, the sponsors, investigators and regulatory authorities should make arrangements for post-trial provisions for the participants who still require a treatment/ intervention identified as beneficial in the trial. This information must also be given to the subjects during the process of obtaining informed consent.

> **Box 13.11** The New Drugs and Clinical Trials Rules, 2019.
>
> **Post trial access.** "Making a new drug or investigational new drug available to a trial subject after completion of clinical trial through which the said drug has been found beneficial to a trial subject during clinical trial for a period as deemed essential by the investigator and the ethics committee".
>
> On the recommendation of investigator and after obtaining EC approval, post trial access of the said drug after trial completion shall be provided by the sponsor to trial subject free of cost if:
> - no alternative therapy is available for the indication being studied and new drug/ IND has demonstrated benefit to trial subject by the investigator;
> - trial subject or his legal heir have given written consent to use new drug or IND in the post-trial period.

2. **Dissemination of results/ Publication ethics (Box 13.12).** Ethics plays an integral role in the process of dissemination of results/ publication. Ethical practices and principles need to be promoted and followed in the publication culture. Few organizations playing important roles in this field are:

   Committee on Publication Ethics (COPE), a voluntary body established in1997, provides education on publication ethics by means of various guidelines for editors, peer reviewers and authors etc.

   World Association of Medical Editors (WAME), a global non-profit voluntary association of editors of peer-reviewed medical journals aiming to:
   - encourage communication among various editors;
   - improve professional standards in editing by means of education and regulation;
   - improve editorial standards.

WAME has issued several policies relating to ethics and professionalism, authors, conflicts of interest, global health and politics, peer review, other publication related issues like impact factor, clinical trial registration etc.

> **Box 13.12** Declaration of Helsinki (2013) on
> *"Publication and Dissemination of results".*
>
> - "Researchers, authors, sponsors, editors and publishers all have ethical commitments with respect to the publication and dissemination of the results of research".
> - All the study results whether positive, negative or inconclusive must be published or otherwise made accessible to general public.

RESEARCH MISCONDUCT

DEFINITION

Research misconduct or ***fraud*** is defined by Office of Science and Technology Policy as *"fabrication, falsification, or plagiarism in proposing, performing, or reviewing research, or in reporting research results."* Another definition of research misconduct as given by the German Rectors' Conference is *"the provision of incorrect information in a scientific context of substantial significance, either intentionally or grossly negligently, the infringement of intellectual property of others or harm done to their research in any other way"*.

MANIFESTATIONS OF RESEARCH MISCONDUCT

- **Fabrication.** Intentional creation of research data or findings/results.
- **Falsification.** Intentional "pruning" to acquire the desired form or "massaging" to obtain the desired results from existing data by using inappropriate methods of data analysis e.g. misrepresentation or deletion of undesired or unfavorable data/results, fraudulent interpretation of results, omission of outliers in data analysis or the disallowed modification of graphics.
- **Plagiarism.** Derived from Latin word plagium meaning 'kidnapping'; deliberate unacknowledged exploitation/ presentation of other person's intellectual property (information or ideas) as one's own achievement. This type of plagiarism is also called "direct plagiarism". *WAME identifies plagiarism as copying six or more consecutive words or use of seven to eleven overlapping words in a set of 30 letters*.
- **Text recycling (Self-plagiarism).** Appearance of the parts of the same text (generally un-attributed) in an author's own multiple publications.
- **Mosaic plagiarism.** Copying someone's ideas or concepts and using them in modified form without attribution.

- **Redundant (duplicate) publication.** A larger problem of repeated publication of data or ideas, multiple or broadly overlapping publishing, often with at least one author in common.
- **Salami slicing.** Publishing the research results in small, multiple subunits.
- **Shot-gunning.** Submitting the manuscripts with two or more publishers.
- **Authorship issues.**
  - *Gift authorship*: listing authors on a publication who do not fulfill the required authorship criteria but as a personal favor or in lieu of payment.
  - *Ghost authorship*: not listing authors who fulfill the requirements for authorship.
  - *Guest authorship*. Listing authors who do not fufill the required authorship criteria but due to their senior status, fame or assumed impact.
  - Listing co-authors against their will.
- **Deception.** The intentional obscuration of a conflict of interest or deliberate inclusion of misguiding statements regarding research funding sources or other documents.

REASONS OF RESEARCH MISCONDUCT/FRAUD (FIGURE 13.4)

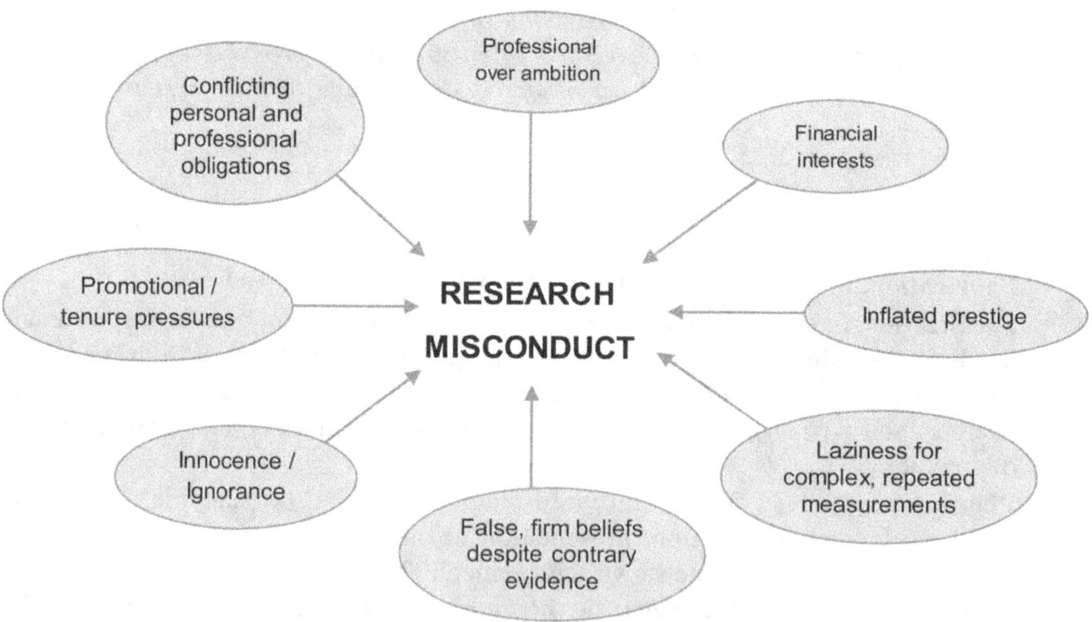

Figure 13.4 Factors responsible for misconduct or fraud in scientific research.

DETECTION OF RESEARCH MISCONDUCT

1. **Vigilant monitoring of data for**

    Debatable/ farfetched trends: e.g. excessive instances of perfect attendance, 100% drug compliance, too good to be true results, implausible data, flat distribution of values, no adverse events etc.

    Different trends at a particular site: e.g. unusually fast recruitment, very few withdrawals, very few adverse events being reported, repeat postponement of meetings etc.

    Practices/behavior at a site: discrepancy between entered and source data, digit preference, same pen used throughout etc.

2. ***Electronic detection of duplicated text.*** Text-matching softwares to detect plagiarism e.g. ithenticate, turnitin etc.

STRATEGIES TO HANDLE OR PREVENT RESEARCH MISCONDUCT

1. *Ensure integrity of scientific research*
    - ✓ Clear standard operating procedures (SOPs).
    - ✓ Educate good clinical and documentation practices.
    - ✓ Strict monitoring.
    - ✓ Ongoing techniques to assess and review research.
    - ✓ Clear reporting policies, procedures and guidelines.
    - ✓ Research governance.
    - ✓ Dummy patients.
    - ✓ Double check data.

2. *Legal actions against involved personnel*
    - ✓ Adopt zero tolerance – any doubtful misconduct should be reported and all claims should be investigated meticulously and impartially.
    - ✓ Warning letters.
    - ✓ Registration/license cancelled.
    - ✓ Blacklisting/restrictions.
    - ✓ Heavy fines, imprisonment.

    Presently, India has no specific law pertaining to scientific fraud.

3. *Handling authorship issues*
    - ✓ Encourage a culture of ethical authorship.
    - ✓ Follow standard guidelines on authorship e.g. International Committee of Medical Journal Editors (ICMJE) (Box 13.13).

> ### Box 13.13 ICMJE Criteria for authorship.
>
> According to ICMJE, there are 4 criteria for assigning authorship:
> - Significant contributions to the inception or planning of the work; or the collection, analysis, or interpretation of data for the work; AND
> - Drafting the work or critically evaluating it for significant intellectual matter; AND
> - Approval of the finalized version for publication; AND
> - Agreement to be answerable for all aspects of the work in making sure that any queries related to the perfection or validity of any part of the work are adequately scrutinized and settled.

ICMR POLICY ON RESEARCH INTEGRITY AND PUBLICATION ETHICS 2019

- The purpose of this policy is to ensure highest ethical and professional standards at various stages of biomedical and health research such as planning, conduct, reporting, reviewing and publishing including authorship issues.
- The policy is applicable to all staff and students in various ICMR centres or institutions across the country.
- Key features included in the policy with respect to reporting and publication of results:
  - ✓ publishing and sharing of results of completed research on public databases, websites or other platforms;
  - ✓ research misconduct in any form is unethical and unacceptable;
  - ✓ ICMJE and COPE guidelines on publication ethics, research integrity, authorship etc. should be followed by all researchers;
  - ✓ avoidance of submitting articles to any predatory journal/s (usually online journals offering incentives e.g. overnight publication, low or free of cost publication etc. and lacking scholarly publishing standards) for publication;
  - ✓ clear identification of contribution of all authors and disallowing ghost and gift authorships.
- The policy also provides procedures for managing research misconduct allegations in a fair, confidential and prompt manner.
- Certain guidelines for avoiding plagiarism as defined in the policy are:
  - ✓ acknowledgement i.e. giving credit to someone else's work;
  - ✓ text taken from another source to be enclosed in quotation marks and citation provided;
  - ✓ reframing of essence of someone else's work in own words and providing citation for the same;
  - ✓ manipulating references to be avoided. Only references directly related to contents should be mentioned in an acceptable format.

Ethics Committee

INTRODUCTION

Ethics Committee (EC) is a board or a committee constituted by an institution to review, grant permission to initiate and periodically review the biomedical research involving humans.

The main responsibilities of EC are:

- ✓ to safeguard the *rights, safety and well being of human participants* enrolled in a clinical trial and to grant public affirmation of that protection,
- ✓ to express judgement on the *clinical trial protocol*, the *appropriateness of the investigators* undertaking the trial and the *availability of adequate facilities*,
- ✓ to review and approve the approaches and documents to be used to obtain the *informed consent* of trial participants, and
- ✓ to ensure adequacy of *confidentiality safeguards*

Various synonyms used for Ethics Committees:

- ✓ IRB- Institutional Review Board
- ✓ REC – Research Ethics Committee
- ✓ ERB- Ethics Review Board
- ✓ ERC – Ethics Review Committee
- ✓ IEC- Institutional Ethics Committee

COMPOSITION OF EC

General considerations

- Important attributes of an EC are *independence* and *competence.*
- *Multidisciplinary* and *Multi-sectorial* in composition.
- *Chairman* should be from outside the Institution to ensure independence of the Committee.
- The *Member Secretary* should be from the same Institution and be responsible for conducting the business of the Committee.
- There should be an adequate representation of *age and gender.*
- The composition of EC should be reasonable with respect to number of members; a minimum of *five* persons is necessary to form the quorum in the absence of which any important decision pertaining to research should not be taken.
- There should be at least one member with nonscientific background/ area of interest and at least one member should be independent of the institution/ trial site.

Table 14.1 gives a comparative overview of Schedule Y, Indian GCP and ICMR guidelines related to ECs.

Table 14.1 Comparison of various guidelines on EC.

	The New Drugs and Clinical Trials Rules, 2019	Indian GCP	ICMR
Total members	At least 7	5-7	7-15
Minimum quorum	Five	Five	Five
Composition	• Chairperson • Member Secretary At least 5 members with following representations: • basic medical scientists (preferably 1 pharmacologist). • Clinicians • legal expert • social scientist/ representation of non-governmental voluntary agency / philosopher / ethicist / theologian or similar person • lay person from the community.	• Chairperson • Member Secretary • 1-2 basic medical scientists (preferably one pharmacologist). • 1-2 clinicians • 1 legal expert or retired judge • 1 social scientist / representative of non-governmental voluntary agency • 1 philosopher / ethicist / theologian • 1 lay person from the community	• Chairperson/ Vice Chairperson (optional) • Member Secretary/Alternate Member Secretary (optional) • basic medical scientist(s) • clinician(s) • legal expert(s) • social scientist/ philosopher/ethicist/ theologian • lay person
Record keeping	Not specified	For a period of 5 years after trial completion	For a period of 3 years after trial completion

- The EC members should collectively possess the qualifications and experience to review and assess the science, ethics and medical characteristics of research protocols; members should be conversant with GCP, The New Drugs and Clinical Trials Rules, 2019 and ethical guidelines for conduct of human research.
- ***Subject experts*** could be called for to express their opinion. The inclusion of representatives from specific patient groups may also be considered depending on the needs of particular research area e.g. HIV/ AIDS, genetic disorders etc.

SPECIAL SITUATIONS FOR ECs

- Large institutions/universities having large number of proposals may have multiple constituted IECs for handling different research areas.
- Small institutions can form alliance with other IECs or approach any registered IEC.
- A sub-committee of the main IEC may be formed for reviewing proposals submitted by undergraduate or postgraduate students.
- Institutions not having their own IEC (user institution) may utilize the services of IEC from an adjoining institution (host institution) after entering into a MoU (Memorandum of understanding). In such a case, EC of host institution can carry out site monitoring visits and will have access to all research records.
- Institutional committee for stem cell research (IC-SCR) will review and approve the research proposals on stem cells before submission to EC.
- Subcommittees, reporting to the main EC, like expedited review sub-committee or SAE subcommittee can be constituted comprising of Chairperson/Member Secretary and 1-2 designated members as specified in SOPs of the EC.
- A separate committee for SAE including 1 or 2 members of EC can also be formed, the report of which will be reviewed by main EC.

REVIEW PROCEDURES

EC is responsible to conduct the review of research proposals on scientific and ethical grounds:
- *Scientific review*: scientific validity of the protocol, risks to subjects, and expected benefits.
- *Ethical review:* ethical implications of the chosen research design and methodology.

Depending on the degree of risk to participants involved, the review procedures can be categorized into exempted from review, expedited review and full review (Figure 14.1).

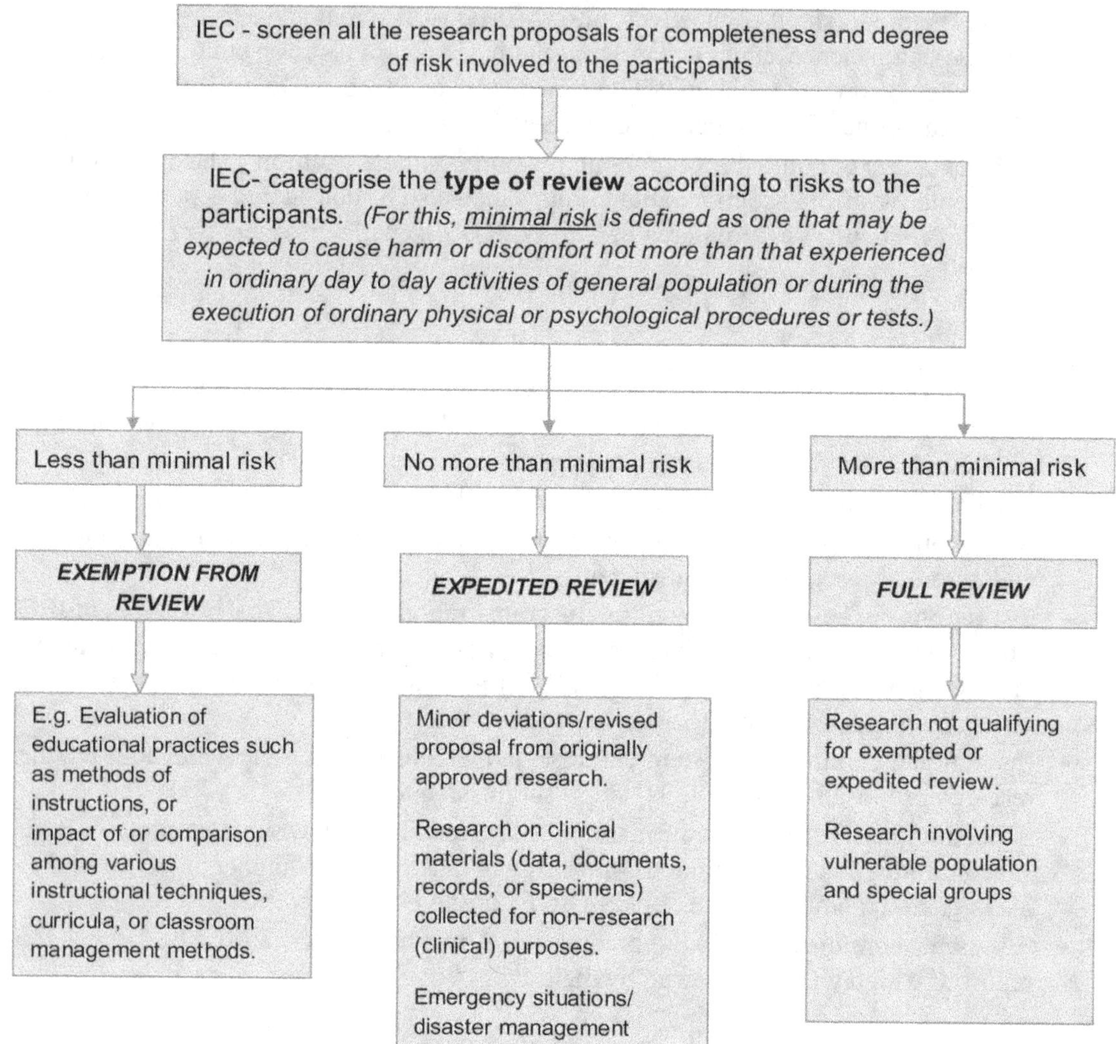

Figure 14.1 Types of ethics committee review procedures.

CONFLICT OF INTEREST (COI) IN ECs

Conflict of interest is a set of situations when professional judgement regarding a primary interest is unduly influenced by some secondary interest. In the context of clinical research, it can arise when judgement concerning subject's safety and welfare or research validity is influenced by a financial or non-financial interest. It can be present at the level of researchers, EC members, sponsors or institutions.

TYPES OF COI FOR EC MEMBERS (FIGURE 14.2)

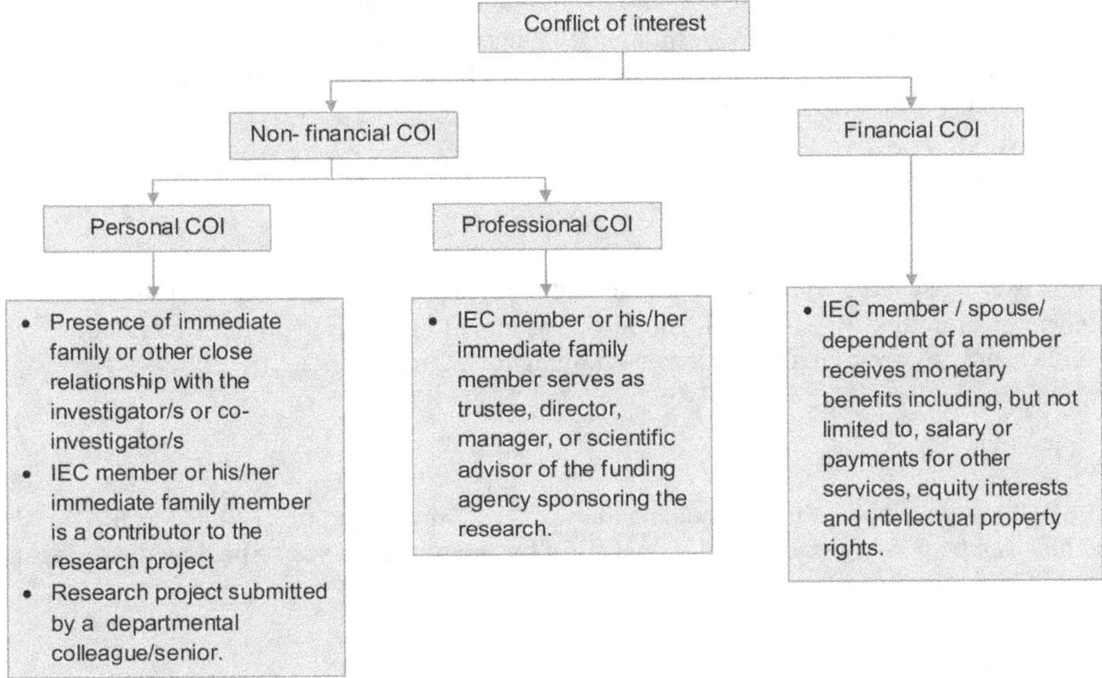

Figure 14.2 Types of COI for EC members.

MANAGING COI AMONG EC MEMBERS

❖ ***Standard operating procedures:*** The declaration and management of COI within the EC should be as per the standard operating procedures (SOPs) of that EC.

❖ ***Voluntary disclosure of COI by EC member:*** If a member has a COI in a research proposal, he should not be involved in decision making process, a prior disclosure to the Chairman should be done and the same should be recorded in minutes of meeting. He/she may be present in the meeting room only to clear any queries about the research but should leave the meeting room during discussion of the study (Box 14.1).

Box 14.1 Note.
EC member who declares COI and does not attend the meeting is not counted towards the quorum for vote. His/ her absence under such situation is referred to as *recusal*, and not abstention or absence.

❖ ***COI form/ declaration form***
   All EC members should sign COI form/ declaration form.
❖ The final authority for determining whether a COI has been managed or eliminated properly lies with the IEC Chairperson. Any clinical research study where the COI has not been eliminated, should not be approved by EC.

FORUM FOR ETHICS REVIEW COMMITTEE IN INDIA (FERCI)

This is a registered society set up as the National Chapter of FERCAP (Forum for Ethics Review Committee in Asia Pacific) in India. The aim of FERCI is to promote ethics review in India mainly by providing education and training for EC members.

SOPs FOR IECs

FERCI has developed a list of model generic SOPs (comprising of 21 SOPs: SOP 1 to 21) which can be personalized by individual IECs for their use. These can be downloaded from http://ferci.org/sops/

CReATE-FERCI INITIATIVE (BOX 14.2)

Box 14.2 CReATE-FERCI initiative.
Under CReATE-FERCI initiative, a suite of five cloud- based software tools have been developed jointly by FERCI and PATH (an international global health organization aiming to improve health) for improving, strengthening and capacity building of clinical researchers and ECs. These tools are: 1. *Simplifier*: an electronic database of a glossary of "simplified" key terms used in consent forms to enhance comprehension for lay persons. 2. *Interpreter*: database with simple "interpretations" of terms used in informed consent documents in vernacular Indian languages. It helps in minimizing errors during translations. 3. *CheckEthix*: a questionnaire based tool to evaluate the ethical soundness of clinical study protocols and informed consent documents; helps to decrease the workload of ECs and researchers to self-score the documents prior to submission. 4. *Regulert*: is a free subscription service providing notifications and other information from various stakeholders like national and international regulatory bodies; helps in keeping the researchers updated with latest global developments in areas of research ethics.

Box 14.2 *Contd...*

> 5. *eEC*: an online document management system comprising of CREaTE Platform for submission of protocols, conduct of ethics reviews, communications and online tracking of status of submissions; helpful in increasing efficiency of ECs and managing high paper burden.
>
> The CReATE software suite is free of cost and can be accessed through a web-based interface.

ACCREDITATION OF ETHICS COMMITTEES

Accreditation of ECs is an independent and systematic examination of the documents, functioning and procedures of ECs by an external accreditation body; with an aim to assess their performance against a set of established standards.

NEED FOR ACCREDITATION

- ✓ To ensure that
- ♦ EC is constituted and functions according to applicable regulations.
- ♦ Members are conversant with their roles and responsibilities and current rules and regulations.
- ♦ The EC has essential SOPs in place which are practised.
- ♦ EC has appropriate policies for declaration and management of conflict of interest.
- ✓ To promote standards for quality.
- ✓ To encourage commitment of the institutions for conducting scientifically and ethically sound research with continual improvement.

MANDATORY ACCREDITATION OF ECs (BOX 14.3).

Box 14.3 Mandatory accreditation of ECs.

The accreditation of ethics committees involved in supervision of clinical trials has been made mandatory by the Ministry of Health and Family Welfare with effect from 1ˢᵗ January, 2018.

BENEFITS OF ACCREDITATION

Various benefits of accreditation to different stakeholders including subjects, regulatory bodies, trial site and staff have been described in Table 14.2.

CERTIFYING ORGANIZATIONS

- SIDCER (Strategic Initiative for Developing Capacity in Ethical Review)
- AAHRPP (Association for the Accreditation of Human Research Protection Program)
- National Accreditation Board for Hospitals and Healthcare Providers (NABH)

NABH, a constituent board of Quality Council of India, has been established with an aim to enhance the quality and patient safety in health care system. NABH is responsible to develop and conduct the accreditation program for healthcare organizations and ethics committees.

Table 14.2 Benefits of accreditation.

Subjects/ Participants

- Ensures high quality of subject care and safety.
- Subject care by credential and trained medical staff under investigator's supervision.

Trial sites/ Institutions

- Ensures adherence to regulatory guidelines and standards at the clinical trial sites.
- Provides ownership of clinical trial processes by the ECs.
- Continual improvement in quality care raising subject and community confidence in clinical trials.

Site staff

- Provision of continuous learning and healthy working environment.
- Improvement in overall professional growth of investigator, site staff and researchers.

Regulatory bodies

- Provides an assurance to regulatory authorities that all the research procedures and processes are in accordance with applicable regulatory requirements.

ORGANIZATIONAL STRUCTURE OF NABH (FIGURE 14.3)

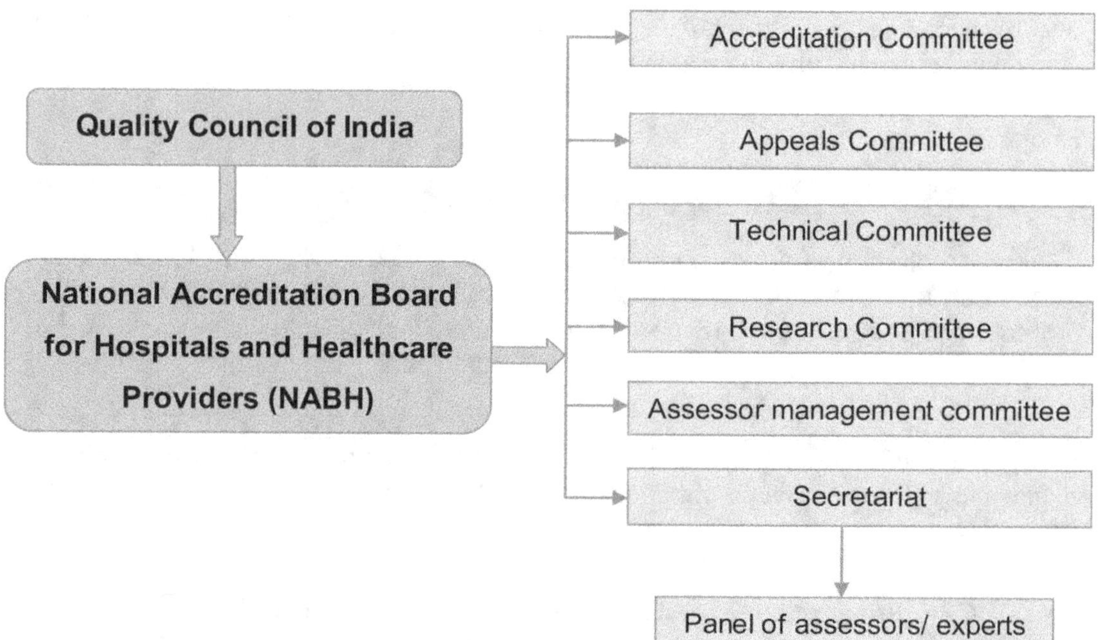

Figure 14.3 Organizational structure of NABH.

NABH STANDARDS FOR ECs ACCREDITATION

NABH has developed standards for ECs accreditation which include 10 standard and 49 objective elements (Annexure IV).

PROCESS OF NABH ACCREDITATION OF ETHICS COMMITTEES (FIGURE 14.4)

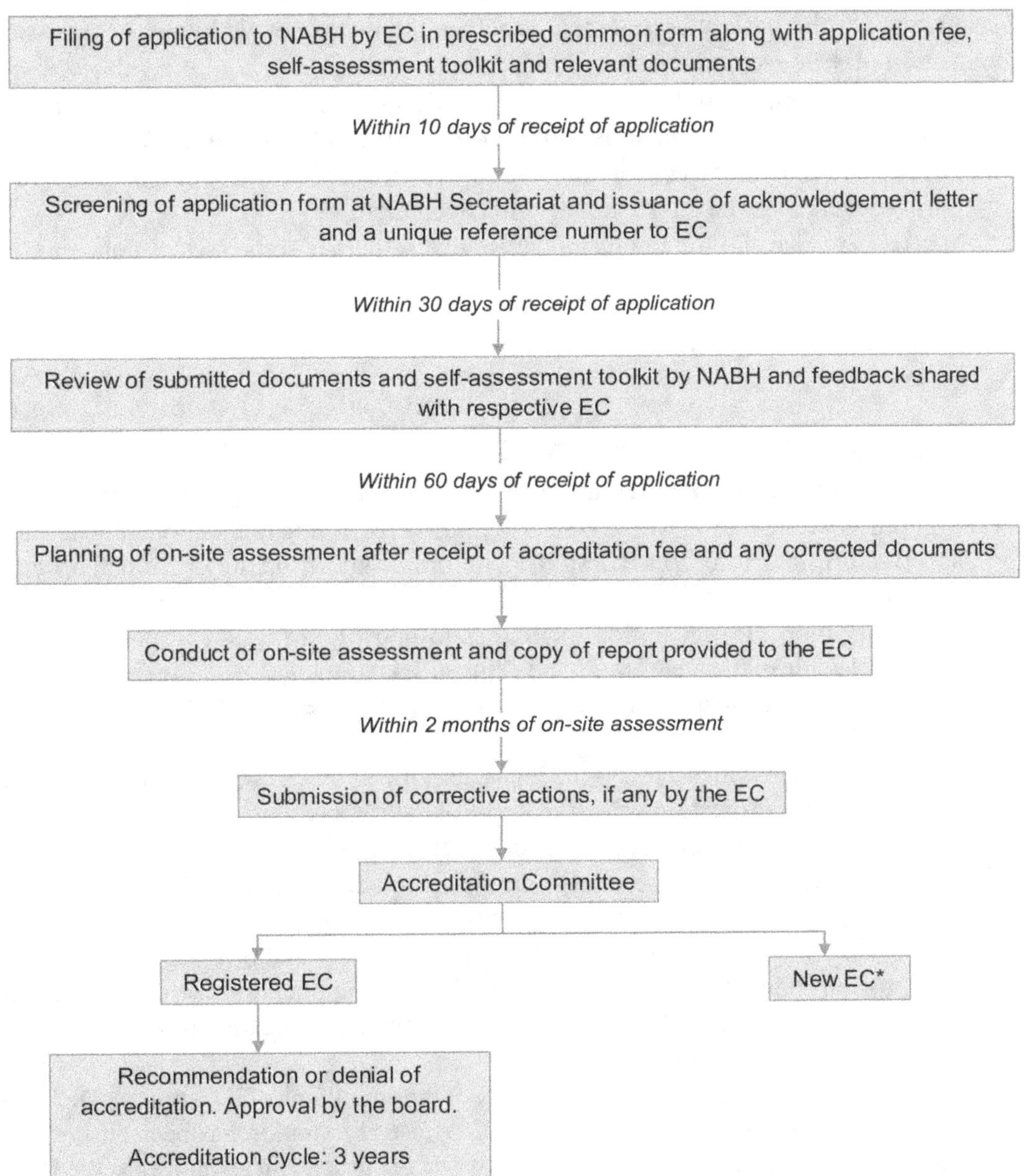

Figure 14.4 Process of NABH accreditation of ECs.

*EC has not initiated the review, monitoring and approval of trials but qualifies for accreditation on the basis of documentation and on-site NABH assessment. ***Provisional accreditation*** may be granted with a maximum validity of 12 months within which EC must begin trial approval process after obtaining prior permission from competent authority failing which accreditation may be withdrawn. EC needs to inform NABH about any contracts with the sponsor/s and trial related activities, so NABH team can visit for verification of implementation of standards. On the basis of assessment report, continuation or withdraw of provisional accreditation may be recommended by NABH.

- EC accreditation is valid for 3 years. An application for renewal of accreditation may be filed by EC at least 6 months before the expiry of validity of accreditation.
- During one accreditation cycle of 3 years, NABH conducts surveillance visit of EC during second year i.e 15-18 months after accreditation.
- NABH may also call for an unannounced visit if there is some serious concern.

RECENT AMENDMENTS IN INDIAN REGULATIONS RELATING TO ETHICS COMMITTEES

- ❖ **G.S.R. 72(E) dated February 8, 2013**
- (i) Insertion of Rule 122 DD: Requirements and guidelines for registration of EC
- ✓ Compulsory registration with CDSCO of all ECs reviewing regulatory clinical trials to approve clinical trials/BABE studies in India within 45 days from the date of commencement of the D & C Rules, 2013;
- ✓ The application for registration of EC has to be made to DCGI as per form CT-01 Eighth schedule of the New Drugs and Clinical Trials Rules, 2019. The registration will be granted within 100 days of receipt of application (as per DCGI office order dated 30 May 2014).
- ✓ The EC shall allow inspectors or officials authorized by CDSCO to enter its premises for carrying out inspection of any records, data or document and provide answers to any queries raised by such inspectors or officials.
- ✓ If there is any change in the constitution or membership of the EC, the information should be passed to the Licensing Authority in written.
- ✓ The registration of ECs unless suspended or cancelled would be valid for a duration of 3 years from the date of issue. In cases where the application for re-registration is submitted to DCGI within 3 months before the expiry, the registration would continue to be in force until fresh orders are passed.
- ✓ If the EC is not successful in abiding by any of the conditions of registration, DCGI may suspend or cancel the registration. The EC whose registration has been suspended or cancelled, may within 90 days of the receipt of the order, file an appeal to the Central Government which may after hearing the appellant confirm, reverse or modify such order.

Information to be submitted by applicants for EC registration

- Name and address of the office of EC
- Authority under which EC constituted
- Requisites regarding membership
- Terms of reference
- Quorum required
- Determinants of appointment
- Procedures of resignation, substitution or dismissal of members
- Brief profile of Chairman and all members
- Details of the supporting staff
- All SOPs in general, SOPs for vulnerable population, training of members and handling conflict of interest
- Training policy for new and existing members
- Audit/ inspection report, if any
- Undertaking by the Committee

For ECs existing before the amendment *(G.S.R. 72(E) dated February 8, 2013)*

- type of clinical research reviewed by the EC
- documents reviewed for every clinical trial
- documentation of minutes of meetings and number of meetings concerning clinical trials
- SAEs reviewed during trials conduct.

(ii) For medical members of ECs (medical scientists and clinicians), post graduate qualification and adequate experience in their respective fields made mandatory.

(iii) Mandatory training of new and existing EC members on GCP guidelines, clinical trials provisions under D & C Rules and other regulatory requirements to protect the rights, safety and well-being of trial subjects. EC to make policy for the same.

(iv) ECs to have separate SOPs (standard operating procedures) on review of studies involving vulnerable populations, training of EC members and strategies to handle conflict of interest.

(v) Archival of EC documents for at least 5 years from the date of trial completion or termination. Both hard and soft copies should be archived.

❖ **G.S.R. 53 (E) dated January 30ᵗʰ, 2013 and G.S.R. 889 (E) dated December 12, 2014**

Insertion of Rule 122 DAB: Compensation in case of injury or death during clinical trial

Responsibility of Ethics Committee in the SAE reporting process and payment of financial compensation:

In case of any SAE (death/ other than death) reported in a clinical trial subject, the Ethics Committee, after receiving the reports from Sponsor and Investigator, shall analyze the report and forward its report to DCGI accompanied by its opinion on financial compensation to be paid by the Sponsor within 30 days of the occurrence of event.

❖ **Independent Ethics Committees (IndECs)**

As per the notification from DCGI in 2013, the IndECs registered under CDSCO can give clearance for and oversee only BA/BE studies *(File no. ECR/Misc/Indt.EC/007/2013; July 30, 2013)*.

❖ **Newer responsibilities on ECs consigned by DCGI (Circulars by CDSCO; August 2016)**

✓ IECs given the power *to decide the suitability of clinical trial site* irrespective of the number of beds. However, it was suggested that sites must have emergency rescue and care arrangements.

✓ IECs empowered to *determine the limit for number of trials per investigator* on the basis of complexity and requirements of the particular study and facilities at the site.

✓ For *addition/deletion of site/s and investigators*, only IEC permission would be required. Sponsor needs to inform about any such addition/deletion and obtain No Objection Certificate from DCGI.

❖ **Re-registration of ECs (2016)**

CDSCO released a new checklist for re-registration of ECs in 2016 which has stricter requirements as:

- Mandatory to submit evidence (e.g. training records or certificates) that all members of ECs have been adequately trained in GCP guidelines and clinical trial provisions as per D & C Rules.

- ECs need to submit a brief description of the methods used by the committee for the monitoring of clinical trials.

- SAE review details to be submitted- Information regarding review of SAEs reported during trial conduct (provide protocol title and list of SAEs other than death) and SAE-death reported protocol wise.

- **Academic non-regulatory studies (G.S.R. 313 (E), dated March 16, 2016)**

  For academic clinical trial with an approved drug tested for off-label indication or new route of administration, only IEC approval is mandatory and no permission from DCGI is required and the data obtained is not intended to be submitted to DCGI.

Recommentations related to ECs in the New Drugs and Clinical Trials Rules, 2019 (Box 14.4).

Box 14.4 The New Drugs and Clinical Trials Rules, 2019.

As per the New Drugs and Clinical Trials Rules, 2019, two types of Ethics Committees have been defined:

❖ EC for Clinical trial, Bioavailability and Bioequivalence study

❖ EC for biomedical and health research

Box 14.4 *Contd...*

EC for Clinical trial, Bioavailability and Bioequivalence study

- _Composition_: minimum of 7 members, at least 50 percent non-affiliated members, mandatory to have at least one woman member.
- _Training requirements of EC members:_ All members of the Ethics Committee need to undergo such training and development programmes as defined by by the Central Licencing Authority from time to time.

  In case a member has not successfully completed such training and developmental programmes, he/she may be disqualified from holding the post of member of the Ethics Committee and shall cease to be a member of such committee.
- _Functioning of EC_: as per Indian GCP guidelines.
- _Registration of EC_ : with DCGI
- The application for registration has to be made in Form CT-01. The registration of EC shall be granted in Form CT-02 within a period of 45 working days from the date of receipt of application.
- The CLA should be informed regarding any modification in the constitution or membership of registered EC within 30 working days.
- An EC whose application for registration has been rejected by DCGI, may file an appeal to the Central Government, MoHFW within 60 working days from the date of receipt of rejection order. The Central Government shall dispose of the appeal within 60 working days from the date of filing the appeal.
- Registration shall be valid for a period of 5 years from the date of its issue, unless suspended or cancelled by the Central licensing authority.
- On expiry of validity period of registration, an application for renewal of registration shall be made by EC 90 days prior to the date of expiry.
- _Maintenance of records:_ All the records, data, registers and other documents pertaining to functioning and review of clinical trial and BA/BE study shall be maintained by EC for a period of 5 years after trial completion.
- Additional records to be maintained by EC _(not specified in previous regulations)_:
- ✓ recommendation given by Ethics Committee for determination of compensation;
- ✓ records related to the serious adverse event, medical management of trial subjects and compensation paid.

EC for biomedical and health research: Key features

- Any institution or organization planning to conduct biomedical and health research needs to have an Ethics Committee for reviewing and overseeing the conduct of such research as detailed in National ethical guidelines for biomedical and health research involving human participants.

Box 14.4 _Contd..._

- The composition and functioning of EC shall be according to the National ethical guidelines for biomedical and health research involving human participants as specified by ICMR.
- EC should get registered with an authority designated by the Central Government, MoHFW, and Department of Health research.
- Provisional registration shall initially be granted with validity for a period of 2 years subsequent to which final registration may be granted which will remain valid for a period of 5 years from the date of issue.
- In case of suspension or cancellation of registration of EC, an appeal to the Central Government may be made within a period of 45 working days of the receipt of the order.

CHAPTER 15

Informed Consent

OVERVIEW

INTRODUCTION

Informed consent is a choice made by a competent person to take part in research after obtaining the required information and without being subjected to constraint, inappropriate influence, temptation or intimidation. It can also be defined as decision making by research participants having legal and intellectual capability to make such choices in their own right. Informed consent safeguards the subject's freedom of making decision and respect for autonomy. Appropriate information about the research is given to the study subject in a simple, clear and easy to understand language in a document known as the *"Informed Consent Document (ICD)"* comprising of informed consent form (ICF) and participant/ patient information sheet (PIS). Subjects, their legally acceptable representatives (LARs) or guardians must be given sufficient time and opportunity to make inquiries related to study and all queries are resolved to their satisfaction. Both the patient information sheet and the informed consent form should be approved by the ethics committee and submitted to the regulatory authority. If any modifications are made in ICD, the same need to be approved by EC and submitted to the regulatory authority before their implementation.

INFORMED CONSENT: COMPONENTS (FIGURE 15.1)

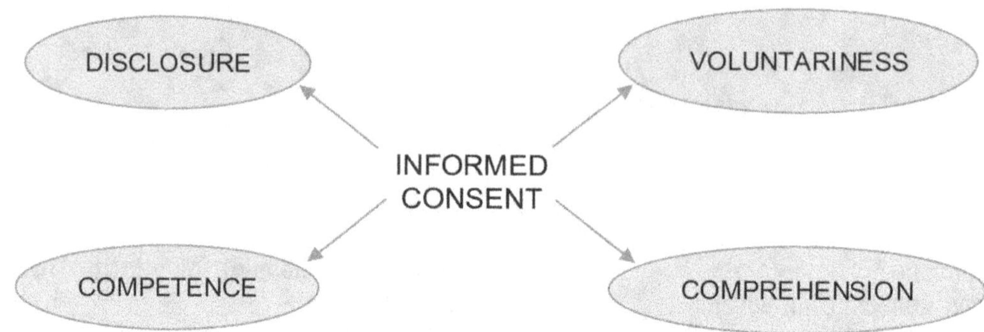

Figure 15.1 Components of informed consent.

INFORMED CONSENT PROCESS IN CHILDREN

The process of taking informed consent in pediatric studies varies according to the age of the children to be included.

Age of child: < 7 years	Age of child: 7-12 years	Age of child: 12-18 years
Parental consent	Verbal / Oral assent of child in the presence of parent/LAR	Written assent of child Parent/LAR's counter signature on the assent form

- *Assent* is the child's agreement for participation in research. The age for giving assent is 7-18 years. It is important to note that absence of disagreement should not be interpreted as assent.
- Adolescents, although have mental ability to consent, but since legal age to provide consent is not yet attained, the process of obtaining their agreement is termed as assent.
- The content and language of the assent form should be designed keeping in mind the understanding capacity, developmental level, social and emotional status of the children.
- In long duration studies, fresh assent or re-assent may need to be taken as the child grows up. Also, if the child attains 18 years of age during the course of trial, fresh consent should be taken.
- The study team must always respect the dissent or refusal of child to participate.
- Whether the consent of one or both parents is required before enrolling the child, has to be determined by the Ethics Committee. Generally, if the research involves greater than minimal risk or high risk to the child, consent of both parents should be obtained.
- In pediatric ethics, informed consent combines informed parental permission and (when appropriate) the assent of child.
- Since children are being considered as vulnerable group, it is mandatory to have audio-visual recording of the informed consent process.

WAIVER OF ASSENT

Waiver of assent may be provided by EC under certain situations as:

- When the research is assumed to provide direct benefit to the child which cannot be obtained otherwise; here the child's dissent can be overruled.
- Research involving children with mental retardation and other developmental disorders where the child is not capable on developmental and intellectual grounds to give assent.
- Other similar conditions (given below) when informed consent of adults is waived off.

INFORMED CONSENT PROCESS IN SPECIAL CASES (BOX 15.1 AND FIGURE 15.2)

Box 15.1 Informed Consent Process In Special Cases.

Inability of the subject to give informed consent (e.g. due to unconsciousness or presence of severe mental illness or disorder): In such a case, consent may be taken from a legally acceptable representative (LAR; a legally acceptable representative is an individual who can give consent for or authorize an intervention in the subject as permitted by the law(s) of India).

Illiterate subject or his/her legally acceptable representative: the entire informed consent process should be performed in the presence of an impartial witness who should put his signatures in the consent form. In such a case, thumb impression of the subject or his/her LAR may be taken along with.

Vulnerable population: Special focus should be made on ensuring the freedom of consent obtained from vulnerable population. The mode of consent must be duly considered and approved by the ethics committee. Also, audio-visual recording of the informed consent process is mandatory in case of vulnerable population.

Surrogate consent may be taken from

- authorized person or legal custodian *if participant loses consciousness or competence to consent during the research period* as in Alzheimer's disease or psychiatric conditions,
- authorized relative or legal custodian or the institutional head in the case of *abandoned institutionalized individuals or wards under judicial custody*

Informed consent in non-therapeutic study: In such a case, the consent should always be obtained from the subject. However, studies with no therapeutic objective may be carried out in subjects with consent of LAR provided all of the below mentioned criteria are met:

- objective of the trial demands involvement of subject(s) who can personally give the informed consent;
- the anticipated risks to the subject(s) are less and
- Ethics Committee's written approval is obtained for including such subject(s).

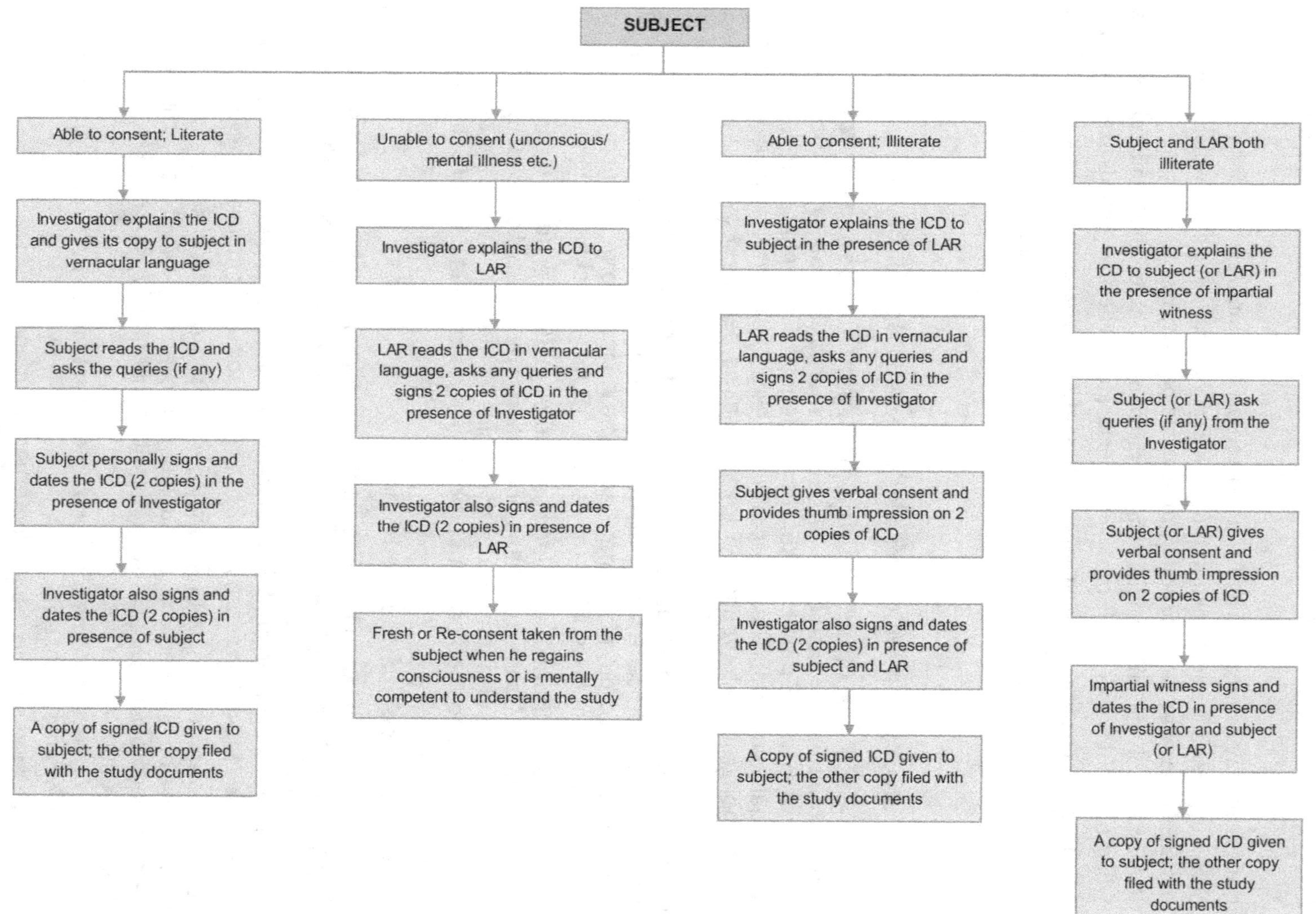

Figure 15.2 Flowchart depicting the informed consent process in various situations.

WAIVER OF CONSENT

Voluntary informed consent is always mandatory for every research proposal. However, this requirement can be waived in the presence of adequate justification of research exposing the subjects to not more than minimal risk. If such studies provide safeguard for privacy and confidentiality, and do not breach the rights of subjects then IECs may waive off the need for informed consent under following circumstances:

- When objective of research is a sensitive issue e.g. study on disease burden of HIV/AIDS.
- Research on freely accessible information, documents, records and archived materials, certain types of studies e.g. study on quality assurance, consumer acceptance and third party interviews.
- Research on anonymised biological materials from expired persons, remaining samples after biochemical or other examinations, cell lines or cell free derivatives like viral isolates, DNA or RNA from recognised institutions or qualified investigators, samples or data from repositories or registries etc.
- Under emergency circumstances when it is not possible to obtain surrogate consent.

FRESH OR RE-CONSENT

This should be obtained under following circumstances:

- When some new information is available necessitating deviation of protocol.
- Attainment of consciousness from state of being unconscious in a research participant or attainment of mental competence to understand the study. In case such an event is expected *a priori*, procedures to handle it should be mentioned in the informed consent form.
- When study is extended further or long follow up is planned at a later stage.
- When there is change of procedures, site visits.
- Change of LAR
- Prior to publication, in case there are chances of disclosure of identity through data presentation or photographs these should be camouflaged appropriately.
- Possibility of carrying out future research on stored biological samples if not anonymized.

RECENT AMENDMENTS IN DRUGS AND COSMETIC RULES REGARDING INFORMED CONSENT (BOX 15.2)

> **Box 15.2** Recent Amendments in Drugs and Cosmetics Rules Regarding Informed Consent Form (ICF) (GSR. 53 (E) dated 30th January 2013).
>
> ❖ Amendment of essential elements of ICF to include statements that
> ♦ In case of an injury experienced by a clinical trial participant, such participant would be provided *free medical management* upto the duration required.
> ♦ In case of a trial related injury or death, the sponsor or his representative are liable to provide *financial compensation*.
> ❖ Amendments in the format of ICF to include
> ♦ Address of the subject
> ♦ Qualification
> ♦ Occupation: Student/ Self-employed/ Service/ Housewife/ Others
> ♦ Annual income of the subject
> ♦ Name and address of the nominee(s) and his relation to the subject (for the purpose of compensation in case of trial related death)
> ❖ Obligatory for investigator to hand over a copy of duly filled ICF to the subject or his/ her attendant.

AUDIO-VISUAL RECORDING OF INFORMED CONSENT PROCESS

Audio-visual recording of informed consent process in clinical trials made mandatory (G.S.R. 364 (E), dated June 7, 2013)

In 2014, CDSCO issued draft guidance on audio-visual recording of informed consent process according to which in all clinical trials including global clinical trials, in addition to the need of taking written informed consent, audio-visual recording of the informed consent process of each research participant, including the process of explaining the details to the participant and his/her understanding/ comprehension of informed consent is mandatory while ensuring the maintenance of confidentiality.

Advantages

- Safeguarding the stakeholders (patients, investigator, EC, sponsor)
- Simplification of the consent process
- Reliability
- Transparency
- Improvement in conduct of informed consent process
- Confirmation of informed decision

Challenges

- Lack of infrastructure at government institutions
- Interpretation of patient's behavior on camera

- Compromising confidentiality
- Risk of tampering the records
- Cost implications
- Issues with practical feasibility
- Impact on subject recruitment

Facilities required for AV recording of informed consent process (Box 15.3)

> **Box 15.3** Facilities required to conduct audio-visual recording of informed consent process.
>
> - An adequately designated area which is free from any external disturbance /s, well-lit, comfortable for subject and ensures subject's privacy.
> - Camera having video facility with
>   - ✓ good resolution (at least 1280x720 pixels)
>   - ✓ sufficient memory (at least 4 GB)
>   - ✓ sufficient battery back up (at least 2 hours)
>   - ✓ shows non editable date & time on video (preferably)
> - Mike system
> - Computer with CD/DVD writer
> - Blank CDs/DVDs with cover
> External Hard disk (at least 1 TB)

Current recommendations by CDSCO on AV recording of informed consent process (Box 15.4)

> **Box 15.4** Note.
>
> In view of the various challenges faced with AV recording of informed consent process, a new notification was released by CDSCO in 2015 *(G.S.R. 611 (E), dated July 31, 2015)* which has been incorporated in the New Drugs and Clinical Trials Rules, 2019. As per the notification,
>
> ❖ Audio-visual recording of the consent process is mandatory only in case of vulnerable populations in studies involving 'NCE' or 'NME'; the records of audio-visual process and the participant's understanding on such consent shall be preserved by the investigator.
> ❖ In case of clinical trial on anti-HIV and anti-leprosy drugs, only audio recording of the informed consent process is essential.

PATIENT COMPREHENSION OF INFORMED CONSENT DOCUMENT

Due to diverse educational qualifications, level of understanding etc. the comprehension of ICD by participants can be quite variable and unpredictable. Hence, assessment of the participant comprehension becomes important (Table 15.1).

Table 15.1 Methods to test patient comprehension of ICD.
• Teach-back method: patients asked to describe in their own words what has been told.
• Questionnaires to test understanding.
• Tools to test comprehension e.g. Deaconess Informed Consent Comprehension Test

ELECTRONIC INFORMED CONSENT (eIC)

In December 2016, US Food and Drug Administration (USFDA) released a guidance document with recommendations regarding the application of electronic media and technologies for obtaining informed consent. As per this guidance, ***electronic informed consent (eIC)*** refers to using electronic systems and processes employing various multimedia components to communicate study related information to trial subjects and to obtain and document informed consent. Electronic IC provides the same information as paper IC but in an electronic format.

eIC MULTIMEDIA COMPONENTS (FIGURE 15.3)

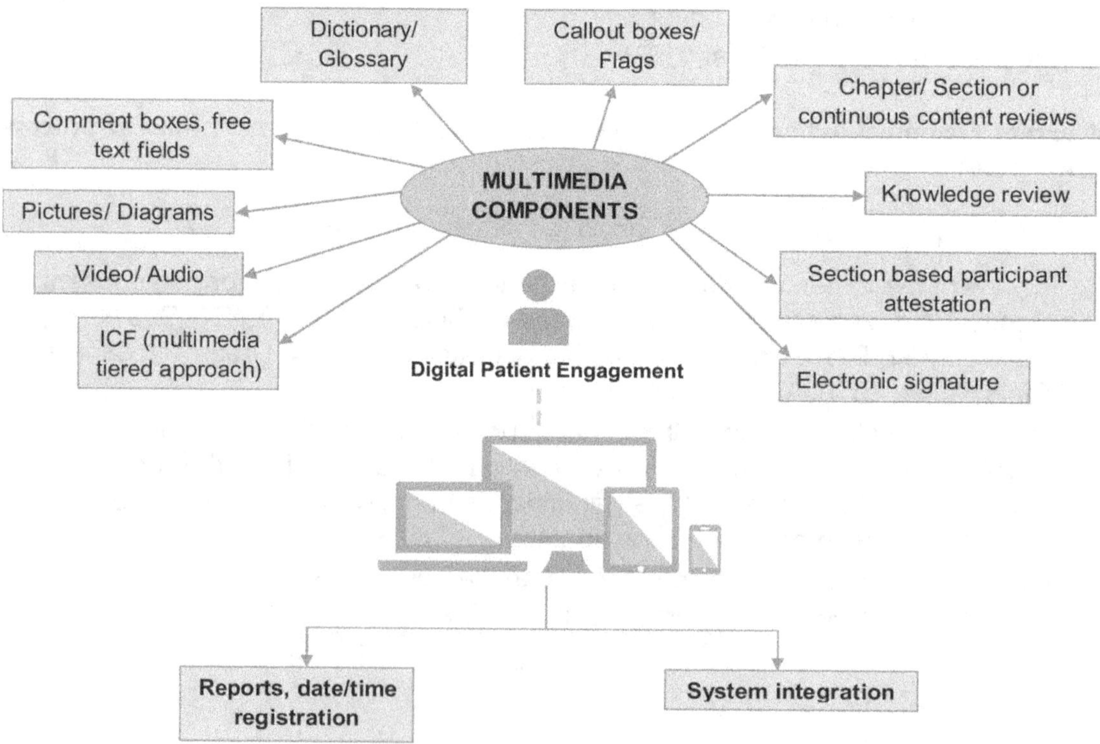

Figure 15.3 Multimedia components of eIC.

❖ *Multimedia tiered consent*

It comprises of a concise main section (containing essential elements) and later sub-sections with information in more detail (optional for subject). Such multimedia format allows study subjects to navigate between various sections to gain information on specific items (by means of enhancements like hyperlinks) as required. The tiered consent is structured to ensure that the main section is viewed and the e-consent tool may potentially record the time spent in each section.

What will happen if you participate in this study?

The expected duration of your participation in this study is 3 months. On being randomized to one of the treatment arms, you will receive the respective drug. After that, you need to come to medicine outpatient department for follow up visits every 3 weeks for 12 weeks (a total of 4 follow up visits). You need to bring your medicine container with remaining pills at each visit. During the visits, activities conducted will be:

- discussion with investigator regarding any relevant history
- general physical examination
- compliance checking (pill count)
- ECG
- Blood sample drawn
- Questionnaire about your health

For more information, please refer to the **detailed study treatment visit schedule**

Procedure	Baseline Visit 0 week	Visit 1 3 week	Visit 2 6 week	Visit 3 9 week	Visit 4 12 week
History	X	X	X	X	X
Physical examination	X	X	X	X	X
Pill count		X	X	X	X
ECG	X	X	X	X	X
Blood sampling	X		X		X
Health questionnaire	X				X
Approximate blood drawn (mL)	10		10		10

❖ *Video*

Video is mainly used to provide a visual and potentially auditory overview of the study and facilitate the subject's understanding of the content. Videos may include general videos like "What is clinical research?" or specific videos on disease, trial procedures, study summary video etc.

An example of a video can be visualized at www.takeandtell.org/#video

❖ *Audio*

The audio components which may be used are voiceover of:
- consent document as an alternative to reading,
- video content to promote better understanding,
- other components e.g. instructions, call out boxes etc.

❖ *Pictures and diagrams (Figure 15.4)*

These are the visual aids to help explain certain study related aspects. Examples may include study procedures, adverse event incidences etc.

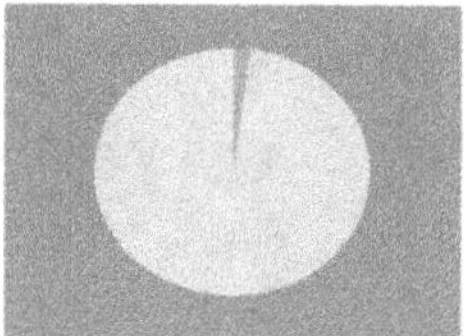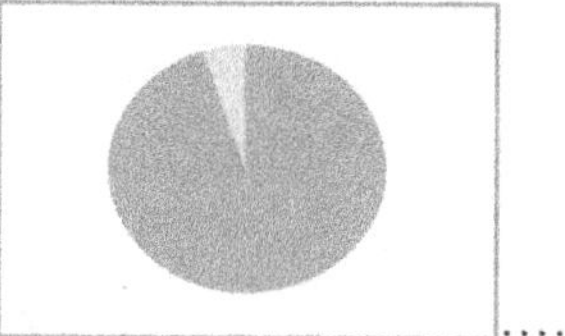

Nausea : 2/100 people; gastric upset: 5/100 people

Figure 4. Example of a diagram showing incidence of adverse events

Figure 15.4 Example of a diagram showing incidence of adverse events.

❖ *Comment boxes, free text fields (Figure 15.5)*

Addition of comment boxes or free text fields may facilitate e-consent to become source document for various elements of informed consent.

Figure 15.5 Example of comment box.

❖ *Dictionary/ Glossary*
- A dictionary includes definitions of general words maintained independently of the specific clinical trial.
- A glossary includes a set of words specifically defined by sponsor/ vendor relevant to specific study.

  These may be provided as standard user interface cues like hover-over, highlight or in pop-up boxes.

❖ *Callout boxes (Figure 15.6)*

These can be highlighted text within the document or text boxes summarizing key information in few simple sentences to reinforce important points.

❖ *Chapter/ Section or continuous content reviews*

The content of the consent document may be divided into different sections or available as a single document.

> Your participation in the study is purely voluntary and you can withdraw anytime without your medical care and legal rights being affected

Figure 15.6 Example of callout box.

❖ *Knowledge review (Figure 15.7)*

This consists of short set of questions the subject is asked to answer to highlight key information. Some useful aspects include:

- Promotion of subject's active engagement in the consent process,
- Assessment of subject's comprehension,
- In case of incorrect answers, the subject is directed to pertinent information in the document,
- Study staff gets information regarding the areas which need direct discussion with subject.

Question 1 of 5

If I experience any injury during the study, ...

    (i)   I can contact the Investigator

    (ii)   I will receive free medical management

    (iii)   I may get compensation in the form of money

    (iv)   All of the above

Figure 15.7 Example of knowledge review.

❖ *Section based participant attestation*

This includes receiving subject's acknowledgement/s regarding understanding of various sections. Usually, there is a sliding tool at the end of each section for the participant to indicate:

"Yes, I understand" OR "No, I have a question".

❖ *Electronic signature*

It is an electronic method of authentication and may be obtained by using e.g. computer-readable ID cards, biometrics, digital signatures, username and password combinations etc.

IMPORTANT CONSIDERATIONS WHILE OBTAINING ELECTRONIC INFORMED CONSENT

1. *eIC as a supplement or replacement to paper-based IC process*

Depending on the subject's needs and choices, eIC can be used to supplement or replace paper based IC. For example, some subjects may have issues like impaired eye-sight, poor motor skills, lack of familiarity etc. and may experience difficulty in navigating through electronic systems.

2. *Place of conduct and operation*

The consent process may be conducted at *study site* with both subject and investigator at same location or *remotely* (at subject's home or other suitable place). In case of conduct remotely, measures should be incorporated to ensure that the subject signing the document is the one actually going to participate or is the subject's LAR.

3. *Answering the subject's questions*

Sufficient opportunity should be provided to prospective study participants to ask any questions before signing the document. There should be provisions for in-person discussion with study personnel, video-conferencing, telephone calls, electronic messaging, live chats with remotely located investigator etc.

4. *Verification of identity of the person signing an eIC*

This can be done with the help of other official identifications e.g. birth certificate, driving license, passport, security questions etc.

5. *Copy of eIC document to study subjects*

A paper or electronic copy (electronic storage device or via email) of the document may be provided to subject. If the eIC contains hyperlinks or websites to convey information, the details given there should be included in a printed hard copy, if provided.

6. *Data confidentiality in eIC process*

The electronic system supporting the eIC should be secure with restricted access to ensure data confidentiality.

PROCESS FLOW FOR EXECUTING eIC (FIGURE 15.8)

Figure 15.8 Step wise process for executing electronic informed consent.

ADVANTAGES OF eIC PROCESS

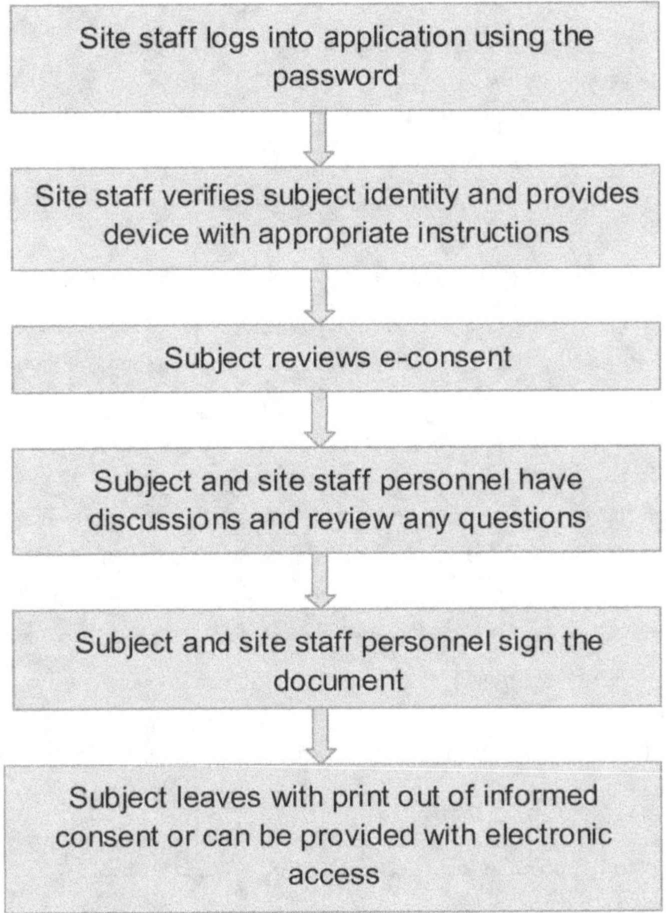

An e IC is expected to streamline enrolment, provide real time enrolment statistics, and greatly improve quality and ethical concerns. Table 15.2 gives a list of advantages offered by eIC to various stakeholders i.e. patients, clinical trial sites, ethics committee/health authorities and sponsor/CROs.

POTENTIAL BARRIERS TO IMPLEMENTATION OF eIC

♦ Huge investment costs and intensive need of resources.

<table>
<tr><td colspan="1">Table 15.2 Advantages of eIC to different stakeholders.</td></tr>
</table>

Subjects

- Relatively easy understanding
- Presentation in a consistent and simplified manner
- Interactive interface to ensure active subject involvement
- Better retention and comprehension of information
- Absence of any pressure; can be proceeded at one's own pace
- Tailored to individual learning style

Clinical trial sites

- Easier to check subject understanding
- Able to focus on subject's questions and issues of concern
- Timely entry of eIC data to study database
- Alert messages to sites in case of e-consent errors or need to take e-consent again
- Complements risk-based monitoring by providing more information (glossary etc.)
- Reduced administrative time (paperless system, links with other systems)

Sponsor/CRO

- Improved data quality and consistency
- Improved timely identification of any consenting issues
- Enhanced efficiency by reducing time in monitoring ICFs during site visit
- Potential improvement of subject retention due to better understanding
- Rapid notifications to subjects of any amendments or new information
- Complements risk-based monitoring by providing more information (glossary etc.)
- Improved continuous oversight

EC/ Health authorities

- Few significant findings during inspections/ audits e.g. related to new versions, missing signatures etc.
- Increased transparency
- Enhanced protection of subjects due to improved ongoing insights

♦ Study subject's limited experience with electronic systems
♦ Relatively more time consuming set-up process
♦ Non-uniformity in acceptance of certain components in different countries e.g. e-signature
♦ Need for back-up system in case of failure
♦ Technically more demanding
♦ Greater up-front work to tailor the eIC to special subject populations
♦ Insufficient existing guidance

CHAPTER 16

Compensation Issues in Clinical Trials

OVERVIEW

INTRODUCTION

ICH-GCP ON COMPENSATION

- In compliance with the applicable regulatory requirement(s), the sponsor is liable to provide insurance or compensation (legal and financial cover) to the investigator/ institution against claims emerging from the trial, except those occurring due to misconduct and/or negligence.
- The sponsor's strategies and procedures should address the costs of medical management of trial participants in the event of trial-related injuries as per the applicable regulatory requirement(s).
- The procedure and manner of providing compensation to trial participants should be as per the applicable regulatory requirement(s).

DECLARATION OF HELSINKI ON COMPENSATION (BOX 16.1)

Box 16.1 Declaration of Helsinki on *"Compensation"*.

Adequate compensation and medical management for subjects being injured or harmed as a consequence of their involvement in research must be ensured.

❖ ***Compensation for Accidental Injury***

The trial participants experiencing any physical injury due to their involvement in clinical trials are eligible to receive financial or other support as compensation corresponding to any temporary or permanent impairment or disability subject to approval from IEC. In case of death, the dependents of subjects are entitled to material compensation.

Sponsor's obligation to pay :

Before the research is initiated, the sponsor whether a drug manufacturing company, an institution, a government or any other party as the case may be, should agree to provide compensation in case any research participant experiences a serious physical or mental injury or agree to provide insurance coverage in case of an unforeseen injury whenever possible.

COMPENSATION IN INVESTIGATOR INITIATED RESEARCH

These studies may include academic studies, student research or research funded by extramural agencies (national/international, government/ non-Government). For compensation issues in case of research related injury or harm in these studies:

- The sponsor is the investigator/ the host institution where the study is being conducted.
- The primary responsibility to provide compensation and/ or insurance lies with the host institution which can have a corpus fund created for such purposes.
- In case of funded research, a budgetary provision for compensation and /or insurance cover should be made while applying for research grants.

RECENT AMENDMENTS IN DRUGS AND COSMETICS RULES REGARDING COMPENSATION

(G.S.R. 53 (E) dated 30th January 2013)

(G.S.R. 889 (E) dated December 12, 2014; effective June 2015)

Insertion of Rule 122 DAB: Compensation in case of injury or death during clinical trial.

(i)   In case of *an injury experienced by a clinical trial subject during its conduct,* free medical management would be provided up to the required duration or till the time of establishment of injury not being related to clinical trial, whichever is earlier.

(ii) In case the *injury is related to clinical trial,* the trial subject is entitled for financial compensation over and above any expenses incurred on the medical management.

(iii) In case of non- permanent injury, the quantum of compensation shall correspond to nature of the non-permanent injury and loss of wages of the subject.

(iv) In case of *clinical trial related death* of the subject, his/her nominee would be entitled for financial compensation which will be over and above any expenses sustained on the medical management of subject.

(v) Definition of *clinical trial related injury or death* (Box 16.2).

Clinical trial related injury or death has been defined as any injury or death or permanent disability experienced by a subject during its conduct because of below mentioned factors:

- adverse effect of study intervention(s)
- any non-compliance to approved trial protocol, scientific misconduct or negligence by the sponsor / his representative / investigator
- failure of study intervention to produce proposed therapeutic effect where, the subject was deprived of available standard treatment according to trial protocol
- use of placebo in a placebo controlled trial where, the subject was deprived of available standard treatment according to trial protocol
- adverse effects due to concomitantly administered drug/s other than standard treatment, but required according to trial protocol
- for injury to a child in-utero because of the enrolment of parent/s in clinical trial
- any procedures during the conduct of clinical trial

Box 16.2 The New Drugs and Clinical Trials Rules, 2019.

Clinical trial or BA/BE study related injury or death or permanent disability

The term Clinical trial related injury or death has been expanded to "Clinical trial or BA/BE study related injury or death or permanent disability"; the criteria for considering this are albeit the same as mentioned above.

(vi) *Expansion of responsibilities of Sponsor, Investigator and Ethics Committee.*

These mainly pertain to adverse event reporting to various concerned authorities within stipulated timelines and have been discussed below under "Procedure for payment of financial compensation".

Additionally, the responsibility of investigator is to keep the trial subject informed through informed consent process about:

- ✓ the essential elements of clinical trial,
- ✓ subject's right to claim compensation if there is any trial related injury or death,
- ✓ subject's or his/her legal nominee's right to contact the sponsor or his representative if there is any trial related injury or death.

(vii) Definition of Serious adverse events (SAEs)

A serious adverse event is defined as an untoward medical occurrence during clinical trial that is associated with:

- Death,

- In-patient hospitalization (in case the study is conducted on out-patients),
- Prolongation of hospitalization (in case the study is conducted on in-patients),
- Persistent or significant disability or incapacity,
- A congenital anomaly or birth defect,
- Is life-threatening.

PROCEDURE FOR PAYMENT OF FINANCIAL COMPENSATION

PROCEDURE FOR PAYMENT OF FINANCIAL COMPENSATION IN CASE OF SAE OF DEATH (FIGURE 16.1 AND BOX 16.3)

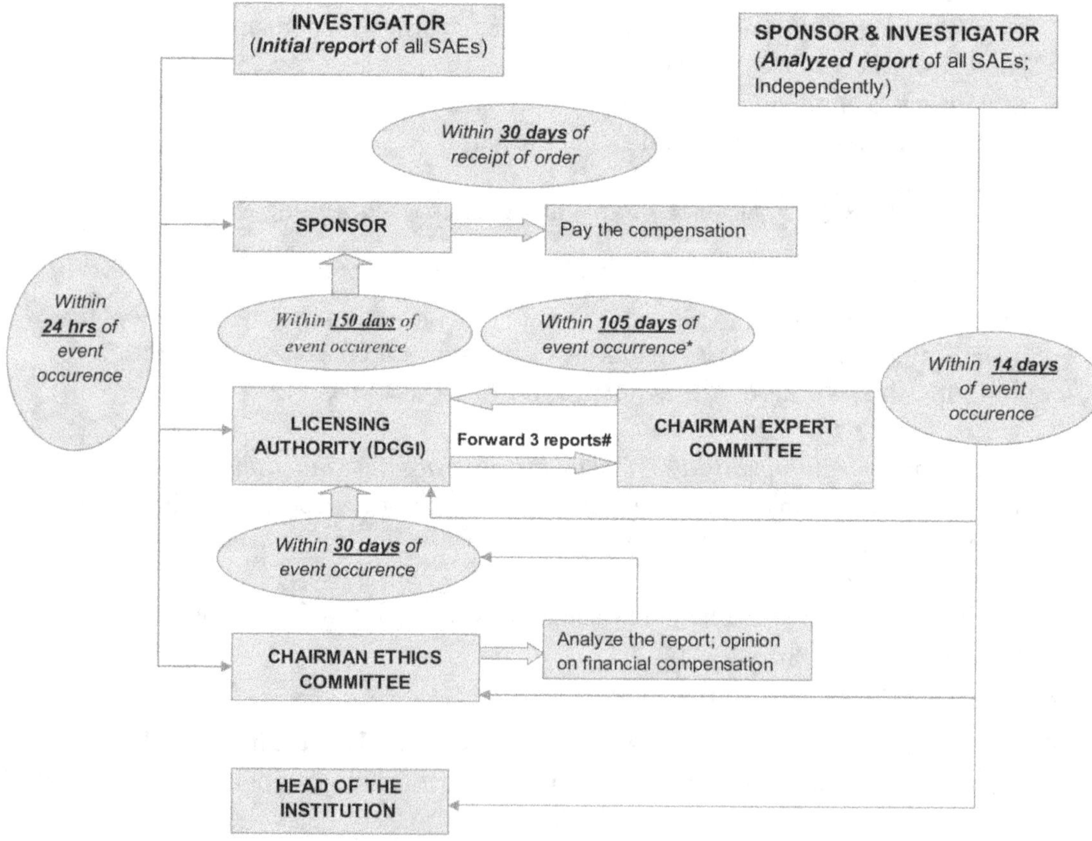

Figure 16.1 Procedure for payment of financial compensation in case of SAE of death.

> **Box 16.3** The New Drugs and Clinical Trials Rules, 2019.
>
> **Procedure for payment of financial compensation in case of SAE of death**
> - The Investigator shall report all SAEs to the CLA, EC and sponsor within 24 hours of their occurrence.
> - The Sponsor/its representative and the investigator should forward their analyzed reports on SAE of death to the CLA and head of the institution where clinical trial or BA/BE study was conducted within 14 days of the knowledge of occurrence of SAE of death.
> - The EC shall forward its report on SAE of death after analyzing in detail accompanied by its opinion on financial compensation to the CLA within a period of 30 days of receiving the SAE report of death from the investigator.
> - The CLA shall forward the 3 reports viz. report of the investigator, sponsor or its representative and the Ethics Committee to the Chairperson of the expert committee.
> - The Expert Committee after examination of the reports of SAE of death shall give its recommendations to Licensing authority on the cause of death and quantum of compensation within 60 days from the receipt of the report of SAE.
> - The CLA shall, after contemplating the recommendations of expert committee, decide the quantum of compensation as per the specified formula to be paid by sponsor or his representative, pass orders within 90 days from the receipt of the report of SAE.
> - The sponsor or his representative shall pay the compensation as specified in the orders from the CLA within 30 days of receiving such order.

PROCEDURE FOR PAYMENT OF FINANCIAL COMPENSATION IN CASE OF SAE OTHER THAN DEATH (FIGURE 16.2 AND BOX 16.4)

- ❖ In case of failure of the investigator to report an SAE within the specified time period, he needs to give explanation for the same to licensing authority along with SAE report.
- ❖ All the expenses for medical management and financial compensation shall be borne by the **sponsor** of the clinical trial.
- ❖ Sponsor or his representative shall give an **undertaking** accompanying the clinical trial application to provide compensation in the event of clinical trial related injury or death.
- ❖ In case of **failure to provide** medical management/ financial compensation
  - clinical trial or BA/BE study can be suspended/ cancelled;
  - sponsor can be debarred from conducting future clinical trials or BA/BE studies;

- any other action can be taken for such period as considered appropriate depending on the particular case.

❖ **Penalty for failure to provide compensation** *(as per the Drugs and Cosmetics Amendment Bill, 2015; Section 4Q).* Whoever is liable to provide compensation for clinical trial related injury, disability or death if fails to do so, shall be liable for punishment with imprisonment extending upto one year and fine amounting to not less than twice the amount of compensation.

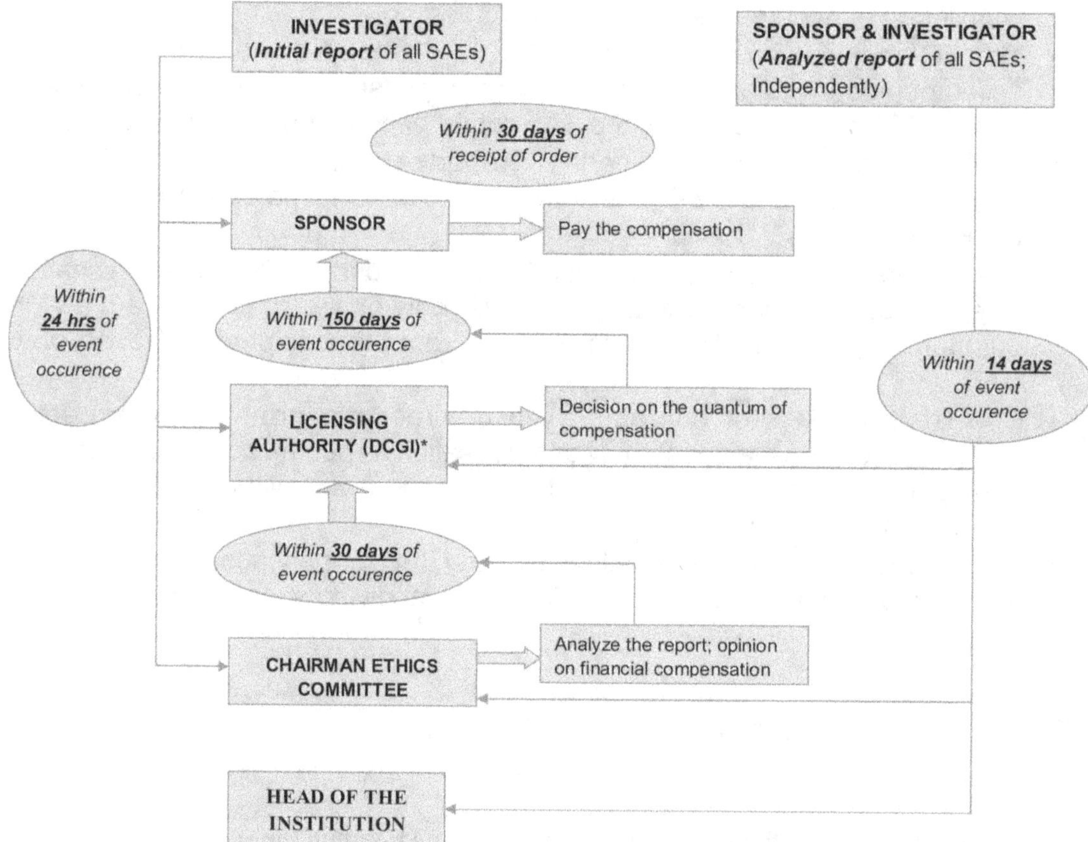

Figure 16.2 Procedure for payment of financial compensation in case of SAE other than death.

Box 16.4 The New Drugs and Clinical Trials Rules, 2019.

Procedure for payment of financial compensation in case of SAE of permanent disability or any other injury other than death

- The Investigator shall report all SAEs to the CLA, EC and sponsor within 24 hours of their occurrence.
- The Sponsor/its representative and the Investigator should forward their analyzed reports on SAE to the Central Licensing Authority, Chairperson of the EC and head of the institution where clinical trial or BA/BE study was conducted within 14 days of the reporting of SAE.
- The EC shall forward its report on SAE of permanent disability or any other injury other than death after analyzing in detail accompanied by its opinion on financial compensation to the CLA within a period of 30 days of receiving the report of SAE
- The CLA shall determine the cause of injury and pass order or may constitute an independent expert committee, whenever deemed necessary to examine such SAE of injury.
- The expert committee after examination of the reports of SAE shall give its recommendations to licensing authority on the cause of SAE and quantum of compensation within 60 days from the receipt of the report of SAE.
- The CLA shall decide the quantum of compensation as per the specified formula to be paid by sponsor or his representative, and pass orders within 90 days from the receipt of the report of SAE.
- The sponsor or his representative shall pay the compensation as specified in the orders from the Central Licensing Authority within 30 days of receiving such order.

Compensation for injury or death related to biomedical and health research (Box 16.5).

Box 16.5 The New Drugs and Clinical Trials Rules, 2019.

"Medical management and compensation for injury or death relating to biomedical and health research overseen by an EC for biomedical and health research shall be in accordance with the National Ethical Guidelines for Biomedical and Health Research Involving Human Participants specified by the ICMR from time to time".

QUANTUM OF COMPENSATION

In the New Drugs and Clinical Trials Rules, 2019, formulae for determining the quantum of compensation have been incorporated (Box 16.6).

Box 16.6 The New Drugs and Clinical Trials Rules, 2019.

Seventh Schedule: "Formulae to determine the quantum of compensation in the cases of clinical trial related injury or death (described below)".

---

1. **Formula in case of clinical trial related death**

$$\text{Compensation} = (B \times F \times R) / 99.37$$

where

B = Base amount (i.e. 8 lacs)

F = Age factor i.e. factor depending on the age of trial subject based on Workmen compensation act (Annexure IX).

{An age factor ranging from *99.37 for 65 years and above* to a maximum of *228.54 for 16 years and less* has been fixed}

R = Risk factor; determined on a scale of 0.5 to 4 on the basis of subject's condition (e.g. seriousness, severity and duration of disease, any co-morbidities etc.) at the time of enrolment in clinical trial;

Risk factor	Patient risk
0.5	Terminally ill patient (expected survival not more than (NMT) 6 months)
1	High risk (expected survival 6-24 months)
2	Moderate risk
3	Low risk
4	Healthy volunteers; no risk

However, subjects having likelihood of mortality equal to or greater than 90% within 30 days should be provided a fixed amount of Rs. 2 lacs.

2. **Formula in case of clinical trial related injury (other than death)**

(i) **Compensation formula for SAE causing permanent disability**

♦ If *<100% disability*;

$$\text{Compensation} = (D \times C \times 90) / 100 \times 100$$

where,

D = percentage disability experienced by the subject

C = quantum of compensation in case of death of subject

♦ If *100% disability*;

   Compensation = 90% of compensation due to death

(ii) Compensation for SAE leading to congenital anomaly or birth defect

Congenital anomaly or birth defect may present as or give rise to :

✓ still birth

✓ anomaly leading to early death

✓ deformity; reversible with adequate intervention

✓ irreversible disability (mental or physical)

♦ Compensation in such cases would be a lump sum amount such that if that amount is kept by fixed deposit, monthly interest is approximately half of minimum wage of unskilled worker in Delhi (corresponds to half of the base amount in case of compensation in death case i.e. approximately 4 lacs).

♦ If SAE leads to permanent/temporary disability in the child, medical management till the duration needed would be provided by the sponsor which will be over and above the financial compensation.

(iii) Chronic life threatening disease; and

(iv) Reversible SAE in case it is resolved

$$\text{Compensation} = 2 \times W \times N$$

where,

W = minimum wage per day of an unskilled worker (in Delhi)

N = Number of days of hospitalization

SECTION – F

CLINICAL RESEARCH: AN OVERVIEW

CONTENTS

CHAPTER 17

Types and Principles of Clinical Research

OVERVIEW

INTRODUCTION

Clinical research encompasses the experimental/ observational studies involving humans as participants. The objectives of conducting clinical research are manifold and include development of new drugs or interventions, identification of disease etio-pathogenesis, study of any trends, or evaluation of relationship of disease conditions to genetics.

CLINICAL RESEARCH VERSUS CLINICAL PRACTICE

Clinical research differs from clinical practice with respect to many aspects as explained in table 17.1.

TYPES OF CLINICAL RESEARCH

Broadly, clinical research is classified into experimental and observational on the basis of whether the subjects are exposed to any intervention as part of the research (Figure 17.1).

EXPERIMENTAL STUDIES

CLINICAL TRIALS

This is a category of experimental/ interventional study conducted with the purpose to evaluate the response of a subject or population (as in the case of clinical trials studying groups) to treatment/s allocated by the study investigator (Box 17.1).

Table 17.1 Comparison of clinical research with clinical practice.	
Clinical research	**Clinical practice**
The main goal of investigator/ researcher is to gain knowledge about disease condition of interest or treatment.	The main goal of physician is to provide treatment to the patients.
The researcher has to follow standardized procedures as laid down in the study plan.	The physician can take his own decisions as per the need.
The researcher randomly assigns the subjects to treatment or control group.	The physician usually offers standard treatment to the patients.
Costs of the treatment are usually covered, and subjects may receive additional compensation.	Costs of the treatment are borne by the patient himself or insurance company.
The results of the research may be helpful in developing new therapeutic interventions/ modalities and may be published to disseminate the knowledge gained.	The treatment is directed to improve the patient's condition and results are not used in research.
The researcher may check in with the patient's physicians to learn about the patient's conditions and treatments.	The physician usually doesn't share the patient's information with researchers.
Clinical research serves the common or collective good; individual participant may or may not be benefitted.	Clinical practice is designed to enhance the well being of individual patients.

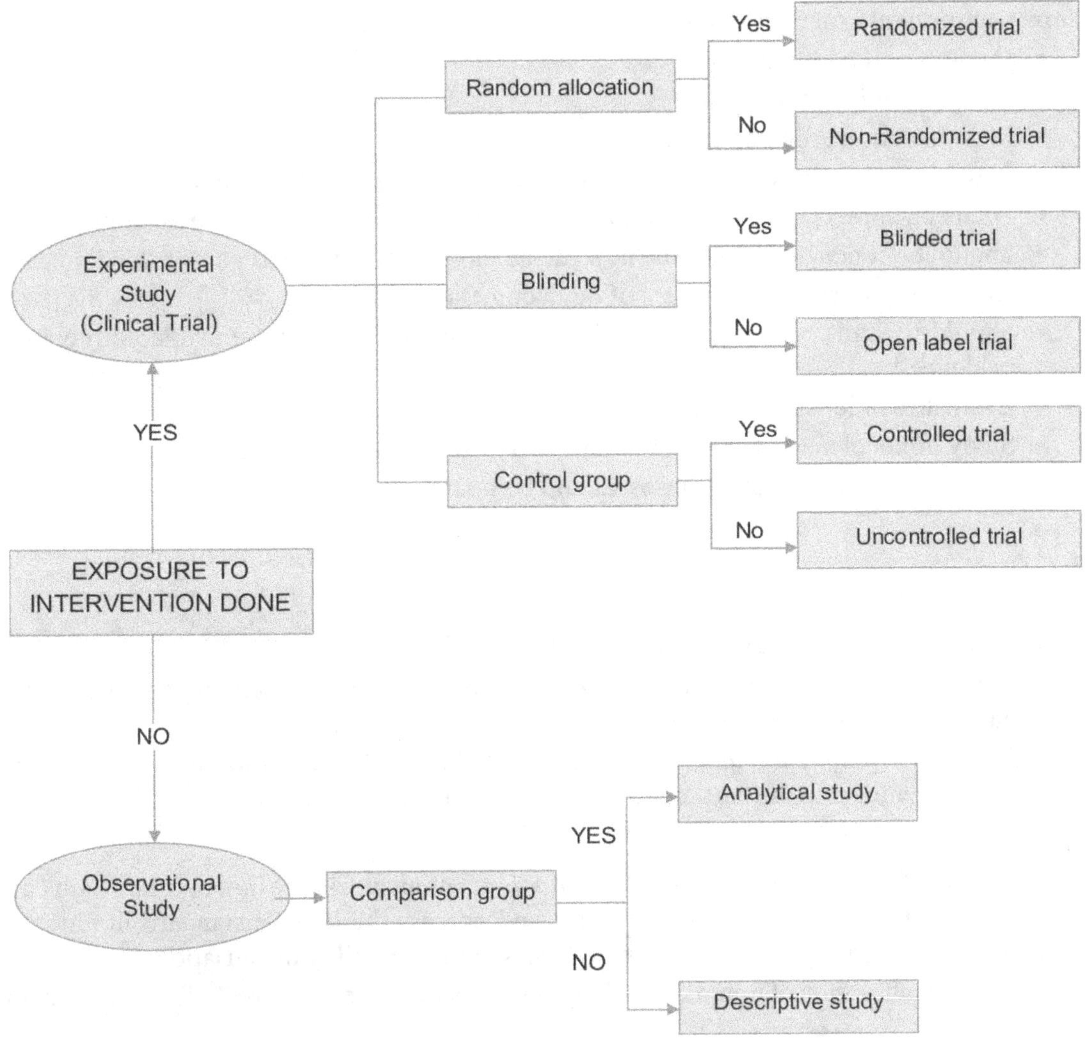

Figure 17.1 Types of clinical research.

Box 17.1 The New Drugs and Clinical Trials Rules, 2019.

Definition of clinical trial

"Clinical trial in relation to a new drug or investigational new drug means any systematic study of such new drug or investigational new drug in human subjects to generate data for discovering or verifying its (i) clinical or; (ii) pharmacological including pharmacodynamics, pharmacokinetics or; (iii) adverse effects, with the objective of determining the safety, efficacy or tolerance of such new drug or investigational new drug".

Core Components of Clinical Trials
- Involvement of human subjects.
- Prospective in nature.
- Most include a group acting as comparison/ control.
- Should employ some method/ technique to measure the response to intervention.
- Focus on aspects not known so far e.g. efficacy or safety of new medications.
- Should be conducted before the new medication is considered as part of standard care.
- Undertaken during early stages of development of treatments.
- Should be built on strong scientific background and review the available literature evidence.
- Evaluate a rational/ suitable hypothesis.
- Study protocol must be ethically sound and justified.
- Any assumed or potential biases should be taken care of.

TYPES OF CLINICAL TRIALS

❖ ***Randomized versus Non-randomized clinical trials***

Clinical trials can be either randomized or non-randomized depending on whether the participants are randomly allocated to treatment arms.

Randomized clinical trials (RCTs): The hallmark of RCTs is allotment of exposures or interventions to the participants entirely by the play of chance.

Strengths of RCTs
- ✓ The RCT is considered as the *'gold-standard'* clinical trial design and its results are adequately assumed to be most robust and possess the highest standard in terms of level of scientific evidence generated (maximum probability of causation).
- ✓ Random allocation of treatments, if appropriately done, helps in precluding the selection bias.
- ✓ RCTs decrease the chances of bias in assessment of outcomes.
- ✓ RCTs usually involve blinding of involved personnel to the intervention assigned to study subjects, in an effort to reduce information bias.
- ✓ Another strength of RCTs is elimination of confounding bias.
- ✓ RCTs tend to be statistically efficient.

Drawbacks of RCTs
- ✓ External validity. Whereas the RCT, if properly conducted, possess good internal validity i.e. it evaluates what it aims to do, however, external validity in RCT i.e. generalizability of study results to a larger population may be compromised.
- ✓ The randomized controlled trial includes only those subjects who are found suitable after going through a screening process before their enrolment in study. This is however different from observational studies where no strict screening process is done.

✓ Another limitation is that RCTs cannot be conducted under some situations, e.g. where the study involves exposure of participants to harmful agents like toxins, or other noxious substances which would be unethical.

✓ RCTs can be very expensive. Indeed, the expense of large RCTs can go up to billions of US dollars.

Cohort multiple randomised controlled trial (cmRCT) (Box 17.2).

Box 17.2 Cohort Multiple Randomized Controlled Trial (cm RCT).

This is a relatively newer concept in which a large cohort is identified and followed using routine data collection. The identified cohort can be utilized to test multiple treatments/ interventions; each treatment being randomly assigned to a sample of patients fulfilling eligibility criteria for that treatment; this sample of patients is then compared with the remaining eligible patients from cohort who are being given the standard care. Few advantages of cmRCTs over conventional RCTs are simplified design, low cost involved in the recruitment of comparison group, exploitation of same cohort for multiple trials and the evaluation of interventions in real world environment.

❖ ***Open label versus blinded clinical trials*** depending on whether and which group/s of personnel conducting/ taking part in trial are aware/unaware of the intervention being assigned to study participants.

❖ ***Controlled versus Uncontrolled clinical trials*** based on the presence/ absence of a group against which the study intervention is compared.

Examples of comparators/controls include:

♦ Placebo
♦ Active standard treatment
♦ Different doses of the same drug
♦ No treatment at all given to the control group
♦ Historical controls
♦ External controls

❖ ***Efficacy versus Effectiveness trials (Table 17.2)***
This classification of clinical trials is based on different aspects of the interventions they explore.

❖ ***Superiority versus Equivalence/ Non inferiority trials***
Superiority trials. The primary objective of these trials is to demonstrate that the response to investigational agent is superior to comparator (usually placebo).
Equivalence/ Non inferiority trials. These are designed to demonstrate the equivalence of two treatments, or perhaps better stated that a new treatment is not inferior to a standard one. The primary objective of these trials is demonstration of clinically insignificant difference in response to two or more interventions.

Table 17.2 Key differences between efficacy and effectiveness trials.

Efficacy (Explanatory) trials	Effectiveness (Pragmatic) trials
Aim: To examine the efficacy of a treatment/ intervention in a controlled environment.	To test the effectiveness of an intervention in a broad routine clinical practice.
Designed: to ensure control of the potential biases and confounding factors, so that the study intervention produces maximal and uninterrupted effect.	To assess interventions in real world in order to generate applicable and generalizable results.
Research question: if and how an intervention works	Whether the intervention produces actual effect in real life scenario
Study population: Homogenous; strict inclusion/ exclusion criteria	Heterogeneous; Looser inclusion/exclusion criteria
Outcomes: measurable symptoms or markers (clinical or biological)	Usually patient-centered outcomes e.g. quality of life
Comparator: placebo or another active treatment established in routine practice settings	Active treatment (same or different class)
Internal Validity: High internal validity	Low internal validity
External validity/ Generalizability : Low	High
Phase of clinical trial: Mostly Phase II-III	Mostly Phase IV

❖ Based on the number of participants

♦ *N-of-1 trials/ Single patient trials/ Individual patient trials.* In these, a single patient is intensively evaluated in a double-blind, carefully controlled manner. Patients serve as their own controls and often receive two or more treatments on multiple occasions, with each treatment presented in a randomized order. These are applicable for situations like:

- Rare disease –very few patients available for clinical trials.
- Condition where the treatment has been evaluated in studies that include very different patients.
- Individual variations in intervention responses are common e.g. attention deficit and hyperactivity disorder.
- Patients with certain problems differ in important ways from others with similar conditions e.g. physically disabled, mentally retarded.

Advantages:
- ✓ Simpler patient recruitment
- ✓ Less expense
- ✓ More rapid trial completion
- ✓ Less complex data processing and statistical analysis
- ✓ Easier interpretation of results

Disadvantages:
- ✓ Greater difficulty in extrapolating data to other patients
- ✓ Applicability limited to certain circumstances only e.g. chronic disease with stable course over the clinical trial duration, treatment effect manifested within short time, rapidly reversible treatment effect, absence of period effect, most appropriate efficacy parameters chosen etc.
- ✓ Not suitable for new medicine development
- ♦ *Mega trials.* Randomised trials conducted on a large scale and enrolling large number of participants.

Advantages:
- ✓ Increase statistical power
- ✓ Remove or minimise bias

Disadvantages:
- ✓ The results of mega-trials cannot readily be generalised because their conclusions are observations, not causal hypotheses
- ✓ Mega-trials can be repeated but cannot be replicated
- ✓ In a mega-trial, analysis is only meaningful at the group level and not at individual level.

The New Drugs and Clinical Trials Rules 2019 have incorporated few new definitions related to clinical research (Table 17.3).

Box 17.3 The New Drugs and Clinical Trials Rules, 2019.

New definitions included:
- **Biomedical and health research:** "research including studies on basic, applied and operational research or clinical research, designed primarily to increase scientific knowledge about diseases and conditions (physical or socio-behavioral); their detection and cause; and evolving strategies for health promotion, prevention, or amelioration of disease and rehabilitation but does not include clinical trial".
- **Academic clinical trial:** "a clinical trial of a drug already approved for a certain claim and initiated by any investigator, academic or research institution for a new indication or new route of administration or new dose or new dosage form, where the results of such a trial are used only for academic or research purposes and not for seeking approval of the Central Licensing Authority or regulatory authority of any country for marketing or commercial purpose".

Box 17.3 Contd...

- **Global clinical trial:** "a clinical trial conducted as part of the clinical development of a drug in more than one country".
- **Efficacy:** "efficacy in relation to a drug means its ability to achieve the desired effect in a controlled clinical setting".
- **Clinical trial site:** "any hospital or institute or any other clinical establishment having the required facilities to conduct a clinical trial".
- **Trial subject:** "a person who is either a patient or a healthy person to whom investigational product is administered for the purposes of a clinical trial".

PRINCIPLES OF CLINICAL RESEARCH

❖ **Weigh the benefits of new intervention against other forms of treatment** i.e. compare one or more treatments in comparable subjects under comparable circumstances. The comparators used may vary depending on the proposed aims and objectives of the study.

❖ **Formulate a single, precise and realistic question** *a priori* **to be answered by the clinical trial.** Aiming to answer too many questions from a single trial is associated with multiple problems like:
  - Questionable quality of generated data.
  - Trial difficult to conduct.
  - Trial may not be completed.
  - Complicate protocol.
  - Greater chances of error i.e. false differences.
  - Probability calculations are distorted.
  - Difficult to estimate the degree of error.

  It is further to be noted that the question asked must be simple so that the answer will be clear and readily interpretable. Further, the question must be realistic and compatible with patient recruitment and with the human and material resources available.

❖ **Reason in terms of groups and not in terms of individuals.** The chances of variability between individuals are usually high due to demographic and physiological characteristics of the subjects, differences in their response to treatment, environmental and other external factors, characteristics of the disorder being treated, associated illnesses and treatments thereof etc. Appropriate measures should be taken to reduce inter-individual variability among the groups and hence ensure homogeneity.

❖ **Define inclusion and exclusion criteria strictly.** The eligibility criteria for inclusion/ exclusion of patients need to be clearly defined. Also, special measures need to be in place to ensure homogeneity of the groups since greater the difference between groups, the more variable the response to therapy. The influence of variability due to recognizable factors can be minimized by:
  - randomization

- increasing the sample size
- standardizing the conditions of conduct and monitoring of trial like recruitment of subjects, assessment criteria etc.

❖ **Statistical reasoning.**

♦ Null hypothesis and alternate hypothesis. In a trial designed to prove a difference between two treatments, "null hypothesis" stating no difference between them, needs to be rejected. Similarly, the alternate hypothesis which states that there is a difference between the two interventions is rejected in trials showing no difference between them.

♦ Minimize type 1 and type 2 errors

o Type 1 or α-error: How big a risk can be taken that the two treatments are incorrectly designated as significantly different i.e. effect erroneously attributed to drug. Type 1 error or $\alpha = 0.05$ is commonly accepted.

o Type II or β-error: How big a risk can be taken that the two treatments are incorrectly designated as not significantly different i.e. not detecting the difference in spite of presence of difference. Type II error or β is normally kept at 0.10 or 0.20.

♦ Study should have sufficient power $(1-\beta)$

❖ **External validity/ generalizability of the trial results.** Results of trial can only be generalized to a specific population from which the sample was drawn or populations having characteristics similar to the trial population.

❖ **A trial can only answer the question for which it was formulated.** If other findings are significant, these help in hypothesis generation for subsequent clinical trials.

❖ **Statistical vs clinical significance.** Results obtained may be statistically significant but not clinically significant. Clinical significance of results depends on:

o Quality of study.

o Magnitude of results obtained.

o Probability of the effect being a true one.

❖ The trials should be conducted in accordance with the applicable **ethical and regulatory guidelines**.

Key rules helpful in obtaining significant results in a clinical trial are enumerated in box 17.4.

Box 17.4 Golden rules to generate significant results in a clinical trial.

✓ Variability amongst groups is kept to a minimum
✓ Sources of bias are recognized and accounted for in the design and analysis of results
✓ Conditions of trial are standardized
✓ Sample size is large enough
✓ Study is powerful enough to minimize type 1 and type 2 errors

---

OBSERVATIONAL STUDIES

Please refer to the Chapter on "Pharmaco-epidemiology" for details.

SECTION – G

CLINICAL TRIALS: METHODOLOGICAL ASPECTS

CONTENTS

CHAPTER 18

Good Clinical Practice

OVERVIEW

Introduction
Essential Elements of GCP
GCP- Responsible Parties
ICH-GCP Guidelines
Structure of ICH-GCP
13 Cardinal Principles of ICH-GCP
ICH-GCP Guidelines on IEC/IRB

ICH-GCP Guidelines on Investigator
ICH-GCP Guidelines on Sponsor
ICH E6: GCP (R2) Addendum
Indian GCP Guidelines
Structure of Indian GCP
Differences between Indian GCP and ICH-GCP
Essential Documents

INTRODUCTION

Good Clinical Practice (GCP) is a set of standards applicable to different stages of clinical trials including planning, executing, managing, monitoring, analyzing and reporting to ensure quality in various scientific and ethical aspects. Compliance with GCP helps to ensure that:

♦ the rights, safety and welfare of trial subjects are safeguarded, in accordance with the principles laid down in the Declaration of Helsinki and

♦ the data generated are valid and accurate

ESSENTIAL ELEMENTS OF GCP (FIGURE 18.1)

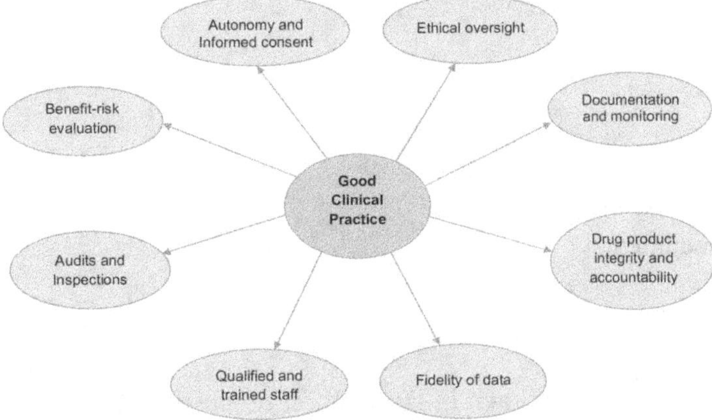

Figure 18.1 Essential elements of Good Clinical Practice (GCP).

GCP- RESPONSIBLE PARTIES

The responsibility of complying with GCP lies with all the parties involved in conducting clinical trials (Figure 18.2).

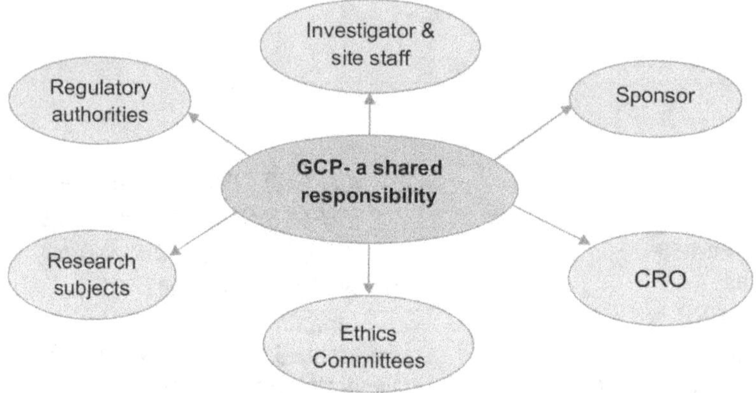

Figure 18.2 GCP - a shared responsibility (CRO: Contract Research Organization).

ICH-GCP GUIDELINES

ICH-GCP [E6 (R1)] guidelines were formulated in 1996 with an objective to lay down a uniform standard for the US, EU and Japan to promote the mutual approval of clinical trial data by the regulatory agencies in these regions.

STRUCTURE OF ICH-GCP

- Glossary
- Principles
- IRB/IEC
- Investigator
- Sponsor
- Protocol
- Investigators' Brochure
- Essential Documents

13 CARDINAL PRINCIPLES OF ICH-GCP

- Ethical principles as laid down in Declaration of Helsinki to be duly followed while conducting clinical trials.

- Trial should be conducted only in situations where the anticipated benefits outweigh the potential risks.
- The rights, safety and welfare of trial participants should be given priority over societal interest.
- Adequate information on the investigational product from preclinical and clinical data should be available to sustain the conduct of proposed clinical trial.
- The details about clinical trials should be explained in a comprehensible protocol with scientific justification.
- The trial protocol should be approved a priori by IRB/IEC.
- A qualified physician should take responsibility of providing health care to trial participants.
- All the personnel involved in trial conduct should be adequately qualified, trained and experienced.
- It is mandatory to obtain informed consent from all the participants before their enrolment in trial.
- The data generated should be documented, managed and archived in a manner facilitating its precise reporting, explanation and authentication.
- Steps must be taken to maintain the privacy and confidentiality of trial participants.
- The Good Manufacturing Practices (GMP) guidelines as applicable must be followed to manufacture, handle and store the investigational products.
- Systems and procedures should be implemented in order to ensure good quality during various aspects of trial.

ICH-GCP GUIDELINES ON IEC/IRB

❖ *Responsibilities of IEC/IRB*

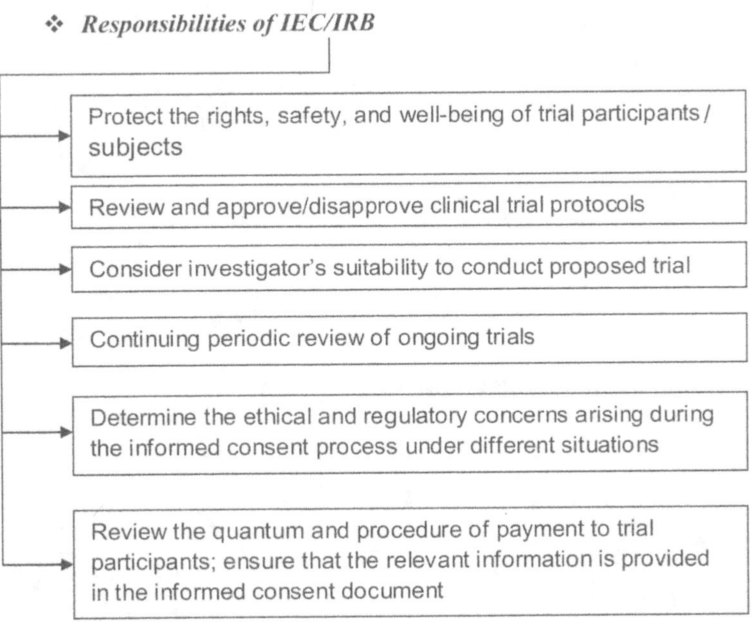

Figure 18.3 Responsibilities of IEC/IRB according to ICH-GCP guidelines.

❖ ***Composition, functions and operations***
- Reasonable number of members with adequate qualifications and experience; a minimum of 5 members (at least 1 member with non-scientific background and 1 member from outside the institution/ trial site).
- Functions according to written SOPs.
- Retention of all relevant records for a minimum duration of 3 years after the trial is over.

❖ ***Responsibilities of IEC/ IRB*** (Figure 18.3).

ICH-GCP GUIDELINES ON INVESTIGATOR

❖ ***Qualifications and agreements***
- Adequately qualified, trained and experienced
- Should have a thorough knowledge of the investigational product (IP) as described in protocol and investigator's brochure (IB).

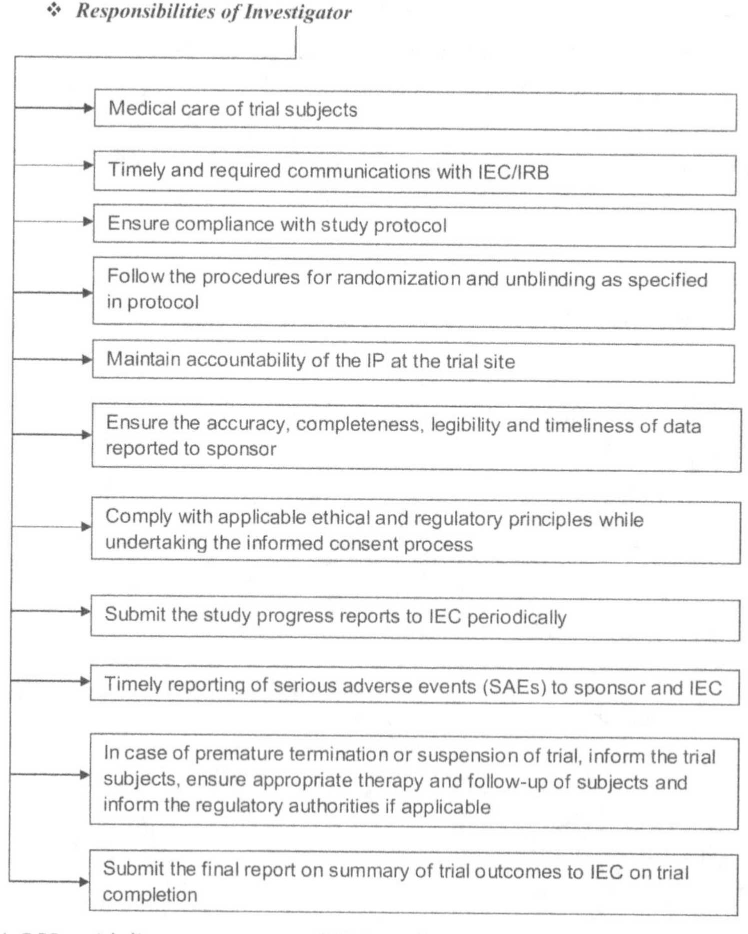

Figure 18.4 ICH-GCP guidelines on responsibilities of study investigator.

- Awareness and compliance with GCP and other applicable regulatory guidelines.
- Maintain a record of suitably qualified personnel who have been delegated trial related duties by him.
- Should permit the conduct of monitoring, audit and inspections at the trial site
- Should have adequate resources (patient load, sufficient time, qualified and trained staff, facilities etc.) for proper and safe execution of the trial.

❖ ***Responsibilities of the Investigator*** **(Figure 18.4).**

ICH-GCP GUIDELINES ON SPONSOR

❖ ***Responsibilities of sponsor*** **(Figure 18.5).**

ICH E6: GCP (R2) ADDENDUM

In November 2016, revised version of GCP guidelines (R2) was released as an integrated addendum to ICH E6 (R1). Changes incorporated in the revised version are as described below:

1. ***Introduction.*** Rationale of having addendum E6 (R2) is included and described as:
- Increased clinical trial scale, complexity and costs.
- Increased efficiency by technology.
- Evolution of risk management process.
- In order to enforce sponsors to implement improved oversight and management of clinical trials.
- Enhance electronic data recording and reporting.
- Enhance e-record standards to increase clinical trial quality and efficiency.
2. ***Chapter 1. Glossary.*** Inclusion of three new definitions (total number of definitions now=65) as:
- **Certified Copy.** "A copy (irrespective of the type of media used) of the original record that has been authenticated (i.e. by a dated signature or generation by means of a validated procedure) to have the same information, including data that describe the context, content, and structure, as the original".
- **Monitoring Plan.** "A document that describes the strategy, methods, responsibilities, and requirements for monitoring the trial".
- **Validation of Computerized Systems.** "A process of establishing and documenting that the specified requirements of a computerized system can be consistently fulfilled from design until decommissioning of the system or transition to a new system. The approach to validation should be based on a risk assessment that takes into consideration the intended use of the system and the potential of the system to affect human subject protection and reliability of trial results".

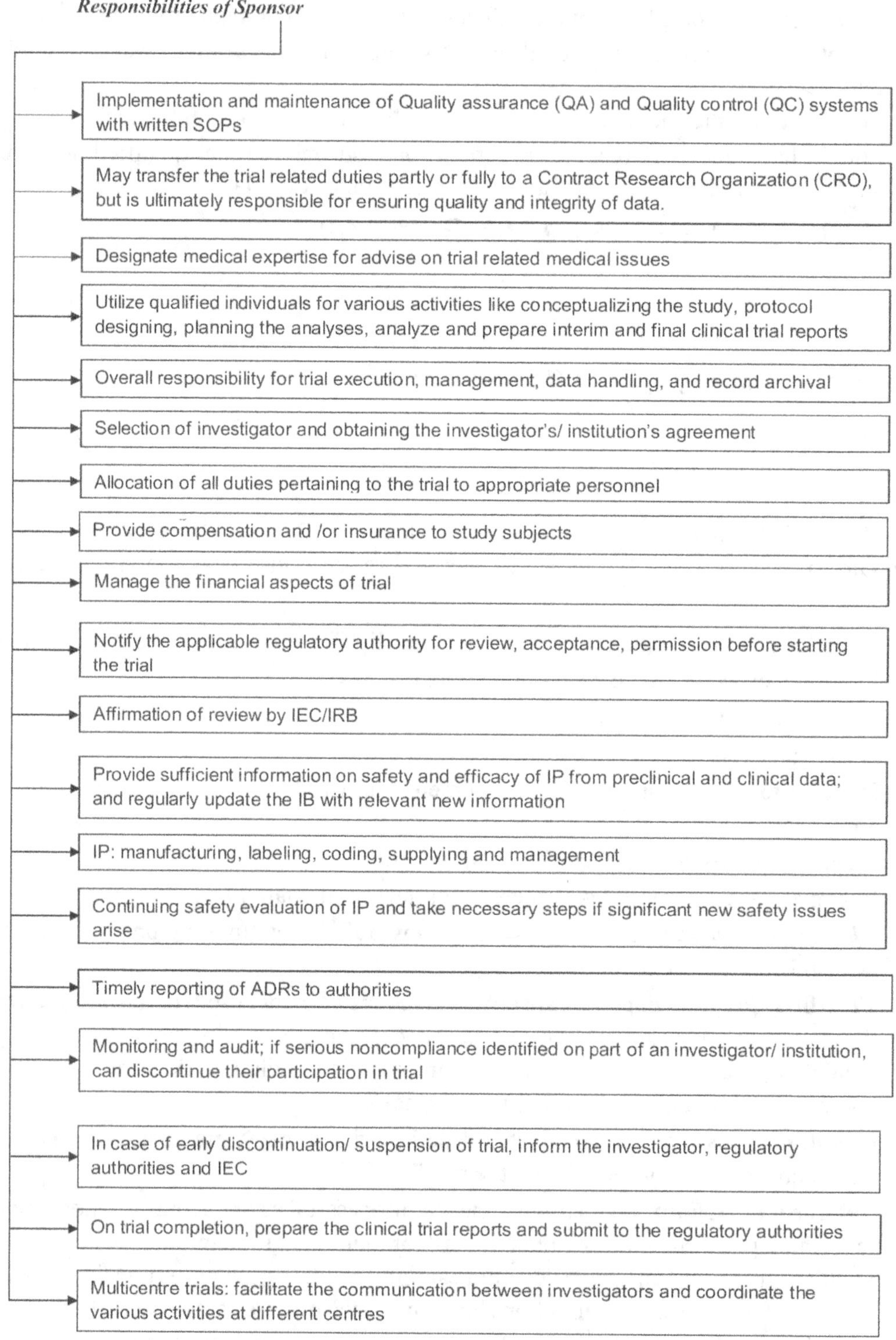

Figure 18.5 ICH-GCP guidelines on responsibilities of study sponsor.

3. **Chapter 2. Principles of GCP.** The addendum clarifies that ICH GCP standards should apply to all trial information, paper or electronic and it indicates that computerized system procedures should be implemented to ensure trial quality (human subjects protection and data integrity).

4. **Chapter 4. Investigator.**

- Responsibilities of Investigator/Institution to maintain supervision of individuals or party performing delegated tasks, is now stipulated in the addendum.

- Requirement is also added for investigators to keep all source documents and/or records with ALCOA+C (Attributable, Legible, Contemporaneous, Original, Accurate and Complete) standards and modifications if any traceable via audit trail.

5. **Chapter 5. Sponsor.** This section is impacted the most with this addendum.

- GCP (R2) now stipulates for the sponsor to establish a comprehensive quality management system (QMS) to capture and categorize risks with an oversight process that synthesizes review across all functions (*Risk-based Quality management system*), focusing on critical data integrity, trial subject protection and safety. This approach should be customized to the specific data collected in the trial and should define exactly how and when high-risk data will be reviewed.

- Sponsor's responsibility on oversight when trial related duties are delegated to Contract research organizations (CROs) and their subcontractors.

- Risk based approach on system validation including standard operating procedures (SOPs) covering the complete system lifecycle as well as responsibilities and training.

- Risk based approach to monitoring i.e. RBM (centralized and/or on-site monitoring) as well as requirements for associated monitoring reports introduced.

- On-site and centralized monitoring requirements introduced.

- Monitoring plan mandatory (outlining content requirements).

- Non-compliance requirements for root cause and corrective and preventive actions for major issues, a follow-up of issues to resolution and visibility of all involved staff.

6. **Chapter 8. Essential documents.** The importance of maintaining records on site, version control, retrieval and search of essential documents for sponsor and investigators/institutions are specified in the addendum.

- Essential documents can be supplemented/ may be reduced where justified prior to study initiation.

- Sponsor to ensure the investigator control of/ continuous access to e-CRF data before, during and after the trial, and no exclusive sponsor control of those data.

- Copies used to replace original documents should fulfill certified copies requirements (i.e. dated signature or generation through a validated process).

INDIAN GCP GUIDELINES

The Indian GCP guidelines were formulated by an expert committee constituted by CDSCO in 2001. At present, Indian GCP is under the process of revision. The adoption of these guidelines has been endorsed by the Drug Technical Advisory Board (DTAB) for streamlining clinical studies/ trials in India.

STRUCTURE OF INDIAN GCP

- Definitions.
- Pre-requisites.
- Responsibilities.
- Records & Data.
- Quality Assurance.
- Statistics.
- Special Concerns.
- Appendices.

The Indian GCP guidelines are based on ICH-GCP, but there are few differences between the two (Table 18.1).

DIFFERENCES BETWEEN INDIAN GCP AND ICH-GCP

Table 18.1 Differences between Indian GCP and ICH-GCP.

	Indian GCP	ICH GCP
Investigator qualifications	Investigator should be qualified as per the requirement of Medical Council of India (MCI) (3.3.1)	Not mentioned
Investigator responsibility	To sign and forward the data like CRF, results and interpretations, analysis and reports etc. from his centre to sponsor and ethics committee (3.3.8)	To provide a summary of the outcome of trial to ethics committee (4.13)
Investigator and Sponsor SOPs	Mandatory for investigator and sponsor to sign a copy of SOPs (3.1.3)	Investigator and his staff have to be aware of and comply with SOPs; compliance to SOPs checked by monitors and auditors
Powers of IEC	IEC can order trial discontinuation if goals have been achieved or unequivocal results obtained (2.4.2.6)	Independent Data Monitoring Committee (IDMC) constituted by sponsor holds this responsibility (5.5.2)
Essential elements for informed consent	Issues of biological samples covered in the informed consent form (2.4.3.2)	No information regarding biological samples in informed consent form

Table 18.1 Contd...

Informed consent process	Investigator should sign the consent form (2.4.3.1)	Any one designated by the Investigator to conduct the consent process and sign the form (4.8.8)
Labeling of the drug product(s) in study protocol	The label should contain the information as: the words - "For Clinical Studies only", the name or a code number of the study, name and contact numbers of the investigator, name of the institution, subject's identification code (2.3.1.6)	Not explained
Document retention	Study related documents/materials should be safeguarded by the sponsor for 3 years. (3.1.5)	Sponsor specific essential documents to be retained for a minimum of 2 years after the last marketing approval in an ICH region and until no pending marketing applications in an ICH region or for a minimum of 2 years after formal discontinuation of clinical development of IP (5.5.11)

The New Drugs and Clinical Trials Rules 2019 have incorporated the definition of GCP guidelines as given in Box 18.1.

Box 18.1 The New Drugs and Clinical Trials Rules, 2019, India.

New definition included:

Good Clinical Practices Guidelines: the Good Clinical Practices Guidelines for conduct of clinical studies in India, formulated by the Central Drugs Standard Control Organization and adopted by the Drugs Technical Advisory Board.

ESSENTIAL DOCUMENTS

These are the documents which independently and collectively help in evaluating the execution of a clinical trial and quality of the data generated. They are required during the audits and inspections.

As per Indian GCP guidelines, these are classified into three groups on the basis of different stages of study:
- Before the commencement of clinical phase of study;
- During the clinical conduct of study;
- After the study completion or termination.

Practical Considerations in Designing and Conducting Clinical Trials

---

OVERVIEW

Introduction
Study Subjects
*Defining the Study Population
(Eligibility Criteria)*
Recruitment of Subjects
Retention of Study Subjects

Selection of Study Endpoints
Qualities of Endpoints
Classification of Endpoints
Selection of Efficacy Criteria
Types of Efficacy Criteria
Desirable Characteristics of an Efficacy Criterion
Hurdles in the Way of Clinical Trials

INTRODUCTION

Randomized controlled trials (RCTs) constitute the keystone of evidence based medicine. RCTs play an extremely crucial role in providing genuine evidence of the efficacy of interventions, their safety aspects, impact on quality of life, cost effectiveness etc. In order to be feasible, the trials should be uncomplicated, broadly applicable and close to normal clinical practice. However, the researchers involved in planning and conducting trials face numerous problems, and the situation has further been complicated by the introduction of various regulations related to designing and conducting clinical trials. This chapter summarizes various practical problems faced by those planning and conducting clinical trials and suggests some strategies to handle them.

Table 19.1 enlists various practical issues faced by researchers at the planning stage of clinical trials.

ELEMENT	DESCRIPTION
Table 19.1 Various practical issues of concern while planning a clinical trial.	
Research question	Defines the study objective. Characteristics of a good research question: FINER (**F**easible, **I**nteresting, **N**ovel, **E**thical and **R**elevant)
Background and significance	Sets the context of proposed study and gives its rationale. Should describe: What is known about the topic? (citing previous relevant research) What is the relevance of research question? (problems with previous research and uncertainties) What kind of answers are expected from the study? (how the findings of the proposed study will provide solution to uncertain issues, generate new information and influence practice guidelines or public health policy).
Design	How is the study structured? e.g. settings, randomized /non-randomised, blinded/open label, choice of control group, between/within subject comparisons, duration etc.
Study subjects	Defining the study/ target population (inclusion/ exclusion criteria) Methods of recruitment
Study end-points	Primary/secondary, hard/soft, direct/surrogate, composite end points etc.
Efficacy criteria	Based on the treatment and objective of the trial/measurement
Statistical issues	Specifying the Null hypothesis Sample size calculation Descriptive/analytical statistics Type of analysis: Intention to treat (ITT)/ Modified ITT/ Per Protocol Measures to handle missing data

STUDY SUBJECTS

Figure 19.1 gives a diagrammatic representation of relationship of study sample to study population and population with condition as a whole.

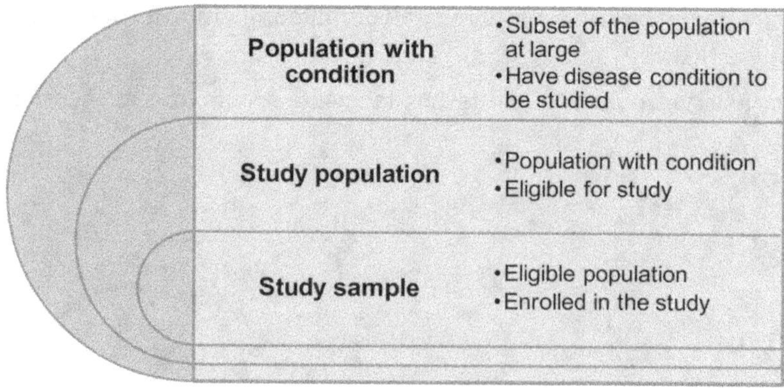

Figure 19.1 General representation of study sample, study population and population as a whole.

❖ **Defining the study population (eligibility criteria)**

Study eligibility criteria need to be well-defined in order to eliminate/diminish bias and variability and escalate the power of study.

Eligibility criteria are based on:

♦ *Patient characteristics* e.g. age, sex, weight, race/ethnic background, use of tobacco/alcohol etc., diet and nutritional status, hypersensitivity to clinical trial medicine or test, other medicine or non medicine allergies, physiological limitations, willingness of patient to participate etc.

♦ *Disease characteristics* e.g. disease being evaluated, duration or severity of disease, concomitant and past diseases and medicines, previous treatments received.

♦ *Environmental and other factors* e.g. patient recruitment and cooperation, participation in other clinical trial, geographical location, institutional status etc.

♦ *Results of screening examinations.*

Important points to consider while selecting subjects for clinical trials

♦ The features of the disease condition under study should be such that response to the interventions can be evaluated easily and within the time frame of the study period.

♦ The different groups of subjects should have uniform characteristics with respect to natural history of disease condition and its expected response to treatment.

♦ The groups must be comprised of individuals who are considered 'representative' of the condition studied.

♦ Expected patient accrual should be assessed realistically.

♦ Ethical principles must be followed in case of increased risk to certain groups of trial subjects.

❖ **Recruitment of subjects/participants**

An important consideration when designing a clinical trial is establishing the source from where subjects will be recruited (Table 19.2).

Table 19.2 Sources of participants recruitment.
• Government employees
• Private industry (e.g. clinics in large industries)
• Referred cases from medical/ professional colleagues
• Referrals from clinical laboratories
• Mass media approaches (via newspaper, radio or television advertisements)
• Mass mailings
• Community screening (e.g. health fairs)
• Subjects enrolled in other clinical studies
• Blood banks
• Local advertisements (notices on bulletin boards)
• Other sources (e.g. investigator's own practice or through unsolicited visits by patients to the investigator)

Lasagna's law. It is observed that rate of recruitment is generally over-predicted. The disease condition, assumed to be widely prevalent, suddenly vanishes as soon as one begins seeking for it and then seems to reappear when the trial is completed. This phenomenon is known as Lasagna's law. This can partially be attributed to stringent eligibility criteria for inclusion in the study and declining enthusiasm of the investigators over time.

Factors influencing participation in clinical trials

Various factors determine the decision to participate in clinical trials by either favoring/ serving as barriers (Figure 19.2).

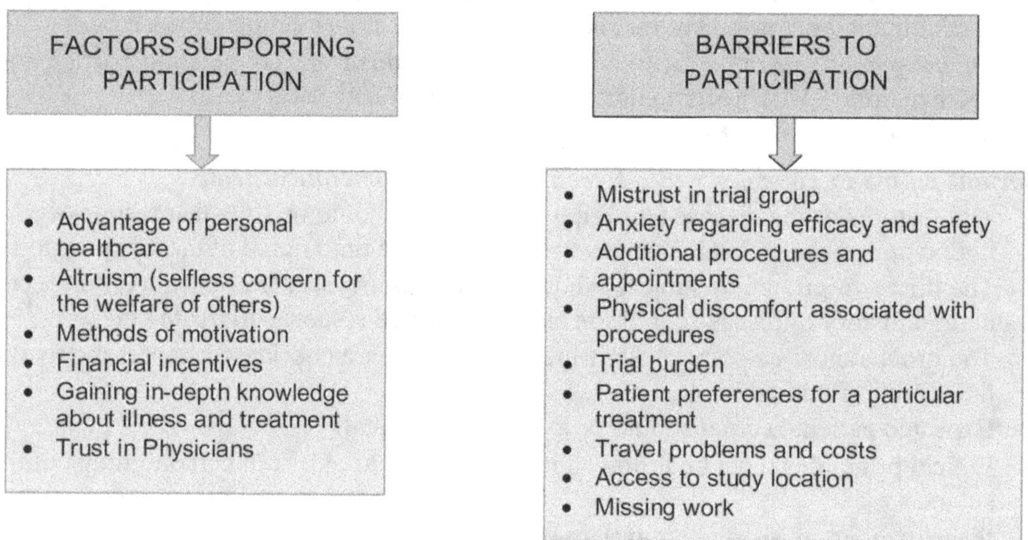

Figure 19.2 Factors influencing participation in clinical trials.

Misconceptions among participants

Some misconceptions commonly prevail among the potential study subjects which can influence their participation or later on withdrawal from the study (Table 19.3). It is always better to clear any doubts/ misconceptions among participants before enrolment in study.

Table 19.3 Common misconceptions among study participants.

- Everyone will get active treatment
- Study carries minimal risk
- Participation in the study will not interfere with patient's daily routine
- The patient's regular physician will be the study physician
- Compensation and other benefits will be great
- Everything will be free of cost
- Patients will have unlimited access to study personnel

Strategies to increase participants recruitment
- ✓ Increase the accessible participants population. e.g. by increasing the time duration of study or the number of trial sites etc.
- ✓ Relax inclusion/exclusion criteria
- ✓ Relax the demands of the protocol e.g. elimination of disagreeable tests, less number of follow-up visits
- ✓ Wider publicity.
- ✓ Financial incentives for sites and clinical investigators exceeding enrolment targets.
- ✓ Coercion / Punishment for below target enrolment e.g. threat to stop the clinical trial (CT) by CT managers, financial penalties for poor enrollment, black-listing such sites for future CT's, informing institutional management about poor performance of clinical investigator.

Risks associated with rapid recruitment
- ✓ Incomplete documentation
- ✓ Compromise on ethical aspects
- ✓ Impact on patient's rights, safety and well-being
- ✓ Impact on quality
- ✓ Potential for protocol deviation/violation
- ✓ High likelihood of regulatory inspection

❖ **Retention of study subjects**

It is a very common observation that during the clinical trial conduct, 30-40 percent of subjects on an average, drop-out or are lost to follow up. A deeper understanding of the factors associated can be instrumental in planning strategies to be implemented to increase the retention rates.

Causes of participants drop-outs/ loss to follow-up
- ♦ *Treatment related causes*
  - Recovery or sufficient improvement
  - Poor acceptance of treatment (inconvenient or unpleasant)
  - Poor tolerability (appearance of side effects)
  - A preliminary therapeutic efficacy considered to be inadequate
- ♦ *Trial related causes*
  - Too frequent, inconvenient or restrictive procedures
  - Very long observation period
  - Study procedures interfering with patient's lifestyle
  - Cold attitude of the investigator/ study personnel

♦ ***Random events related causes***
- Accident/ intercurrent illness/ emergency surgery of subject
- Relocation
- Forgetfulness to come for appointment
- Transportation strike

Strategies to facilitate retention of study subjects
- Select the subjects who are able and willing to cooperate
- Motivation of subjects by clearly explaining all aspects of the trial, and welcoming them as research partners
- Repetitive, inconvenient or unpleasant tests to be reduced to a minimum
- Describe in detail the study procedures and duration of commitment at the time of enrollment
- Discuss and solve transportation issues
- Involve the family members of subjects during discussions
- Maintain a good moral communication with subject's primary care physician
- Give the instructions to subjects in easy-to-carry and easy-to-understand manner.
- Provisions to make follow-up visits convenient like effective organization of appointments, minimal waiting time, reminder letters or telephone calls, ensuring the availability of Investigator/ coordinator during follow-up visits.
- Provide subjects with appointment card/ study calendar with appointment schedule
- Establish a tracking system for follow-up visits: scheduled, completed, missed.
- Contact the subject if he misses the appointment/ there is a long interval between scheduled visits
- Treat the subjects with respect and make them feel comfortable to ask any queries
- Adjustment of sample size at the planning phase to compensate for attrition.

SELECTION OF STUDY ENDPOINTS

An endpoint is described as a measure which permits us to make decision regarding acceptance or rejection of the null hypothesis in a clinical trial.

While selecting endpoints for a clinical trial, it is critical to assure that they:
- carry clinical significance in relation to the disease process
- are able to answer the queries of the trial
- have practical and feasible methods for assessment
- have good enough frequency to ensure adequate statistical power of the study.

QUALITIES OF ENDPOINTS

VALID. Study's ability to actually measure the characteristic it aims to measure

RELIABLE. Consistent results upon subsequent administrations

OBJECTIVE. Based on instrumentation requiring little or no evaluator judgement

CLINICALLY RELEVANT. Should influence the decisions by physicians and patients.

CLASSIFICATION OF ENDPOINTS

1. **Primary vs. secondary endpoints:** Primary endpoints evaluate the outcomes which help in answering the primary (or most relevant) research question in a particular trial, such as whether the test intervention is superior in terms of providing protection against disease-related death than the standard therapy. It serves as a basis for trial design, sample size estimation, power & data analysis & trial reporting. The rationale for its selection is crucial and should be stated clearly to satisfy regulatory authorities. Preferably a single primary endpoint should be chosen in a study.

   Secondary endpoints evaluate the other relevant outcomes in the same study; for example, presence of any effect on disease measures apart from death, evaluating efficacy in key subgroups of patients, evaluating the underlying mechanism of action of the drug, evaluating safety features, such as adverse effects, drug interactions, or reasons for discontinuation of therapy, evaluating the impact of therapy on quality-of-life measures or whether the new intervention is more cost-effective. In cases where secondary end points hold significance as good as primary end points, they are considered as co-primary endpoints.

2. **Hard vs. soft endpoints:** Hard end points are measured by observation and are quantitative in nature e.g., fall in ESR following treatment with an anti-rheumatoid drug; in cardiovascular studies, death or MI.

   Soft end points are often qualitative in nature and are more subjective e.g., reduction in morning stiffness is a soft end point, quality of life parameters. These are equally important in the final assessment of the therapeutic effectiveness/ safety.

3. **Direct vs. surrogate endpoints:** Direct endpoints indicate the therapeutic effect itself e.g. sleep, eradication of infection.

   Surrogate endpoint is a factor reliably related to the therapeutic effect, a surrogate effect e.g. blood lipids or glucose, or blood pressure.

4. **Composite endpoints:** This refers to a conglomerate of individual endpoints which together constitute a 'single' endpoint for that trial. According to the ICH, if it is difficult to assign a single primary variable from multiple parameters related to the primary objective, a useful approach is to integrate or combine the various parameters into a single "composite" end-point.

Examples of composite endpoints:

- In cardiovascular diseases: time to first event of MI, stroke, CABG, hospitalization, death.
- In asthma: asthma symptom scores which combine symptoms of wheezing, coughing and spasms into a single range.
- In diabetic nephropathy: time to decreased renal function, end stage renal disease, death.
- In colon carcinoma: composite of clinical (symptoms related to defecation), pathologic (histo-pathologic examination of colon biopsy specimen), visual (assessment of tumor size endoscopically) and biochemical (laboratory estimation of tumor markers or hepatic involvement due to secondary tumors) endpoints.

Rationale of choosing composite endpoints

- ✓ Statistical issues. An endpoint having multiple outcomes denotes observation of more outcome events in total. Since the sample size in a clinical trial is inversely proportional to the number of events observed in control group, a composite endpoint helps to reduce the sample size, thereby, decreasing the trial duration and expenses.
- ✓ Allows more comprehensive evaluation of a treatment effect than just one outcome.

Drawbacks of composite endpoints

- ✓ The selection of a composite endpoint is based on the assumption that all individual outcome parameters are associated with the disease under study and are equally relevant, which, although might not be the case always.
- ✓ Benefits accrued due to an intervention are presumed to be related to all the parameters of composite end points.
- ✓ There may be inconsistent results, with improvement in certain outcomes and deterioration in others, complicating the overall interpretation of study results. Hence, the relative importance of various parameters of composite end-points need to be ascertained while designing the study.

SELECTION OF EFFICACY CRITERIA

TYPES OF EFFICACY CRITERIA

Table 19.4 enlists various criteria used to evaluate the efficacy of study intervention/s in clinical trials.

Table 19.4 Types of efficacy criteria.

Depending on the treatment and objective of the trial

1. Preventive treatment

   - *Incidence*

   - *Time of onset of disease event*

2. Curative treatment

   - *Duration of the disease*

   - *Incidence of complications or fatal outcome*

3. Symptomatic treatment

   - *Severity of the symptom*

   - *Duration of effect obtained*

   - *Incidence of episodes during a defined time period*

4. Palliative treatment

   - *Life table method e.g. 5 year survival*

   - *Median duration of survival*

Depending on the measurement

1. *Presence or absence (i.e. existence) criteria.*

2. *Graded or scaled criteria.* e.g. graded scales (e.g. neurological reflexes graded from 0 to 4, severity of symptoms graded form 1 to 5 etc.) and visual analog scale (VAS).

3. *Relative change criteria.*

4. *Global criteria* (overall evaluation of a patient's disease or change in disease severity; global improvement)

DESIRABLE CHARACTERISTICS OF AN EFFICACY CRITERION

- ***Sensitivity.*** Ability to detect minor improvements or deteriorations in a condition.
- ***Repeatability.*** Consistency of the results obtained by the same observer operating under the same conditions in a short time span.
- ***Reproducibility.*** Consistency of the results obtained by different observers at different times. Agreement of two observers measuring the same criterion is called "concordance".
- ***Specificity.*** Criterion not influenced by variables other than those which one seeks to measure.
- ***Stability.*** The criterion does not fluctuate "too widely" from one recording to another in the same individual.
- ***Correlation*** with other clinical parameters of interest.
- ***Easy and rapid*** administration as well as interpretation.

HURDLES IN THE WAY OF CLINICAL TRIALS

Figure 19.3 depicts some major hurdles faced by investigators while planning and conducting clinical trials and their potential solutions.

HURDLES

POTENTIAL SOLUTIONS

Lack of resources for randomized trials

- Comparative dearth of resources for clinical research as compared to basic research.
- Lack of funding, or infrastructure to encourage clinical trials.
- Huge increase in trial costs as a result of rising regulatory complexities governing their conduct.

- Allocation of more funds for clinical trials.
- Special organizations may be set up to allocate funds to independent researchers in low to middle income countries.
- Use of appropriate methods to enhance the quality of clinical trials.
- Streamlining regulations and removing unnecessary bureaucracy to help reduce costs.

Complex trial regulations

- Need for multiple approvals (DCGI/ IRBs/ ethics committees etc.).
- Increased complexity of regulatory requirements for obtaining permission to conduct clinical trials/ import new drugs for clinical trials (e.g. drug import licenses).
- Prolonged delays in obtaining regulatory approvals.
- Ethical issues e.g.obtaining informed consent, compensation issues etc.

- Strategies to simplify and standardize the regulatory approval process.
- Defining timelines for obtaining/ granting regulatory approval.
- Following national guidelines focusing on ethical and regulatory aspects.

Limited evidence on how to do trials

- Limited awareness and knowledge about the general methodologies for conducting trials.
- Application of same set of guidelines to all types of clinical trials decreasing the efficient use of resources.
- Lack of training/education of the investigators and other study personnel.

- Formulation of updated guidelines to provide a framework on methodologies relevant to diverse types of clinical trials.
- Conducting workshops and trainings to increase awareness on GCP, ethical and legal aspects, data management etc among investigators and other personnel involved in planning and conducting clinical trials.

Complex trial execution procedures

- Complicated procedures for subject recruitment, randomization, blinding etc.
- Lengthy and time consuming documentation procedures.
- Ensuring a reasonably acceptable compliance.
- Ensure generation of good quality data
- Introduction of bias/es during study planning, conduct or analysis.
- Detailed reporting requirements for adverse events.
- Excessive monitoring visits before, during and after the trials.

- Description of trial related procedures in a detailed, easily understandable, and reproducible manner in the study protocol.
- Implementation of good practices at different stages of the trials viz. Good Clinical Practices (GCP), Good Laboratory Practices (GLP), Good Documentation Practices (GDP) etc.
- Following strategies to evaluate and improve patient compliance.
- Identification of sources of bias and appropriate steps taken to avoid them.
- Standardized guidelines for adverse event reporting.

Figure 19.3 Major hurdles to the conduct of clinical trials.

Designs used in Clinical Trials

INTRODUCTION

One of the critical steps while planning and conducting clinical trials is selection of an appropriate experimental design. Various factors need to be considered while choosing a particular study design like phase of drug development, primary objective of the study, nature of the disease studied (e.g. severity, incidence), type of control groups, study population (e.g. size, distribution, accessibility, customs), merits and demerits of different designs, feasibility concerns with various experimental designs etc.

TYPES OF EXPERIMENTAL DESIGNS

PARALLEL DESIGN

This consists of making as many random groups of trial subjects as there are treatments and subjects receive the same assigned treatment throughout the trial. Usually the number of subjects in each group are kept roughly equal, since the chances of getting efficient statistical comparisons are increased with balanced groups.

Variations of Parallel designs

1. Common parallel design

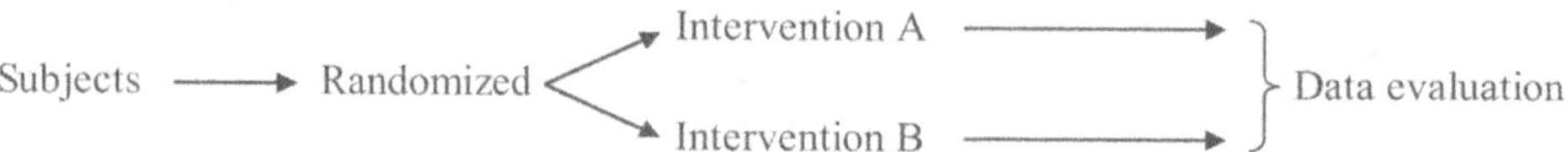

2. Parallel design with placebo initiation

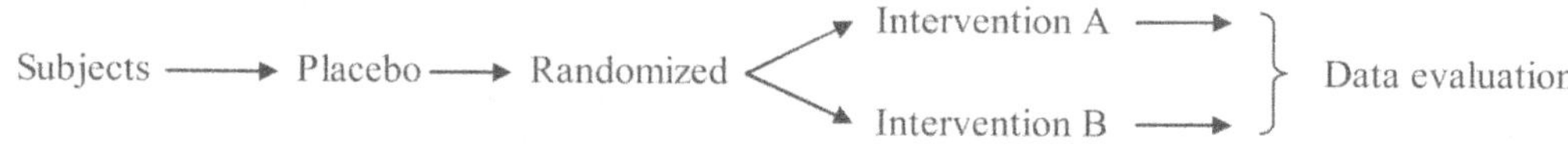

3. Introduction of placebo during treatment

Intervention A ⟶ Placebo ⟶ Intervention A

Intervention B ⟶ Placebo ⟶ Intervention B

4. Multiple doses within each treatment group

Treatment group A ⟶ Dose i —— Dose ii —— Dose iii

Treatment group B ⟶ Dose i' —— Dose ii' —— Dose iii'

Each dose is of a fixed or variable length, and doses may be given in an ascending or random order.

Merits

- Simple organization and analysis

Demerits

- Chances of error arising out of non-comparable treatment groups due to imbalance among various factors at baseline.
- Greater chances of variability in results between randomly selected subjects.

DESIGNS FOR WITHIN-SUBJECT COMPARISONS

Within-subject trials are those in which every subject receives one or more interventions being studied/ compared in succession in random order.

Merits of within-subject comparisons

1. Lesser sample size. As every subject "serves as his or her own control," the sample size required in a within-subject trial is less in contrast to parallel-groups design.
2. Lesser internal variability. In within-subject design, intra-individual variability through different phases of the trial is considered, rather than the inter-individual variability

during the same phase. Hence, data obtained has lesser variability as compared to that in between-patient design.

3. Chances of better recruitment as all subjects receive all treatments under investigation.
4. High sensitivity

Demerits of within-subject comparisons

1. Less robust analysis than parallel design (analysis of data is adversely affected by patient dropouts and missing data).
2. Limited applicability. Certain conditions need to be fulfilled for within-patient comparisons like:
   ✓ Stable (usually chronic) disease during various treatment periods
   ✓ The condition at baseline must be identical at the beginning of each treatment period.
   ✓ Treatments with quickly reversible effect.
3. Carry-over effects. These trials assume that the results of a particular phase of trial are not influenced by the intervention/s administered prior to that phase. However, any delayed/ carry-over/ residual effects need to be considered in circumstances like:
   ✓ Intervention produces an irreversible effect (e.g. clinical cure).
   ✓ Intervention has a delayed effect which may be evident after stoppage of treatment.
   ✓ Slower elimination of drug or its metabolite/s from biological media or receptors.
   Strategies to mitigate the carry-over effects:
   - An *intermediate wash-out period or re-stabilization period* between different treatment phases can be included. The duration of wash-out period should ideally be equal to at least ten half-lives of the drug given.
   - Comparison can be carried out between clinical profile after each treatment period is over and excluding the wash-out period.
   - If there is a suspicion of the presence of carry-over effect, one strategy to salvage data is to analyze the results for first period of trial only as in parallel design, and not considering the following "contaminated" periods.
4. Period effect (treatment by period interaction). Whether a treatment is administered during initial or subsequent period has a bearing on the effect of treatment.
5. Conditioning and learning effect. Conditioning of the subject (for example to efficacy, inefficacy or side effects of treatments given in succession) and learning experience (improved scores in repetitive tests used to assess efficacy). These effects however tend to get cancelled out by randomization of the order of administration.
6. Chances of appearance of a rebound effect after termination of treatment, thus affecting the subsequent phase.
7. Complex analysis as compared to parallel designs.

Classification of within subject experimental designs

(i) **The cross-over trial.** In this design, two interventions or treatments are compared by allocating each intervention to all the subjects in a random order.

The simplest crossover design is a two-treatment, two-period crossover trial in which each participant is administered either the test (A) or reference (B) treatment in the initial study period and the alternative treatment in the subsequent period. These trials are often termed as *2 × 2* or AB/BA trials (Figure 20.1).

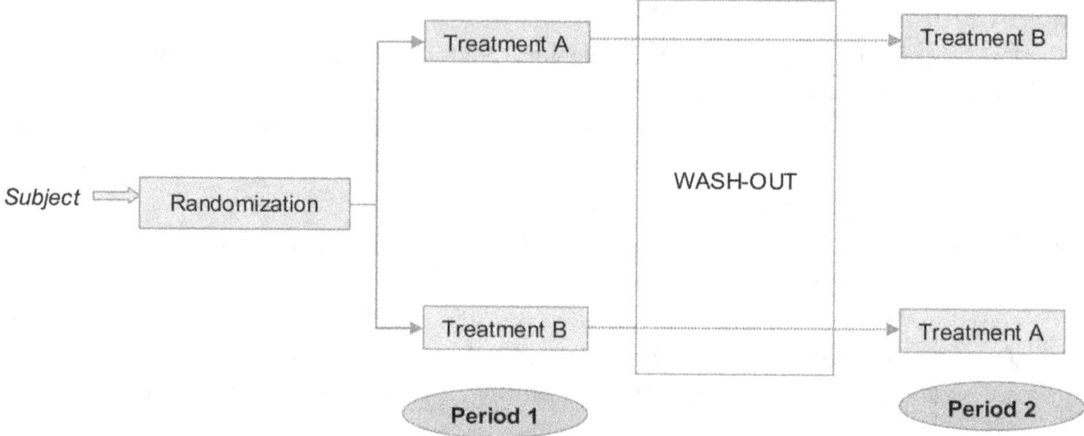

Figure 20.1 A standard two-sequence, two-period cross-over design.

Types of cross-over trials

❖ *Complete cross-over.* Each subject is administered all of the study interventions in randomized order during the study.

❖ *Incomplete cross-over.* A given patient receives some and not all of the study treatments.

❖ *Multiple cross-overs/ Intensive designs.* Each group of subjects receives each treatment for multiple times during the trial e.g. double cross-over (Figure 20.2).

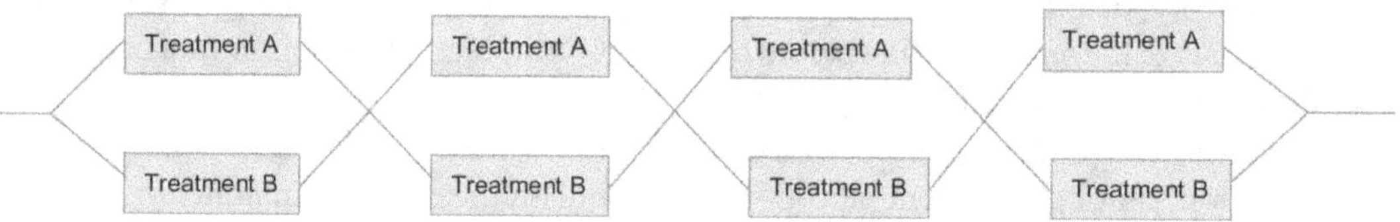

Figure 20.2 Double cross-over design.

❖ *Extra period cross-over.* One treatment is given for an additional period. The extra-period design attempts to avoid carry over effects (Figure 20.3).

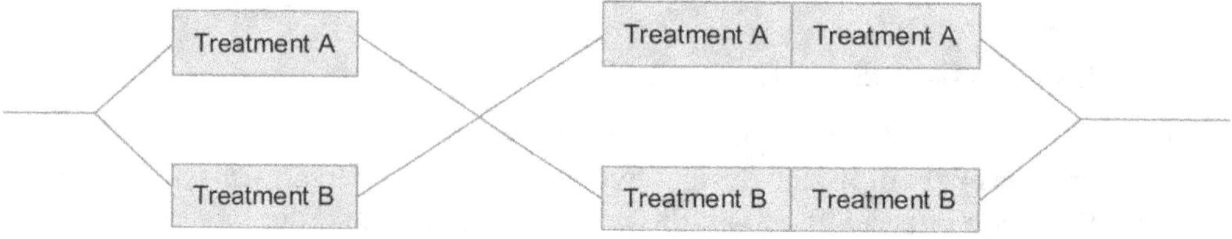

Figure 20.3 Extra period cross-over design

(ii) Latin square design

This design is considered when the trial involves comparison of more than two treatments. The treatments may be allocated in sequence to all the subjects in such a manner that.
- ✓ the number of subjects is equal to or a multiple of the number of treatments compared
- ✓ every subject receives all the treatments in succession.
- ✓ during every period of the trial, at least one of the trial subjects receives each treatment.

Figure 20.4 depicts an example of latin square design with three different treatments A, B and C.

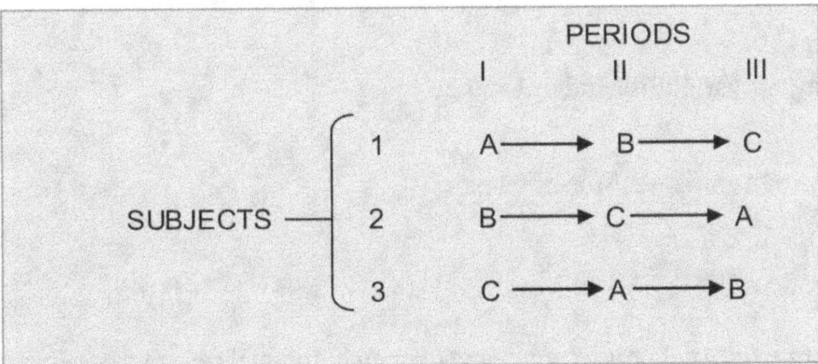

Figure 20.4 Latin square design.

(iii) Greco-latin squares

This design is applicable if in addition to the effect of treatment, the study aims to study the effect of some other factors (which are equal to the number of treatments compared) e.g. concomitant treatment, diet, behavior therapy etc in each subject. These factors can be randomly assigned and two independent or orthogonal latin squares can be superimposed to from a "Greco-latin square" (Figure 20.5).

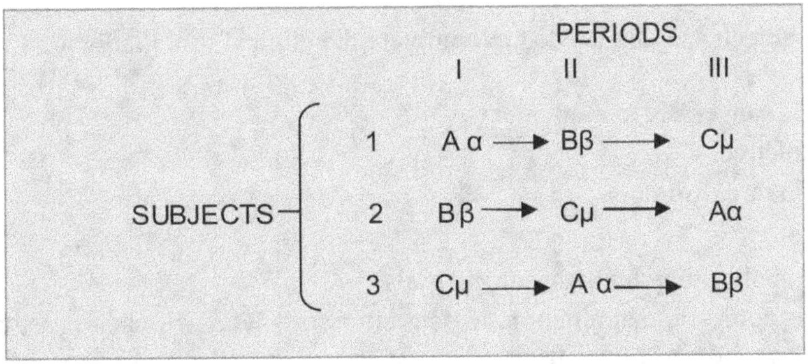

Figure 20.5 Greco-latin square.

MATCHED PAIR DESIGNS

This is a type of design in which pairs of subjects are identified who are "identical" with regard to all pertinent factors and who are expected to show similar response to the treatments. Treatment A is then randomly assigned to one of the members of the matched pair and the other gets treatment B. In practice, pairing is feasible when matching is done for less number of characteristics, all the study participants are familiar before beginning the trial and in trials on homozygous twins.

This design can also be implemented within one individual e.g. one eye, or foot receives one treatment and the other eye or foot receives other treatment.

Merits

- Less intra-pair variability and imbalance.

Demerits

- Difficulty in forming well-matched pairs

SEQUENTIAL DESIGNS

In this design, during the trial progression whenever an individual case or a case per intervention is completed, the data is analyzed; a rule is defined beforehand for terminating the trial rejecting either the null or alternate hypothesis. The major requirements for using this design are:

- ✓ rapid evaluability of subjects: a definitive conclusion about a case must be reached before enrolling more subjects in the trial.
- ✓ short treatment durations: the duration for which individual subjects need to be observed should be less than the interval between subsequent recruitments.
- ✓ clear end point.
- ✓ limited hypothesis to be tested.

Merits

- Fewer subjects may be needed to complete the clinical trial than with a fixed sample size.
- Design is convenient to implement.
- Cost effective.
- Useful in rare disorders.

Demerits

- Limited applicability for most clinical trials.
- Requires complete examination of data after completion of each case, usually with breaking of code in "blind" trials.

Group sequential design. A type of sequential design in which subjects are entered and studied in groups; an interim analysis of the data is conducted and,

✓ if the results are significant or if the treatment groups are totally alike, then the clinical trial is *stopped;*

✓ if the difference between two treatment groups is statistically non-significant, the trial is *continued* further.

The most familiar example of group sequential design is the "3+3" Phase I trial design for determining maximum-tolerated-dose.

FACTORIAL DESIGNS

A factorial design is an experiment that studies the effect of more than one treatment and also permits an assessment of interactions among the treatments.

Applications of factorial designs:

❖ *Comparisons of efficacy of drug combinations with either treatment (A or B) in fixed dosage.*

In this, subjects (number = N) are randomly assigned to treatment in one of four groups:

Treatment A	Treatment B		Subjects
	Present	Absent	
Present	Group 1 (N/4)	Group 2 (N/4)	N/2
Absent	Group 3 (N/4)	Group 4 (N/4)	N/2
Total subjects	N/2	N/2	N

Figure 20.6 A 2 x 2 completely balanced factorial design.

If treatments compared have different routes of administration in double blind trials, e.g. treatment A administered orally to be compared with treatment B administered intramuscularly; the groups can be created as:

Group 1: A (oral) + B (i.m.)

Group 2: A (oral) + Placebo of B (i.m.)

Group 3: B (i.m.) + Placebo of A (oral)

Group 4: Placebo of A (oral) + Placebo of B (i.m.)

Factorial designs may, however, be applied only when different treatments can be administered together without producing any modification (i.e. absence of interference in terms of efficacy or safety between treatments).

Factorial designs are appropriate for treatments acting through different mechanisms e.g. radiotherapy and chemotherapy for tumors.

❖ *To study interactions between different treatments.* The same structural design, as described above, can be used to study the potential interactions between two treatments but the sample size required would be approximately four times larger.

Thus, factorial designs are capable of studying interactions as well as efficiency of combining different treatments, but both objectives cannot be met simultaneously.

Merits of factorial designs

- Lesser number of subjects required to achieve satisfactory inference than separate parallel groups designs.

Demerits

- Complex execution: multiple subgroups, separate random allocation, several drug batches etc.

ADAPTIVE (FLEXIBLE) DESIGNS

These are the designs which permit incorporation of changes in the trial conduct methodology and/or statistical techniques after the beginning of trial without compromising its validity and integrity. According to FDA guidance, an adaptive design clinical trial is defined as "*a study that includes a prospectively planned opportunity for modification of one or more specified aspects of the study design and hypotheses based on analysis of data (usually interim data) from subjects in the study.*" There has been a rising interest in the adoption of adaptive or flexible designs in clinical trials as they are assumed to enhance the drug development process in contrast to traditional non-adaptive methods in a number of ways, for example:

- ✓ increased efficiency in gathering information,
- ✓ increasing the probability of success on the study objective, or
- ✓ yielding greater knowledge regarding efficacy of treatment.

It is to be noted that adaptive designs do not include

- modifications after unexpected/ undesired results in an interim analysis and

- modifications on the basis of information from an external source.

Types of adaptive designs in clinical trials

- ♦ *Adaptation of study eligibility criteria on the basis of analyses of pretreatment (baseline) data.* If the subject recruitment rate is significantly lower than predicted, the screening log can be examined to identify and modify certain noncritical eligibility criteria to increase the likelihood of including screened subjects in the study. Similarly, if on observing the baseline characteristics of accruing study population it is found that expected/ desired subjects are not being enrolled, the eligibility criteria can be modified accordingly.

- ♦ *Adaptations during randomization.* Adaptive randomization methods can be employed which modify the allocation likelihoods as the study progresses to limit the inequalities. These include baseline adaptive and response adaptive randomization. (For details, see the chapter on Randomization).

- *Sample size re-estimation design (SSRD).* If analysis of interim data suggests that the variance of efficacy endpoint is quite less than the initial assumption, the power of study will decrease. In such a case, the sample size can be recalculated (increased) or the study duration may be prolonged to attain the desired power.
- *Drop the loser design.* In this, at the interim analysis, based on pre-specified criteria subjects found to be allocated to inferior treatment are dropped out, the other treatment arm is retained, and a new treatment arm can be added.
- *Group sequential design.* (Described in detail under sequential designs)
- *Biomarker-adaptive design.* This permits adaptation on the basis of responses of biomarkers. It is applied to choose the right subjects for inclusion, study natural course of disease, disease diagnosis at an early stage, optimal screening and establish a validated predictive model.
- *Adaptive treatment-switching design.* This permits the investigator to switch subject's treatment from the one assigned initially to the alternative one. The basis of this design is documented evidence of efficacy or safety during review of accumulated data at preplanned time points.
- *Hypothesis-adaptive design.* Depending on the review of accruing data, this design permits a change in initial hypothesis to the alternate one. For example, change from superiority to non-inferiority hypothesis, modification of study endpoints. Hypothesis-adaptive design is generally finalized prior to database lock or data decoding/unblinding.
- *Adaptive seamless phase II/III design.* This design amalgamates the objectives of isolated Phase IIb and Phase III trials in a single trial. In this design, there is an uninterrupted transition from Phase II to Phase III trial, thereby reducing drug development time. Seamless designs can be of two types: *operationally seamless,* and *inferentially seamless,* which mainly focuses on obtaining final analysis by combining relevant data from Phase II and Phase III parts with the help of new statistical methods.
- *Multiple-adaptive design.* This is a combination of any of the above mentioned adaptive designs. The disadvantage of a multiple adaptive design is difficulties encountered during statistical inference.

Merits of adaptive designs

- No requirement to apply for protocol amendments as potential modifications are approved by regulatory authorities beforehand.
- There is good extent of resilience to react to unexpected events and options are available to make necessary modifications.
- Wider regulatory acceptance, especially in exploratory adaptive design clinical trials
- Enhanced reliability of results particularly with blinded data.
- Helpful to increase the efficiency of drug development process and decrease the attrition rate by allowing earlier detection of any pertinent issues and termination of clinical trial if desired, more efficient use of trial subjects and most appropriate dosage selections.

Demerits of adaptive designs

- Adaptive designs need complex Bayesian approach for statistical analyses.
- Type I error may be difficult to control.
- Risk of compromising the study credibility due to making ad hoc changes on unblinded data.
- Risk of conducting adaptive trials at a very early stage, thereby questioning the overall study findings.

ENRICHMENT DESIGNS

This design involves the incorporation of an additional phase (enrichment phase) in the clinical trial during which testing of new therapeutic agents or manipulation of dose levels is done to identify the subjects showing response. The potential therapeutic responses at various dose levels are assessed and best dose response for each patient is defined in advance in the protocol. After the enrichment phase, the responders enter into a placebo baseline period followed by a randomized double blind parallel group placebo controlled phase. e.g., this design was employed by researchers during the clinical evaluation of transtuzumab; the enrichment strategy demonstrated the efficacy of treatment in a subset of breast cancer subjects overexpressing HER2 receptors on the tumor cells.

RANDOMIZED DISCONTINUATION DESIGN

This uses the enrichment strategy in a two-stage design. In this, all the subjects initially receive the experimental intervention. The subjects showing response continue the same while the subjects not showing any benefit switch to standard therapy; the subjects with stable condition are randomized to experimental or standard treatment (Figure 20.7).

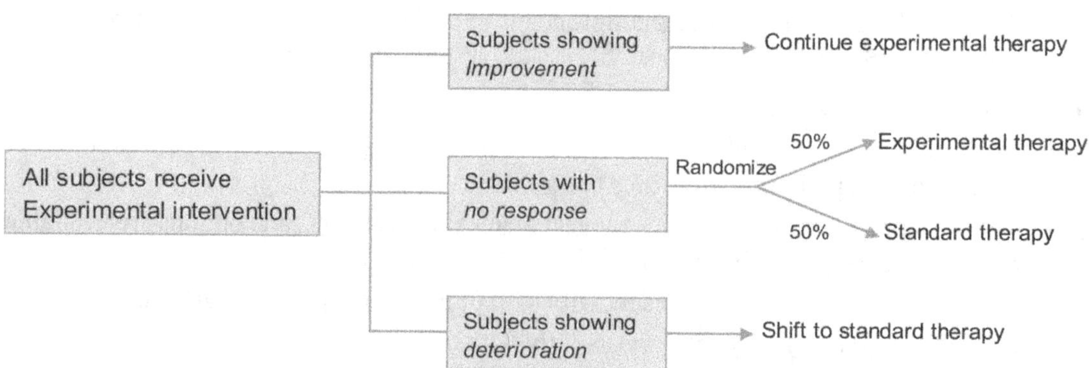

Figure 20.7 Randomized discontinuation design.

EARLY ESCAPE DESIGN

In this, subjects are withdrawn from the study on attainment of a defined level of symptoms or if there is failure of response to a defined level. The withdrawl rate can then be utilized as the measure of efficacy. This design helps in minimizing the participant's duration of exposure to placebo.

PATIENT PREFERENCE DESIGNS

These designs take into consideration the preferences of eligible subjects whether they wish to participate in trial or not. These comprise of at least one group in which the subjects are offered several options available from which they can choose their preferred treatment. Examples of preference designs include:

❖ ***Zelen's design***. In this design, eligible individuals are randomized to standard treatment or an experimental intervention before obtaining their consent for participation in trial. It can be of two subtypes:

♦ *Single randomized consent version*. Subjects randomized to standard treatment arm receive standard treatment and are not communicated about being part of a trial. Subjects who are randomized to experimental intervention arm are given the experimental intervention and told about being part of a trial; if they disagree to participate, they are given the standard treatment but are analysed as if they were randomized to experimental intervention arm (Figure 20.8).

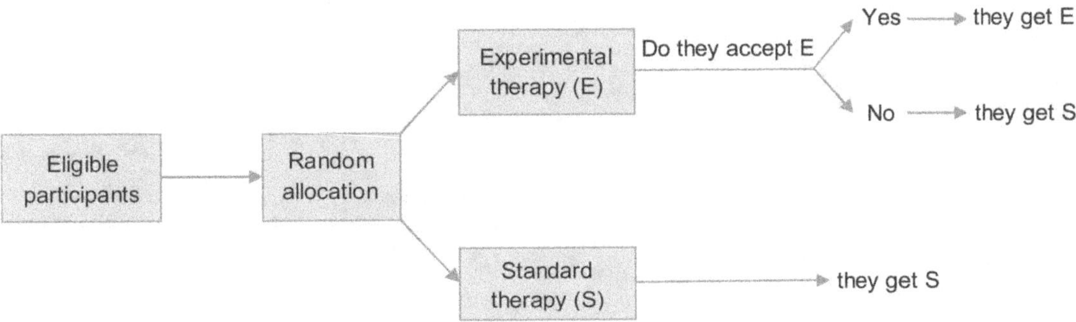

Figure 20.8 Zelen's single randomized consent design.

♦ *Double randomized consent version*. Subjects are initially offered the treatment to which they were randomised; however, if they decline the randomized treatment, they can then be offered alternative therapies—including the experimental treatment (Figure 20.9).

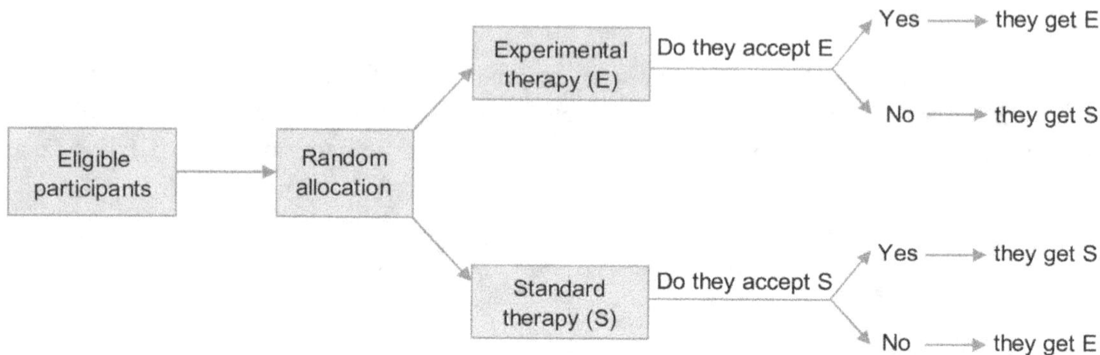

Figure 20.9 Zelen's double randomized consent design.

* ***Comprehensive cohort design.*** In this design, if a person gives consent for randomization, he or she is randomized to one of the study arms- experimental therapy (E) or standard therapy (S). If the person does not give consent to be randomized due to a strong preference for one of the interventions, he receives the preferred intervention and is followed up as if being part of a cohort study. In the end, the outcomes of people enrolled in RCT are compared with those enrolled as part of cohort studies (Figure 20.10).

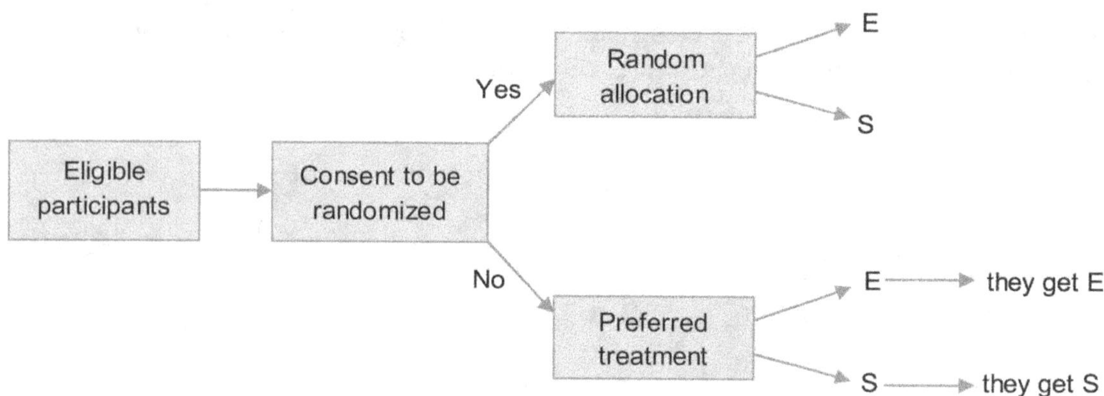

Figure 20.10 Comprehensive cohort design.

❖ **Wennberg's design.** In this, the eligible subjects are randomized to a 'preference group' or an 'RCT group'. Subjects in the preference group are given an option to receive the intervention they prefer, whereas subjects in the RCT group are randomized to any of the study groups (experimental or standard), regardless of their preference. On study completion, the outcomes observed with each intervention in both the groups are compared and the impact of subject's preferences on the outcome are estimated (Figure 20.11).

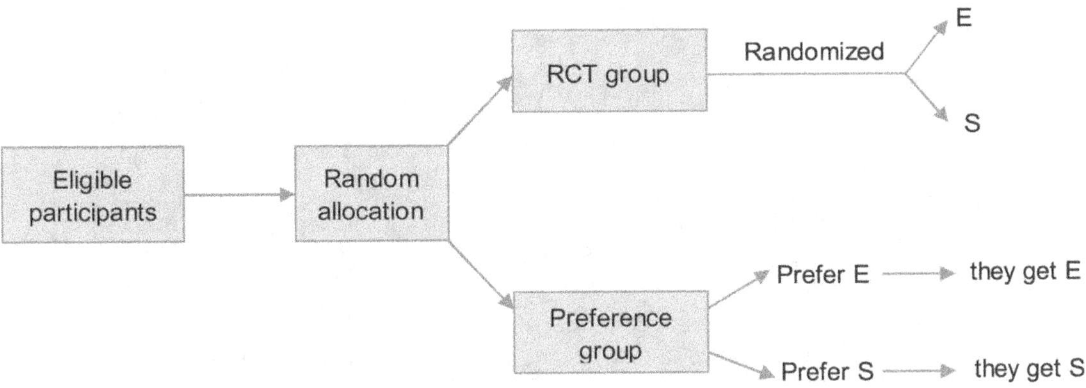

Figure 20.11 Wennberg's design.

CLUSTER / GROUP RANDOMISED DESIGNS

Randomization is performed at cluster level rather than subject level. Cluster is a group of people possessing similar characteristics e.g. school, family, hospital etc. This design is used for assessment of non-therapeutic interventions like lifestyle modification, new educational program for smoking cessation etc.

STEPPED WEDGE DESIGN

This is a pragmatic study design which may be used in trials having individuals as unit of randomization (stepped wedge trial; SWT) but is more commonly used in cluster trials (stepped wedge cluster randomized trial). In this, after an initial non-intervention period, one (or a group of) individual/ cluster is randomly and sequentially crossed over to the test intervention at fixed intervals ("steps"). This process continues till all the individuals/ clusters have been crossed over to the intervention arm. Data is gathered throughout the study so that each individual/ cluster contributes to results under both control and intervention periods (Figure 20.12).

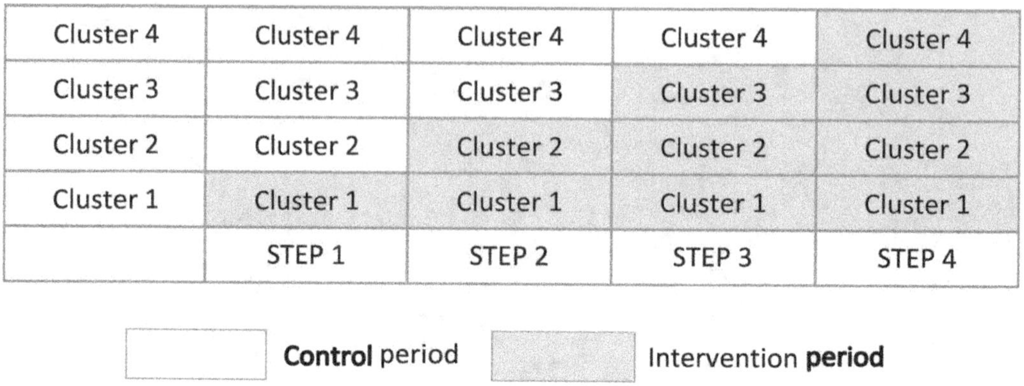

Cluster 4	Cluster 4	Cluster 4	Cluster 4	Cluster 4
Cluster 3	Cluster 3	Cluster 3	Cluster 3	Cluster 3
Cluster 2	Cluster 2	Cluster 2	Cluster 2	Cluster 2
Cluster 1	Cluster 1	Cluster 1	Cluster 1	Cluster 1
	STEP 1	STEP 2	STEP 3	STEP 4

Control period   Intervention **period**

Figure 20.12 Stepped wedge design used in a cluster randomized clinical trial.

Randomization

INTRODUCTION

The term randomization is obtained from "random" meaning chance assignment. Randomization is the process by which patients in a clinical trial are "randomly" assigned to receive one of the treatments being evaluated. As a result of randomization, all the subjects have a similar and independent opportunity of allocation to any of the intervention arms/ groups, and it is not possible to predict *a priori* about the intervention allocated to a particular subject.

Box 21.1 gives a brief history of origin of the concept of randomization in clinical research.

Box 21.1 First randomized controlled trial in history.

The credit of introducing randomization in clinical trials goes to Bradford Hill while conducting streptomycin trial in patients with tuberculosis in 1948. In this trial, a total of 55 patients were randomized to two groups: group 1 received streptomycin along with bed rest and group 2 received bed rest alone. As quoted in a published paper, *"determination of whether a patient would be treated by streptomycin and bed rest (S case) or bed rest alone (C case), was made by reference to a statistical series based on random sampling numbers drawn up for each sex at each center by Professor Bradford Hill; the details of the series were unknown to any of the investigators or to the co-coordinator and were contained in a set of sealed envelopes each bearing on the outside only the name of the hospital and a number. After acceptance of a patient by the panel and before admission to the streptomycin centre, the appropriate numbered envelope was opened at the central office; the card inside told if the patient was to be an S or C cases, and this information was then given to the medical officer at the centre"*. Bradford Hill was later awarded for his contributions in the field of science including the concept of randomization.

MERITS/JUSTIFICATION OF RANDOMIZATION

1. **Unpredictability of treatment.** It is not possible to know which treatment a particular patient will receive.
2. **Avoidance of selection/allocation bias.** Randomization ensures that treatment assignment is not influenced by patient characteristics/prognostic factors.
3. **No correlation between intervention allocation and results.** By eliminating selection bias which can have a bearing on treatment effects and other outcomes, randomization ensures that results are independent of the intervention assigned.
4. **Elimination of systematic error/confounding.** By balancing the groups in a trial for factors like subject characteristics that might bias outcomes.
5. **Consistency with probability theory.** All statistical tests are based on the probability of chance distribution of uncontrolled variables and randomization is the only method which assures this chance distribution.

DEMERITS OF RANDOMIZATION

1. Randomization alone cannot adequately exclude the differences between treatment groups e.g., an equal distribution of risk factors may not truly happen which may seriously challenge the interpretation of results obtained. This can however be minimized by using the technique of stratification.
2. Practical problems in incorporating an appropriate randomization process in a clinical trial.

TIMING OF RANDOMIZATION

The randomization code must be developed *a priori* and the preset list of treatments is utilized to prepare numbered sealed opaque envelopes which are used in sequential order to allocate the treatments. However, there are chances of bias if

- envelopes are not assigned the numbers properly,
- they are not used in pre-decided sequence,
- an envelope is opened in advance,
- any means e.g. trans-illumination are used to guess the contents

Remote allocation (e.g. IVRS - Interactive Voice Response System) helps in overcoming such drawbacks.

RANDOMIZATION TECHNIQUES (FIGURE 21.1)

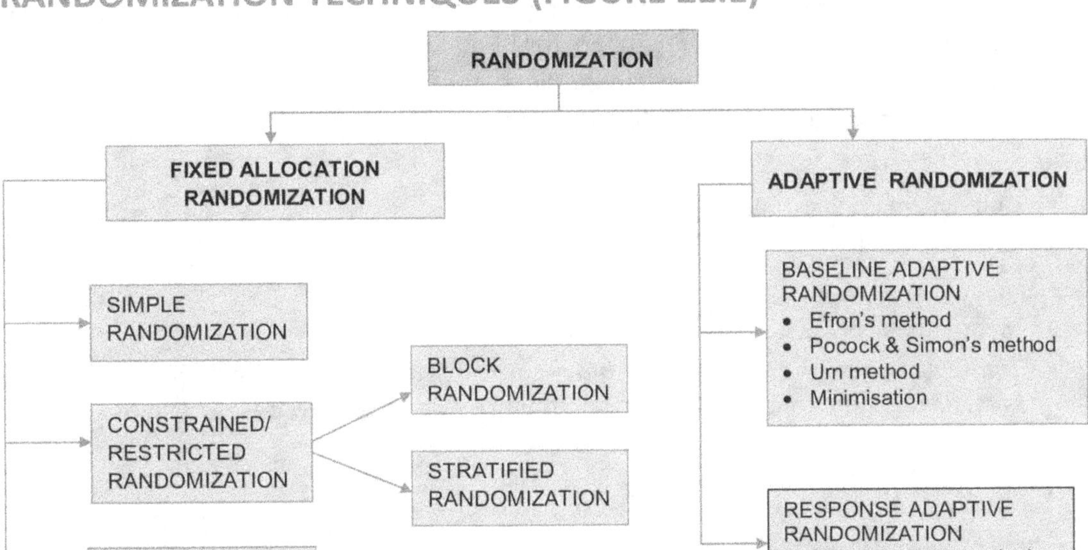

Figure 21.1 Various randomization techniques.

QUASI-RANDOMIZATION

These are some methods of randomization which are not strictly random and are generally unacceptable e.g. alternate assignments, alternate day assignments (patients entering on even number days receive one treatment and on odd days other), heads or tails on coin tosses, cards drawn by the investigator, patient initials, ballots drawn from a hat etc.

FIXED ALLOCATION RANDOMIZATION

SIMPLE RANDOMIZATION

This procedure prepares every new treatment allocation irrespective of the previous ones. The randomization code can be developed using random number tables (e.g. Fisher and Yates) or computer generated random numbers. These tables do not have any atypical sequence (e.g. systematic progression, duplicative figures etc) and all the figures appear for similar number of times on an average.

Prerequisites

- ✓ Define an "*allocation rule*" establishing a correspondence between each treatment and certain figures e.g. even numbers for treatment A.
- ✓ Numbers should always be read in the same direction.
- ✓ Avoid using same part of the table repeatedly.

Merits

- ♦ Convenient implementation
- ♦ Unpredictability

Demerits

- ♦ Inequalities between treatment groups
- ♦ *Time imbalance or chronological bias*- generally it is observed that one intervention is allocated more frequently in the beginning and another towards the end of a trial.

CONSTRAINED/ RESTRICTED RANDOMIZATION

1. Block / Permuted block randomization

This method described by Hill in 1951, helps to introduce balance in the number of subjects assigned to each treatment. A "block" contains a prespecified number and proportion of treatment assignments. The size of each block should be an integer multiple of the number of treatment groups, hence if two treatment strategies are being tested, the block size can be either 2, 4, 6, and so on

Figure 21.2 illustrates various steps required to implement block randomization.

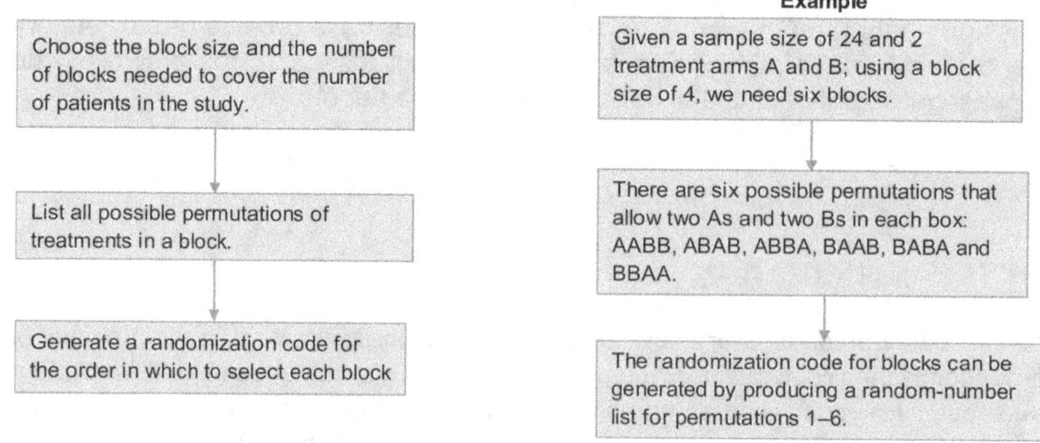

Figure 21.2 Steps in implementation of block randomization.

Merits

- ♦ Ensures balance between study groups which is particularly helpful in multi-centric and sequential design studies.

Demerits
- Complex methodology as compared to simple randomization.
- Risk of predictability: Too-short permutation series (2 or 4) enable prediction of treatment for at least the last patient in case of partial code break in a blinded study which can introduce both selection and ascertainment bias. The risk can be avoided by not reporting the size of blocks in the protocol and/or using variable sizes of the blocks.
- Risk of inequality: Too-long permutation series risk inequality in the number of patients should recruitment stop in the middle of a series.

2. **Stratified Randomization:** Assignment of patients to groups based on an appropriate variable is termed as stratification. Stratified randomization takes into consideration uneven distribution of prognostic/sub-experimental factors which introduce important differences in outcomes not due to treatments per se. The choice of strata may be based on a qualitative (e.g. sex) or a quantitative (e.g. age, blood sugar levels) variable.

Points to be considered while choosing strata
(i) The division of strata should be based on factors or variables which are expected to have a bearing on the outcome of intervention.
(ii) The strata should be independent of each other; there should be no uncertainty regarding the strata to which a subject belongs.
(iii) The boundaries between two adjacent strata must be clearly defined in case of quantitative variables to ensure reproducibility.
(iv) Two different strata should be sufficiently discriminatory i.e. different strata should correspond to supposedly different prognostic groups.
(v) Every stratum must be homogenous with regard to beneficial or adverse effects of treatments compared.
(vi) The choice of stratification factors can be made with the help of surveys, previously conducted trials or a pilot trial.

> *Note:* An ideal situation is to establish the strata and test their **prognostic significance** and **reproducibility** before the commencement of trial.

Multiple Stratification

This technique is useful when multiple relevant prognostic factors have to be included in stratification. For this, different approaches can be used as described in Figure 21.3.

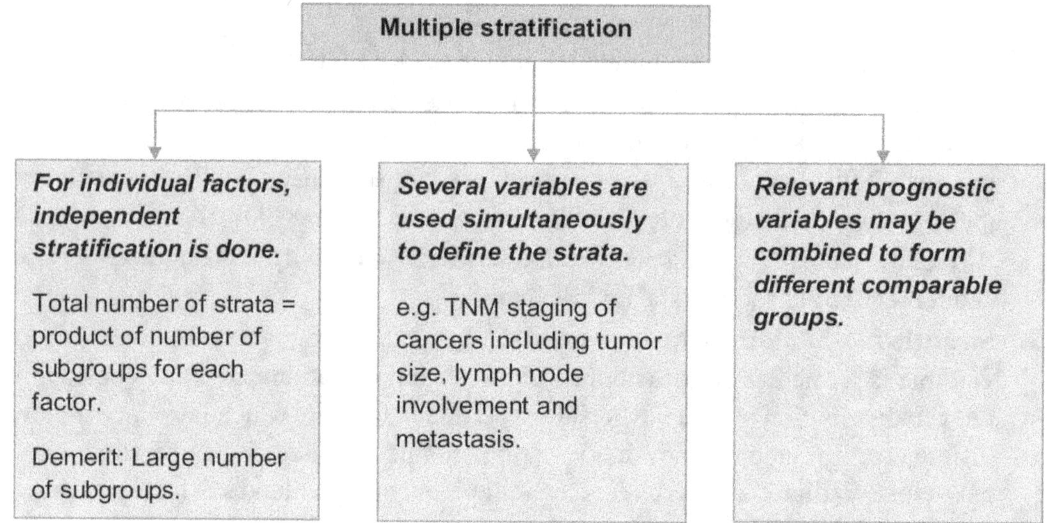

Figure 21.3 Various approaches used in multiple stratification.

Various steps needed in the implementation of stratified randomization are represented in figure 21.4.

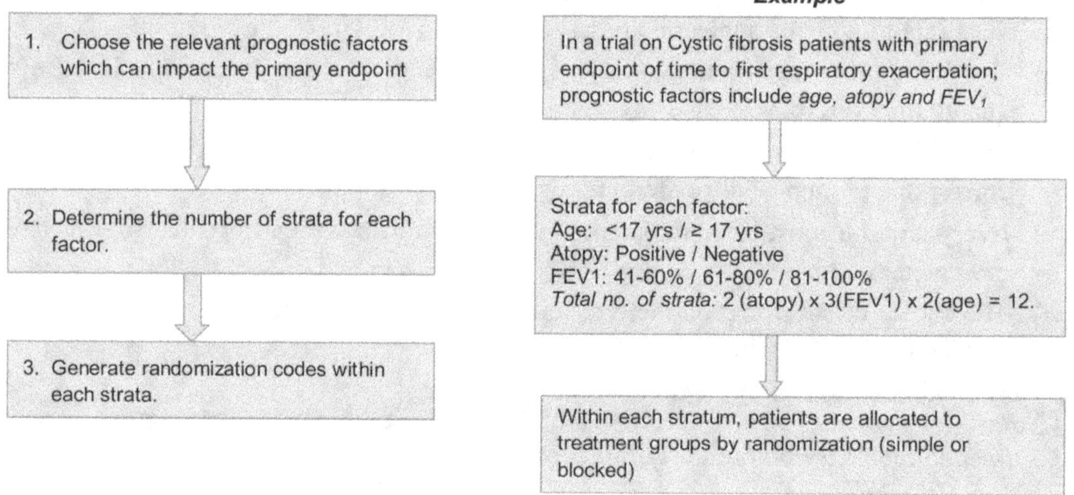

Figure 21.4 Steps in implementation of stratified randomization.

Merits of stratification

- Limits the risk of non-comparability in case of populations having unacceptable variability.
- Easier recruitment due to broader and more heterogenous inclusion.
- Broad representation with greater generalizability of results.
- More sensitive statistical comparison due to reduced variability within each stratum.
- The effect of various factors determining prognosis and their interactions can be additionally studied.

Demerits of stratification
- ♦ Only limited number of strata/ prognostic factors can be assessed.
- ♦ The efficiency of stratification is compromised if certain strata/cells have very less or no subjects. Also there are chances of unbalanced distribution of subjects between different strata.
- ♦ Practical problems like
- ✓ Requirement to separately randomize all the stratified subgroups.
- ✓ Need to prepare drug batches in excess since it is not possible to predict the number of patients in each stratum *a priori*.
- ✓ Higher risk of misallocation

SYSTEMATIC RANDOMIZATION

In this, intervention is allocated to subjects on the basis of (1) a random order in the first block, whose pattern is then repeated in all subsequent blocks; or by (2) a sequential assignment to treatment e.g. assignment of alternate treatments to patients as they are enrolled and giving a different treatment to every nth patient.

ADAPTIVE RANDOMIZATION

These are the methods which modify the likelihood of allocation as the trial proceeds to limit the imbalances.

BASELINE ADAPTIVE RANDOMIZATION

These methods balance the prognostic factors/unequal distribution between different study arms to ensure group comparability.

1. ***Efron's method (Biased coin method)***: This method takes into account a single prognostic factor. For the factor being considered, if a subject enters a stratum having equal distribution of two treatments studied, randomization is done giving each treatment 50% chance of being assigned. If, however, there is an unequal distribution between the treatments, randomization is unbalanced in favor of the group with lesser number of subjects.

2. ***Pocock and Simon's method***: This considers several prognostic factors simultaneously. A calculation (measure of imbalance) is made on the sum of the discrepancies in the number of patients (per intervention) for all the prognostic factors. Unbalanced randomization (e.g. 2:1 or 3:1) is done with precedence given to the treatment with lesser sum.

3. ***Urn method:*** Suppose there is an urn containing a black and a white ball.

   To allocate an intervention a rule is pre-decided, e.g. if on random selection there is a black ball, intervention A is allocated and for white ball, intervention B. After each use, the ball is kept back in the urn. This method is similar to simple randomization with 50% likelihood of being allocated to either intervention.

4. ***Minimization (Taves method/ Dynamic randomization):*** This method excludes formal randomization. Intervention is allocated after a series of calculations which take into consideration the characteristics of all the previously randomized subjects. Every new subject is allocated the imbalanced intervention i.e with lowest number of subjects.

RESPONSE (OUTCOME) ADAPTIVE RANDOMIZATION

These methods aim to augment the number of subjects receiving the most efficacious of the interventions compared, thus providing an ethical advantage.

1. ***Play the winner method:*** This comprises of assigning the same intervention to every new subject as long as it gives successes and switching to other treatment as soon as there is a failure. Instead of just the last result, an account of several of the earlier treatment results can also be taken into consideration ***(Isbeil's method).***

2. ***Two arm bandit method:*** This method constantly updates the likelihood of success as soon as outcome of intervention in each subject is known and assignment to either group is adjusted so that a greater proportion of future subjects would be provided currently better intervention.

CHAPTER 22

Blinding

OVERVIEW

Introduction
Justification for Blinding
Levels of Blinding
Blind Time

Assessing Validity of Double Blind Trial
Breaking the Blind
Limitations of Blinding Methods

INTRODUCTION

'***Blinding***' or '***Masking***' is defined as an experimental technique in which groups of personnel involved in conducting a trial are made unaware of which treatment the participants are assigned to.

JUSTIFICATION FOR BLINDING/MASKING

Reduction of *"bias in favor of the a priori preferred treatment"*.

- Observer bias/Assessment bias. Subjective inference of results and *heterosuggestion* i.e. better therapeutic effect with enthusiastic prescribing physician who firmly believes in worth use of (preferred) treatment.
- Patient or subject bias. Subjective inference of symptoms and *autosuggestion* i.e. therapeutic effect enhanced by 'faith'.

Regardless of study personnel's honesty, a blinded trial is usually more credible than an open label trial due to doubt of proper implementation of randomization in open label trial.

LEVELS OF BLINDING/MASKING (BOX 22.1)

1. **Open label.** No blind is used. Both investigator and patient know the identity of treatment.
2. **Single blind.** Subject or the investigator is blind to treatment (Figure 22.1).
   - ✓ Single blind trials remove only one type of bias: observer or subject bias.

Only the subject is blind/masked	•Subject receives an unknown intervention, ideally identical in appearance to other treatment/s compared, albeit different in terms of therapeutic efficacy.
Only study investigator is blind/masked	•Interventions compared not necessarily exactly indistinguishable. •Requires 2 observers: *Non-blind prescriber* (guides subject on drug administration method), *blind observer* (records data for therapeutic efficacy) •Risk of leaks: Patient may involuntarily divulge vital information to blind observer.

Figure 22.1 Single blind trials.

- ✓ Helpful in providing some degree of control when there are practical constraints in the conduct of a double blind trial.
- ✓ Preparation of perfectly identical drug formulations is technically difficult and may not be feasible always.

3. **Double blind.** Neither the subject nor any personnel in the study team are familiar with the intervention administered till the study is completed. Double blind design is generally believed to generate most credible data from a clinical trial.

   Conditions required for double blind trial
   - Interventions compared should be identical (dosage form, appearance, colour, shape, size, taste, viscosity, excipients) except for the therapeutic efficacy.
   - The code of blinded interventions should be approachable in emergency situations.
   - Stringent measures should be taken to prevent any disclosure.

4. **Triple blind.** Along with the patient and investigator, the statistician is also blind who knows the composition of groups of patients but not of treatments as long as the analysis has not been completed.

> **Box 22.1 Levels of blinding in a clinical trial.**
>
> **Complete double blind** : Keeping all the study personnel blind who come in direct contact with *the subject* (including staff and healthcare personnel etc.)
>
> **Complete triple blind**: Keeping everyone blind who comes in direct contact with *the subject or investigator* (e.g. monitor, statistician, data and safety monitoring board etc.)
>
> **Total clinical trial blind.** Keeping everyone blind who comes in direct contact with *the subject, investigator or the data* (including pathologists, radiologists who interpret the results etc.)

BLIND TIME

This is proposed for

- ❖ **Psychotropic drugs.** Subject's interview is recorded on video tape, successive interviews are then presented to the observer in random order so that he is not influenced from one test to another by knowing the results of the preceding tests.
- ❖ **Pharmacokinetic studies.** Assays are made in coded tubes for which the chronological order of sample collection is not known.

ASSESSING VALIDITY OF DOUBLE BLIND TRIAL

- ✓ *Before the trial initiation,* the blind is "validated" by taking into consideration its implementation and maintenance along with a review of the factors which may challenge or break the blind during the trial. This helps in determining whether a sound system of blinding has been created in the trial.
- ✓ *During the trial conduct,* monitor evaluates how the blinding is maintained. If it is apparent that blinding is not appropriately implemented, amendments or modifications can be incorporated in the protocol to intensify the blind.
- ✓ *After the trial completion,* the subjects and investigators may be asked to predict which intervention was allocated to each subject.

> Generally, it is recommended to conduct an open label trial instead of a hypocritical, inappropriate, poorly validated and poorly maintained double blind trial where the interventions have been made detectable by 'disclosures' or by their peculiar properties.

BREAKING THE BLIND

In emergency situations like attempted suicide or accidental over dosage, need for general anesthesia etc., blind for individual patient needs to be broken. Few methods for breaking the blind are:

Tamper-proof opaque envelopes. A series of numbered envelopes are prepared beforehand to facilitate early identification of the intervention allocated to a particular subject. Hence, breaking the code for one subject will not reveal the intervention given to other subjects. All the envelopes opened should be immediately signed and dated and the concerned authorities be informed. It is however prudent to ensure that envelopes should not be effortlessly opened by steam and closed again and the contents should not be readily evident by trans-illumination.

Advent calendar. Pieces of thin cardboard having numerous, small removable windows each permitting the code to be broken for one subject at a time, can also be used.

LIMITATIONS OF BLINDING METHODS

1. **Problems in blinding of drugs**
  + **Pharmaceutical issues.** The production and matching of placebo and blinded controls with active treatment demands a substantial pharmaceutical effort. A placebo can be made to resemble an active treatment but complications occur when two or more active treatments being compared have non-identical appearance, route or schedule of administration. This problem can be overcome by:

    Reformulation of the drug by altering the pharmaceutical form to resemble another, which however requires demonstration of bioequivalence and is usually not recommended.

    Double-dummy technique. In case of two dissimilar comparators A and B, double blinding can be achieved by administering intervention A with placebo of B, and B with placebo of A. Each subject hence receives two treatments concurrently, an active treatment and a placebo, and the two treatment groups are identical. This technique has the *drawback* of administering an increased number of treatment units to the subjects.
  + **Technical issues.** If one of the study interventions is a drug requiring dosage adjustments according to some predetermined criteria, double blind trial is difficult to be performed. To handle this, adjustment can be made for placebo doses as well or dosage adjustments can be made by a separate non-blind observer.
  + **Regulatory issues.** The stringent laws and regulations regarding the manufacture, quality control and management of marketed drugs are also applicable to placebos, active controls and experimental interventions utilized in clinical trials and should be adequately complied with.

2. Feasibility

- In long duration trials, the problem of maintenance of blind and especially the risk of any disclosures makes the success of a double blind trial more speculative.
- There may be practical issues in blinding the personnel administering the intervention e.g. trials having randomized groups like device implantation versus no device, sham procedure versus actual procedure etc.

Bias

OVERVIEW

INTRODUCTION

Bias is defined as a '*systematic error*' entering into a clinical trial and distorting the data generated. It may be a prejudice or leaning of one's opinion favoring one side of a question or issue too strongly before there are adequate data to support the conclusion or viewpoint. Bias is different from '*random error*' which occurs by chance and can be reduced by increasing sample size. Bias is independent of sample size.

Bias may also be defined as tendency of a sample to be non representative of all patients or data in the trial.

SOURCES OF BIAS IN A CLINICAL TRIAL

- ♦ Bias may enter a trial either because of a factor or belief that is introduced or a factor or belief that is omitted.
- ♦ It may be introduced purposely or may appear due to ignorance.
- ♦ Anyone associated with the clinical trial (sponsor, monitor, investigator, subject) may influence the result and introduce bias.
- ♦ Bias may be introduced into a clinical trial in the planning, conduct or analysis.
- Examining literature.
- Describing and choosing clinical trial sample.

- Administering the experimental intervention.
- Assessment of exposures and outcomes.
- Data analysis and interpretation.
- Publication of results.

PROBLEMS WITH BIAS

- Interpretations of the trial results likely to be challenged.
- Leads to underestimation or overestimation of efficacy or safety.

METHODS TO REDUCE/ AVOID BIAS

- It is essential to recognize bias and decrease or at least recognize the influence it has on interpretation of results.
- Steps to ensure minimization of bias include:
  - Knowledge about the recognizable biases
  - Ability to recognize bias
  - Modification or qualification of interpretations to account for and minimize bias
  - When it is not possible to eliminate bias, define the relevant bias so that it can be considered when conclusions are drawn from a trial
  - Randomized, controlled trial has the greatest probability of reducing bias and should be the preferred design whenever possible
  - Well designed prospective trials yield less biased, more scientifically acceptable data than do comparable retrospective trials
  - Objectivity results in fewer biases than subjectivity

EXAMPLES OF BIAS

An excellent list of biases (57 biases) was assembled by Sackett (1979). Below are mentioned some examples of biases.

1. **Biases in reading up on the field**
- ***Biases of rhetoric:*** Any of the strategies followed to persuade the reader in the absence of a satisfactory reason.
- ***One-sided reference bias:*** Restriction of the references to only those which support them.

- ***Positive results bias:*** Higher likelihood of submitting and accepting positive results than null or negative ones.
- ***Hot stuff bias:*** For current topics, inability to resist publishing additional results even if preliminary or indefinite.

2. Biases in describing and choosing the study sample

- ***Centripetal bias:*** Inclination of the patients with specific disorders towards some reputed clinicians and institutions.
- ***Referral filter bias:*** On referral of ill patients from primary to secondary to tertiary care settings, there is an increase in the number of rare disorders, multiple diagnoses etc.
- ***Diagnostic access bias:*** Variability in access to diagnostic procedures due to geographical, temporal and economic differences.
- ***Diagnostic suspicion bias:*** Knowledge of the individual's previous exposure to an apparent cause may have a bearing on the intensity and outcome of diagnostic procedure.
- ***Diagnostic vogue bias:*** The same disorder may have different diagnostic criteria at different places or different points in time.
- ***Mimicry bias:*** A trivial unidentified exposure may become evident if, instead of causing an illness, it causes a disorder resembling the illness in question.
- ***Wrong sample size bias:*** Too small sample size can prove nothing; too large sample size can prove everything.
- ***Admission rate (Berkson) bias:*** In hospital-based studies, if there is difference in the rate of hospitalization in different exposure disease groups, the relation between exposure and outcome will be deformed and non informatory.
- ***Prevalence-incidence (Neyman) bias:*** A delayed observation of those exposed (or affected) early will omit fatal or other short lasting illnesses.
- ***Missing clinical data bias:*** Clinical data may be missing due to being normal, negative, never evaluated, or evaluated but never documented.
- ***Unacceptable disease bias:*** Disorders associated with social stigma are liable to be underreported.
- ***Migrator bias:*** Systematic differences in migrants from non-migrants.
- ***Volunteer bias:*** Variability in exposures or outcomes between volunteers or 'early comers' and non-volunteers or 'late comers'.
- ***Selection bias:*** Patients may be recruited by the investigator in a manner that introduces bias in data e.g. the recruited subjects may differ from other subjects with the disease in terms of prognosis.

3. Biases in administering the experimental intervention (or exposure)

- ***Contamination bias:*** If subjects in control group accidentally receive the experimental intervention, there may be a systematic diminution of difference in outcomes between experimental and control groups.

- ***Compliance bias:*** In studies demanding a good compliance of subjects to intervention(s) administered, compliance issues may confound the efficacy assessment.
- ***Withdrawal bias:*** Patients being withdrawn from an intervention may have systematic differences from those who continue to receive intervention.
- ***Therapeutic personality bias:*** In open label trials, the investigator's beliefs about efficacy may systematically affect the outcomes (positive personality) as well as their assessment (desire for positive outcome).
- ***Bogus control bias:*** When subjects randomized to an experimental intervention die or worsen clinically before or during its administration and are withdrawn or re-randomized to control group, the experimental intervention will misleadingly appear superior.

4. Biases in the assessment of exposures and outcomes

- ***Insensitive measure bias:*** Incapability of the outcome measures to detect clinically significant changes.
- ***Rumination bias (underlying cause bias):*** Subjects may ruminate (think) about suspected causes for their disorders and thus recall previous exposures differently from controls.
- ***End-digit preference bias:*** During conversion of analog to digital data, there is recording of some terminal digits with an abnormal frequency by the observer.
- ***Apprehension bias:*** Certain variables (pulse, BP) may change systematically from their typical values in anxious subjects.
- ***Unacceptability bias:*** Evasion or refusal of hurting, embarrassing or privacy invading measurements.
- ***Recall bias:*** Questions regarding particular exposures may be asked repeatedly to cases but not to controls.
- ***Instrument bias:*** Errors in instruments' calibration or their maintenance may cause systematized deviations from actual values.
- ***Attention bias:*** Systematic alteration in study subjects behavior if they are aware of being observed.
- ***Obsequiousness bias:*** Systematic alteration in questionnaire responses by subjects towards the investigator' choice.
- ***Information bias:*** The information provided to investigators by subjects is determined by their own beliefs and values.
- ***Observer bias:*** The subjectivity of investigators evaluating the magnitude of subject responses is highly variable, even for tests having objective endpoints.
- ***Interviewer bias:*** The interviewer's expectations, appearance, manner of asking questions, accent etc. often influence the respondent's answers and recording of information.
- ***Regression dilution bias:*** This is related to 'regression to the mean' phenomenon and is seen in longitudinal studies which investigate association between assessment of a continuous variable and risk of occurrence of a given outcome.

5. Biases in data analysis

- ***Post hoc significance bias:*** Selecting the decision levels or tails for alpha and beta after data examination may bias the conclusions.
- ***Data dredging bias (looking for the pony):*** Reviewing the data for all possible associations with no *a priori* hypothesis.
- ***Tidying-up bias:*** Bias arising due to exclusion of outliers or other unclean results; not statistically justified.

6. Biases in interpretation of results

- ***Magnitude bias:*** Interpretation of an observation may be influenced by the scale of measurement.
- ***Significance bias:*** The conflict between statistical significance and clinical or healthcare significance may lead to invalid conclusions.
- ***Cognitive dissonance bias:*** Increased belief in a specific mechanism in the presence of contradictory evidence.

CHAPTER 24

Compliance in Clinical Trials

OVERVIEW

Introduction
Types of Compliance
Reasons for Non-Compliance
Measuring and Evaluating Patient Compliance
  Direct Methods
  Indirect Methods

Consequences of Non-Compliance/
Poor Compliance
Strategies to Improve Compliance
Keeping Compliance into
Consideration during Data Analysis

INTRODUCTION

Patient compliance in clinical trials is described as the adherence of patients to taking their medicines as prescribed as well as avoidance of prohibited substances. The two terms compliance and adherence are usually used interchangeably. *Compliance (with protocol)* may additionally also be described from the perspective of investigators, sponsors or other personnel involved in the clinical trial. It is important to measure compliance of both patients and investigators before the interpretation of results of a clinical trial as negative results can be due to inactive medicine as such or inadequate compliance (patient/study personnel).

TYPES OF COMPLIANCE

Compliance can also be described in terms of problems of omission/ commission (Fig. 24.1).

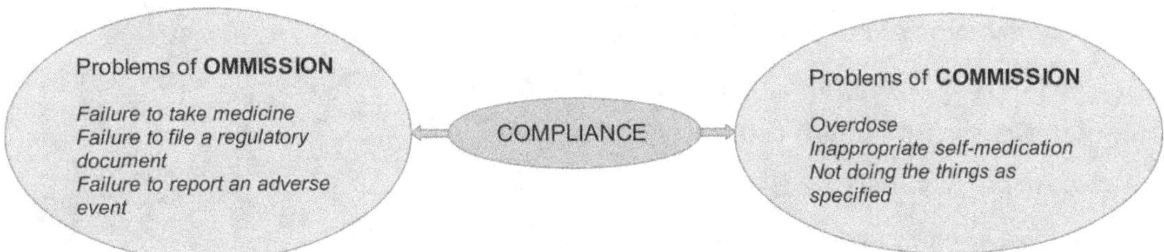

Figure 24.1 Types of Compliance.

REASONS FOR NON-COMPLIANCE

Numerous factors related to disease, patient, treatment, investigator or study may be responsible for inadequate patient compliance (Table 24.1).

Table 24.1 Reasons for poor patient compliance.

1. Disease related reasons

- *Mild condition*
- *Terminal illness accompanied by physical debility*

2. Patient related reasons

- *Forgetfulness*
- *Lack of belief in treatment*
- *Mental illness*
- *Misunderstanding of prescribing instructions*
- *Anger at or dissatisfaction with the investigator or his staff*
- *Multiple comorbidties*

3. Medicine related reasons

- *Poor taste of medicine*
- *Size of tablet or capsules*
- *Cost of therapy*
- *Adverse reactions*

4. Study related reasons

- *Complexity of treatment schedules e.g number of daily doses, number of pills in each dosing*
- *Large number of drugs prescribed*
- *Long duration of therapy*
- *Inconvenient or restrictive precautions*
- *Stressful or demanding protocol requirements*

5. Investigator/Physician related reasons

- *Poor patient-physician relationship*
- *Failure of physician to keep appointment*
- *Long waiting hours for the patient*

MEASURING AND EVALUATING PATIENT COMPLIANCE

Compliance can be measured directly or indirectly.

DIRECT METHODS

1. ***Supervising drug intake.*** The most direct method of assessing compliance is to observe the patients taking their medication.

    Disadvantages:
    - Limited to inpatient trials or those outpatient trials requiring patients to visit to clinic to take medicine.
    - Lack of surety of patient actually swallowing the drug e.g. patient keeping the drug in oral cavity and later spitting it out, self induced vomiting to eliminate the swallowed drug.

2. ***Assaying the drug in biological fluids.*** The levels of drug or metabolite can be measured directly in plasma/ urine or under special circumstances in other biological fluids like sweat, breath or saliva.

    Advantage:
    - More objective method of assessing compliance.
    - Not dependent on patient's memory.

    Disadvantages:
    - Drugs with long half-life (>24 hrs): Presence of drug in biological fluid does not confirm compliance as recent doses might have been skipped.
    - Drugs with short half-life: A non-compliant patient may ingest the drug shortly before clinic visit and thus its presence in blood /urine does not confirm compliance.
    - Not applicable to placebo.
    - Technical difficulties in performing the assay.
    - Inconvenience to the patient.
    - Cost issues

3. ***Biological markers.*** Markers/ tracers added to the drug in small amounts can also serve as means of measuring compliance when assays to estimate the levels of drug/ metabolites are unavailable. The marker used must be
    - ✓ nontoxic at the dose added.
    - ✓ chemically stable in biological fluids.
    - ✓ pharmacologically inert.
    - ✓ easily detected at levels used by methods that are sensitive and specific.
    - ✓ absorption and kinetic parameters similar to the drug to which added.
    - ✓ unaffected by food or other medicines used.
    - ✓ patient should be unaware of its use.

Examples of markers: phenol red, fluorescein, bromide, drugs in trace amounts like riboflavin, phenobarbital, isoniazid, digoxin etc.

Disadvantages:

- Imparts information only regarding the most recent dose taken although that may be the only one taken or only one forgotten.
- Need to prepare a special drug formulation in some cases which carries a risk of altered bioavailability.

4. ***Spot checks on patients.*** In this method, a member of the clinical team makes unannounced visits to patients at their homes and collects the biological fluids for estimating the drug levels. However, the agreement of patients to this procedure should be part of the informed consent.

Disadvantages:

- Potential invasion of patient's privacy.
- Technically feasible only for patients who live relatively close to the clinical trial site.

5. ***Clinic attendance.*** If compliance is assessed in terms of clinic attendance, then examining the records of clinic attendance is a direct method to assess compliance.

INDIRECT METHODS

These methods depend on patient's reports or on data that could be modified by the patient. The extrapolation of acceptable compliance from data gathered with some of these methods may thus be unwarranted.

1. ***Pill counts.*** Most commonly used method. The subjects are provided with bottles containing excess tablets or capsules believing that there should be some remaining at the next visit. The actual number of tablets or capsules in the medicine container used by the patient are counted at each (or selected) clinic visits, and the expected number to be used is also determined.

$$\% \ Compliance \ = \ \frac{Actual \ pill \ use}{Expected \ pill \ use} \times 100$$

Compliance results obtained by pill counts have been reported to demonstrate good agreement with those of tracer studies.

2. ***Electronic counters.*** Electronic counters in the tops of specially prepared medicine bottles have been developed that record the exact day, hour and minute each time the medicine bottle is opened or used.

Advantages:

- The best method to measure compliance in outpatient trials.
- Overall compliance between two visits measured.
- Also assesses the regularity of compliance over time.
- Data are easily quantifiable and expressed.

Disadvantages:

- Does not ensure ingestion of an appropriate number of tablets each time the bottle is opened.
- Patients may purposely fool the system e.g. open the lid large or small number of times.
- Inadvertent invalidation of data by patient e.g. putting medicine in other containers, removing extra medicine for later dosing.
- Expensive approach and hence impractical for large trials.

3. *Medication monitors.* Medicine bottles containing either the precise number of pills for a daily dose or a standard number of pills may be placed into a mechanical device called a "medication monitor" e.g. mechanical dispensers. The patient is advised to operate the machine to obtain medication but is not told that number of bottles is being monitored. This method is generally adopted in inpatient trials.

4. *RFID-enabled computer chip technology.* In this system, a microprocessor is included in the bottle cap. Opening of bottle activates a mechanical spring forming an electronic circuit and the whole process is recorded as an event. When subject brings the package back to the physician, data from the microprocessor can be downloaded onto a computer and thus helps in assessing compliance in an efficient and timely manner. The main drawback includes high cost of technology. MEMS (micro-electro-mechanical systems) caps and smart blister packs e.g. Medicaid, Cypak, Cerepak etc. also work on the same principle.

5. *Assessment based on clinical response.* The patient is assumed to be compliant if he or she improves on the active treatment, or does not improve on placebo.

6. *Physiological markers.* In certain trials, physiological markers may be used as indirect indicators of patient compliance. e.g. measuring heart rate in patients receiving beta-blockers.

7. *Patient interview.* This is the simplest and most unambiguous method to determine the extent to which the drug was taken adequately. The interview should be conducted with judgement and understanding in order to obtain honest answers. An apprehensive attitude of the investigator can generate false answers. The simplest method is to ask the subject "Are you taking all of your medicine?" or "Have you missed taking any of your medicine?". A preset questionnaire may also be used to enhance uniformity.

8. *Pharmacy refills.* Pharmacy records demonstrate whether patients fill and refill their prescriptions at appropriate intervals, thus providing another method to assess compliance. However, obtaining refills of medicine as per a set schedule does not ensure ingestion of those medicines on schedule.

> The most reliable method to measure compliance for research purposes may be a *combination approach* including various strategies together like pill counts, patient self-report/ interview and electronic monitoring.

CONSEQUENCES OF NON-COMPLIANCE/ POOR COMPLIANCE

- *Invalid study results*. An ineffective medicine may be declared effective and vice versa.
- *Introduction of bias* if non-compliance is more common in one treatment group compared to other.
- *Inadequate data on adverse events*.
- *Inappropriate dosage labeling*. Dosage recommendations in package inserts based on patients with average rate of compliance may be inappropriate for patients with total as well as poor compliance.
- *Issues in extrapolation of study results*. Positive data regarding a medicine effectiveness obtained in compliant patients may not be extrapolated to noncompliant patients and vice versa.

STRATEGIES TO IMPROVE COMPLIANCE

1. **Simplification of the treatment. e.g.**
   - ✓ Small number of daily doses.
   - ✓ Flexible dosing regimens.
   - ✓ Simple-to-recognize dosage forms to avoid the risk of confusion with concomitant medications.
   - ✓ Practical unit packaging especially adapted for the treatment prescribed.
2. **Patient motivation**
   - ✓ Convincing the patient regarding the need for treatment.
   - ✓ Create fear about consequences of noncompliance.
   - ✓ Educate patients about their diseases.
   - ✓ Using the LEARN framework: L- Listen with empathy, E- Explore and understand patient belief, A-Acknowledge difference in beliefs between clinician and patient, R-Recommend treatment, N- Negotiate an agreement.
3. **Proper instructions to improve understanding**
   - ✓ Simple instructions in easily understandable language (KISS rule: Keep It Short and Simple).
   - ✓ Asking patients to repeat what they are told to ensure adequate transmission of message.
   - ✓ Provide written instructions particularly for details that cannot be easily remembered.
   - ✓ Provide pictorial instructions for illiterate patients.
   - ✓ Clear labeling of medicine containers and appropriate packaging.

4. **Tailor reminders to patients e.g.**
   - ✓ Memory aids using a calendar with detachable sheets.
   - ✓ Self adhesive labels displayed at an easily accessible site.
   - ✓ Alarms that ring at preset intervals.
   - ✓ Telephone calls from relatives or friends.
   - ✓ Automatic telephone calls with computerized voice reminders.

5. **Feasible study procedures**
   - ✓ Simplify the demands of the protocol on patients.
   - ✓ Minimize the number and duration of unpleasant or painful tests.
   - ✓ Plan patient visits at a mutually convenient time.
   - ✓ Involve the patient's spouse, family, or support group in the trial.

6. **Improve the physician-patient relationship**
   - ✓ Educate physicians about the importance of being sympathetic and caring with the patients.
   - ✓ Maintain relatively frequent contact with the patients especially during emotionally or physically difficult periods.
   - ✓ Have patients see the same physician at each visit.

KEEPING COMPLIANCE INTO CONSIDERATION DURING DATA ANALYSIS

- ♦ *"Intention to treat"* analysis is the gold standard. It is generally not recommended to exclude "non-compliers" from the analysis.
- ♦ Comparison of compliance rates between different intervention groups in the study can be done. This may reveal variability in the acceptance rate of treatments between various groups which may indirectly account for observed differences in efficacy and tolerability.
- ♦ Within each treatment group, efficacy and tolerability can be compared between compliers and non-compliers. For this, a clear definition of compliers (e.g. patients taking at least 75% of the prescribed drug) and non-compliers must be included in the protocol.

Clinical Trial Monitoring

OVERVIEW

Introduction
Purpose of Trial Monitoring
Regulatory Requirements for Monitoring
Monitor/Clinical Research Associate
Qualifications of Monitor
Roles and Responsibilities of Monitor

On-Site Monitoring Visits
Pre-study Visit/Site Feasibility Visit
Periodic Monitoring Visits
during the Study Conduct
Study Initiation Visit
End of Study/Study Close Out/Closure Visit
Documentation of Monitoring Visits

INTRODUCTION

Clinical trial monitoring is an act to supervise a clinical trial through its progress, and to ensure that it is executed, recorded, and reported in compliance with the protocol, standard operating procedures, Good Clinical Practice, and the relevant regulatory requirements.

PURPOSE OF TRIAL MONITORING

To establish and ensure that
- The rights, safety and well being of trial participants are safeguarded.
- The data reported is authentic, complete and consistent with source documents.
- The trial execution is according to the currently approved protocol/amendment(s), GCP, and applicable regulatory requirement(s).

REGULATORY REQUIREMENTS FOR MONITORING

- The sponsors are responsible to ensure an adequate and timely monitoring of the trial in order to assure that the trial is conducted in compliance with the investigational plan and protocol.
- The sponsor appoints a monitor appropriately qualified, trained and experienced to oversee the progress of trial.

MONITOR/CLINICAL RESEARCH ASSOCIATE

A person selected by the sponsor or contract research organization (CRO) to monitor and report the conduct of a clinical trial. The monitor serves as the major communication connection between the sponsor and investigator.

QUALIFICATIONS OF MONITOR

- A monitor should be adequately qualified with respect to relevant medical, pharmaceutical and/or scientific areas and possess appropriate experience in clinical trials.
- He/she should be adequately trained and should have a sound scientific and/or clinical knowledge in order to monitor the trial properly.
- He/she should be conversant with all characteristics of the investigational product and protocol (including its annexes and amendments).

ROLES AND RESPONSIBILITIES OF MONITOR (FIGURE 25.1)

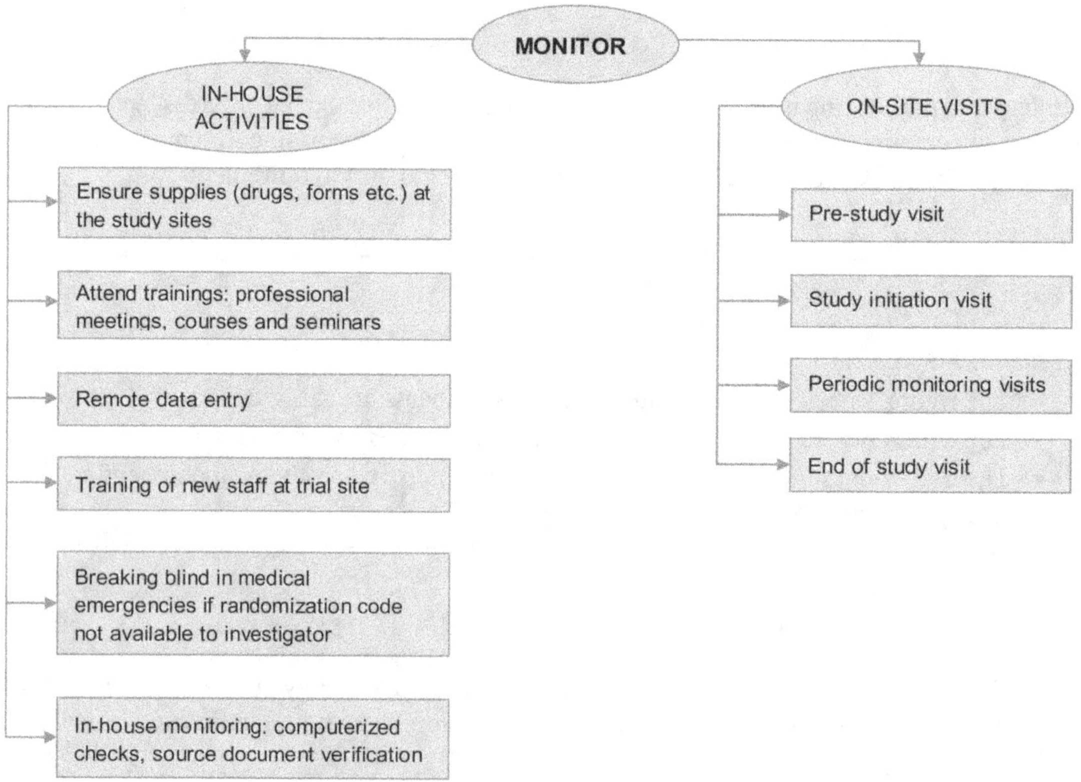

Figure 25.1 Roles and responsibilities of monitor.

ON-SITE MONITORING VISITS

The monitor should perform activites according to a pre- defined written set of SOPs. There should be a written record of the monitor's visits, phone calls and any other communication with the investigators and other involved parties.

- ❖ **Pre-study visit/Site feasibility visit.** A visit that is conducted at the potential study site to assess the qualifications of the potential investigator and his/her study site team, and to determine if the site facilities meet study requirements. During this visit, the monitor should confirm that
  - the investigator(s) have the required qualifications, expertise and facilities to carry out the study.
  - the investigator(s) are available throughout the study period.
  - all personnel providing assistance to the investigator during study conduct are informed about and will abide by the protocol, SOPs and other study details.
  - facilities at the institution for example premises, laboratories, equipment, staff, storage space etc. are adequate to conduct the study in safe and proper manner.
  - reasonable number of subjects are expected to be recruited in the study.
- ❖ **Study initiation visit.** A visit made prior to subject enrollment to verify
  - a study site's readiness to conduct a study,
  - availability of required documentation and supplies,
  - study site team preparedness to enroll subjects and conduct the study according to the protocol.
- ❖ **Periodic monitoring visits during the study conduct.** The monitor should visit the site as early as possible after first subject has been enrolled. The frequency of site visits may depend on:
  - o Study design.
  - o Length and complexity of study.
  - o Recruitment rate.
  - o Site's compliance with protocol.
  - o Site's experience with clinical research.

Various activities conducted by monitor during periodic visits are related to:

Subject/ participant status
- Consider the strategies to recruit subjects.
- Confirm the status of subjects enrolled in study.
- Verify the eligibility of enrolled subjects.
- Ensure the implementation of randomization procedures correctly
- Ensure that blinding to intervention is maintained.
- Check consent forms of all subjects for completeness.

Study supplies, handling, management and accountability

- Ensure adequate availability of study drugs/ interventions.
- Assess the expiry of study drugs/ interventions.
- Ensure completeness and correctness of receiving and dispensing records.
- Meet with personnel dispensing study drugs/interventions for any issues.
- Inspect storage premises and facilities (secured with restricted access).
- Check the process of dose calculation and preparation of dosage forms if required.

Regulatory aspects

- Examine the study files for presence of all essential documents (signed protocol, any protocol amendments, informed consent form, IRB/IEC approval and communication/s).
- Ensure ongoing and periodic IRB/IEC notifications/ reporting as required.
- Assure compliance with informed consent procedures and availability of a valid consent form for every participant.
- Gather any new or revised information pertinent to regulatory issues.

Laboratory aspects

- Assess laboratory requirements as specified in protocol.
- Examine the laboratory certificates for applicable dates.
- Ensure adequate management of all laboratory specimens.
- Resolve any issues regarding collection of samples or functioning of central, site or core laboratories.

Responsibilities of site study staff

- Oversee the responsibilities of site study staff and any changes in staff or responsibilities from last monitoring visit.
- Provide training to site personnel as and when required including new study personnel, any modification in study conduct like a protocol amendment or any modifications introduced in study procedures.

Review of serious adverse events (SAE)

- Assess all SAEs reported at the site.
- Collect additional information on SAEs as required.
- Ensure an accurate and appropriate reporting of all SAEs.

Source document / data review

- Verify the consistency of recorded data with source documents.
- Examine the data for any incorrect entries, omissions and outliers.
- Review the source documents for compliance with protocol.
- In paper- based trials, collect all the original copies of filled data forms.
- Generate pertinent queries related to data.
- Acquire suitable responses to unresolved data queries.

Outstanding matters
- Discuss the actions needed to be taken by site and /or sponsor for outstanding matters.

Meeting with Principal Investigator (PI) and Clinical Research Coordinator (CRC)
- Discuss the overall progression of trial.
- Discuss emerging concerns that may potentially affect subject safety/ trial execution.
- Discuss pending matters and actions needed to be taken by site and/or sponsor.
- Sign the site visit log.
- ❖ **End of study/study close out/closure visit.** The final monitoring visit conducted to discuss closure procedures with the investigator and study staff. This visit takes place in a timely manner after the last subject has completed the study. During a study close-out visit, monitor may:
  - ✓ discuss timeframes and approaches for resolving outstanding issues and queries;
  - ✓ check the return or destruction of unutilized test product/s;
  - ✓ gather the incomplete subject data forms and other forms related to study like site visit log and screening logs;
  - ✓ carry out a final examination of study file documents;
  - ✓ discuss the strategies for record archival;
  - ✓ discuss the approaches to notify principal investigator and participants of study results.

DOCUMENTATION OF MONITORING VISITS

After conducting each site visit, the monitor discusses the observations, problems and areas of concern with the PI and CRC. Prior to leaving the site, the monitor should sign and date the site visit log, the document maintaining a record of monitoring visits at the site. The name of monitor, dates of visit, and the motive of visit (e.g. pre-study, initiation, periodic or end of study visit) are recorded by monitor on the site visit logs which are kept in the site study file.

Site visit report. The monitor should submit an extensive site visit report (also known as a "trip report") to the sponsor or sponsor-assignee after each site visit and after all telephonic communications, letters and other correspondence with the investigator. Monitor's report should include
- ✓ the date,
- ✓ name of site,
- ✓ names of the monitor and the personnel contacted,
- ✓ a synopsis of what was reviewed by the monitor,
- ✓ observations, deviations & deficiencies observed, and
- ✓ any actions taken / proposed to ensure compliance.

The review and follow-up of the monitoring report should be documented by the sponsor or his appointed representative.

Follow-up letter to the PI. The monitor makes a summary of the findings and sends a follow-up letter or progress report to the PI at the study site. The PI and CRC examine the letter to ensure their agreement with the documented observations and recommendations to resolve deficits or remedial measures, if any. The follow-up letter has to be maintained in the site study file.

CHAPTER 26

Data and Safety Monitoring Boards

OVERVIEW

Introduction
Determining the Need for a DSMB
DSMB Establishment and Operation
DSMB Composition
Standard Operating Procedures of DSMB

Responsibilities of DSMB
Interim Monitoring
Other Responsibilities
Independence of the DSMB

INTRODUCTION

A clinical trial data and safety monitoring board (DSMB) is an assembly of experts which periodically reviews the accruing data from single or multiple ongoing clinical trials. DSMB renders advice to the sponsor on matters related to safety of trial participants and credibility and scientific rationale of the trial.

DSMB is also known as Data Monitoring Committee (DMC) or Data and Safety Monitoring Committee (DSMC).

DETERMINING THE NEED FOR A DSMB

There are several factors associated mainly to safety, feasibility and scientific integrity which need to be considered while ascertaining the requirement for establishing DSMB for a particular trial.

- DSMBs are often established for large, multi-centric studies usually aiming to evaluate the interventions assumed to increase life expectancy or diminish the risk of a major adverse event like cardiovascular event.
- DSMBs are usually considered for any controlled trial comparing the rates of mortality or major morbidity.
- DSMBs are not generally required in early studies such as Phase 1 or early Phase 2 studies, or pilot/feasibility studies. However, the need of a DSMB to oversee safety may be considered when the anticipated risks to subjects are unusually high e.g. use of novel approaches in clinical trials.

- They are often not established for trials evaluating less serious outcomes like alleviation of symptoms unless the trial participants are at a higher risk of more severe outcomes.

Currently, establishment of DSMBs in trials is not mandatory as per FDA requirements except in case of research studies conducted in emergency settings where informed consent requirement is waived off.

DSMB ESTABLISHMENT AND OPERATION

DSMB CONSTITUTION

- The process of choosing members of DSMB is extremely crucial since the responsibilities of DSMB relate to the safety and well being of research subjects.
- The sponsor and/or trial steering committee usually nominate members of a DSMB after taking into consideration several factors like adequate expertise, experience in clinical research and in working for any other DSMBs, and absence of serious conflicts of interest.
- The sponsor often nominates the DSMB chair, but may discuss with trial investigators or trial steering committee members. The Chairman of DSMB should be the one who has prior DSMB experience and willingly commits his participation for the entire duration of the trial (or for the term of nomination for chairs of DSMBs monitoring multiple trials).
- The composition of DSMB should ideally be in line with the disciplines and clinical background required to interpret clinical trial data and adequately evaluate subject safety.
- The number of members in DSMB is determined by the phase of clinical trial, diversity of medical matters, complexity in study planning and analysis, and anticipated level of risk. Usually DSMB comprises of three to seven members with a minimum of:
  - ✓ Expert(s) in the clinical field of the condition /subject population being studied;
  - ✓ One or more biostatisticians; and,
  - ✓ Investigators with experience in clinical trials planning, execution and analyses.
- *Ad hoc* specialists may be invited to take part as non-voting members at any time in cases demanding additional expertise. Some trials, depending on study population and nature of intervention, may well include a bioethicist on the DSMB, steering committee, or advisory panel.
- DSMBs for multi-national trials should include representatives from a reasonably defined number of countries or regions taking part in research; it is often not practically possible to have representations from all the participating countries in the DSMB.

Confidentiality of interim data and analyses. In order to minimize bias, maintaining the confidentiality of un-blinded interim analyses is utmost important. Sponsors need to address such confidentiality issues in written agreements between the sponsor and members of the DSMB as well as between the sponsor and investigators.

STANDARD OPERATING PROCEDURES OF DSMB

DSMBs typically function in accordance with a written charter including well-defined standard operating procedures. The sponsor may prepare the charter in agreement with DSMB, or the DSMB may prepare it with subsequent agreement by the sponsor. Issues to be covered generally include

- ✓ schedule and format for meetings,
- ✓ layout for data demonstration,
- ✓ description of the person/s who can have access to interim data and who may participate in all or part of DSMB meetings,
- ✓ methods to assess conflict of interest of prospective DSMB members,
- ✓ the methodology and timelines of providing interim reports to the DSMB, and
- ✓ other issues related to committee functioning.

RESPONSIBILITIES OF DSMB

INTERIM MONITORING

One of the major responsibilities of DSMB is to review and examine the collected study data on periodic basis for subject safety, study execution and management and efficacy of study intervention/s.

Monitoring for effectiveness

- If the emerging data from a placebo controlled trial suggests that subjects in the intervention group are showing better results, DSMB may need to consider early termination of trial provided the data is sufficiently convincing and there is very less probability of a false positive interpretation.
- If the interim data suggests absence of any benefit or superiority to existing treatment with new product or very high rates of non-compliance which may compromise the power of study, a DSMB may determine if study continuation is futile and recommend premature termination of study.

Monitoring for safety

DSMB may recommend premature termination of trial due to safety aspects in situations when the probability of benefits of intervention to outweigh the risks is very less e.g.

- If subjects in the intervention group are assumed to be at higher risk of developing the outcome of interest (e.g., mortality, disease progression, organ damage) earlier than those in the control group.
- Rate of adverse events is significantly high in treatment arm as compared to control arm.

- Serious issues regarding the extent and type of adverse events arise during the study conduct e.g. death or other serious adverse events.

In other circumstances, a DSMB may recommend *measures short of termination* to reduce the risk of adverse outcomes. For example, the DSMB may recommend

- ✓ Modification of eligibility criteria if a particular subgroup seems to be at higher risk.
- ✓ Modification of the product dosage and/or schedule if such an action is assumed to decrease the risk of adverse events.
- ✓ Inclusion of screening methods which could identify subjects having high risk of a specific adverse event.
- ✓ Modify the consent form to add information regarding newly identified safety concerns and in some situations taking re-consent of subjects to continue participation in study.

Monitoring study conduct

A DSMB often reviews data pertaining to overall and by site clinical trial conduct such as:

- Rates of subject enrollment, non-compliance and lost to follow up;
- Extent of protocol violations if any;
- Accuracy and promptness of data;
- Degree of agreement between centralized and site review of events;
- Balance between different intervention groups on critical prognostic factors;
- Accrual within major subgroups.

The DSMB may give recommendations regarding trial conduct if there are concerns related to safety of subjects and study integrity.

Consideration of external data

A DSMB may need to determine the influence of external information on the trial being monitored. Observations from an identical study may impact the design of ongoing study or its continuation. Under certain circumstances, unexpected safety issues reported in related studies may be brought to the notice of DSMB by the sponsor. Such data may give rise to recommendations ranging from study termination to other measures short of termination as mentioned above.

OTHER RESPONSIBILITIES

Making recommendations. One of the fundamental responsibilities of a DSMB is to make recommendations to the sponsor regarding study continuation. Recommendations for any modifications should be submitted along with minimum data required for the sponsor to make a reasonable decision about the recommendation, and the justification for such recommendations should be very clear and precise.

Maintaining meeting records. DSMB should ideally maintain records of minutes of all meetings and issue a written report to the sponsor after each meeting. Also, DSMB or the group writing confidential interim reports on behalf of DSMB should maintain all meeting records and take adequate measures to ensure confidentiality of data generated.

INDEPENDENCE OF THE DSMB

Independence of a DSMB relies on the associations of its members to those involved in trial organization, conduct and regulation. Independence is maximum when members are not involved in trial design and conduct apart from their role in DSMB, and have no connections related to finance or other matters to the sponsor or other trial organizers (other than their compensation for providing services on the DSMB).

CHAPTER 27

Clinical Data Management

OVERVIEW

INTRODUCTION

Clinical data management (CDM) is the collection, assimilation and substantiation of clinical trial data with an aim to ensure well timed delivery of data which is of good quality and compliant with good clinical practice (GCP) as well as analytical and reporting requirements. In other words, it is the process that captures and transforms the 'raw' output from clinical trials, that is data on source documents, into a 'usable' form for statistical analysis and reporting.

DATA FLOW IN A CLINICAL TRIAL

Source data. "All the information present in original records and their certified copies related to clinical observations, or other tasks in a clinical trial required for trial evaluation. Source data are obtained from source documents (original records or certified copies)" (ICH E6 1.51)

Source documents. "All the original documents, data and records (e.g. clinical records and charts, laboratory values, subjects' diaries, medication dispensing records, data recorded from automated instruments, photographs, radiographic images, subject files, pharmacy records etc.) available at the medical and technical departments involved in the conduct of clinical trial" (ICH E6 1.52).

Figure 27.1 represents a flowchart of various steps involved in the process of data flow in a clinical trial.

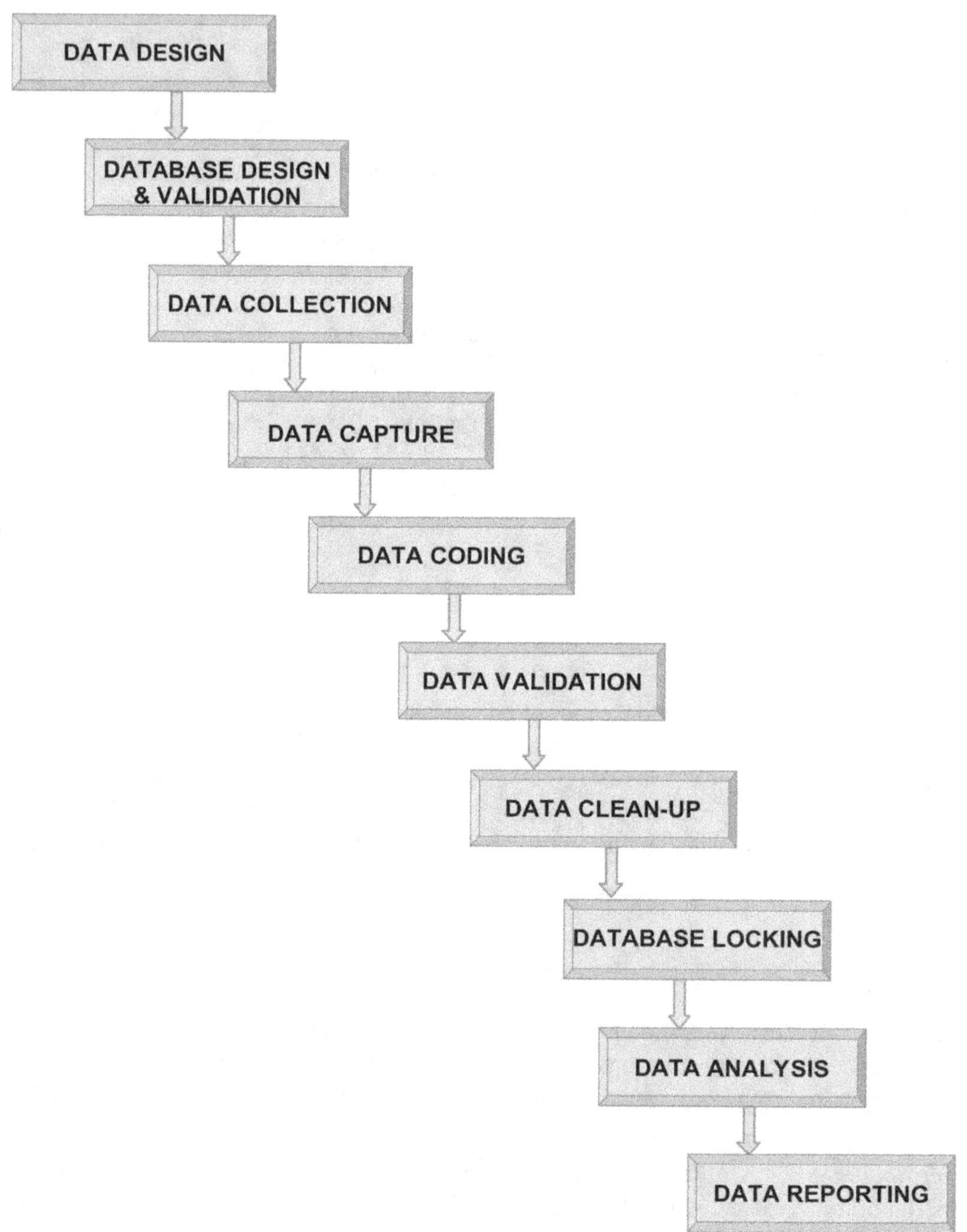

Figure 27.1 Data flow in a clinical trial.

GOOD DOCUMENTATION PRACTICE (GDP)

To ensure the generation of high quality data in a clinical trial, it is imperative to understand and emphasize on the need of good documentation practice. Key attributes for good documentation were described by USFDA in the form of ALCOA (attributable, legible, contemporaneous, original, and accurate); some more letters were added by European association to describe attributes of electronic documentation. Various attributes of a good quality data are shown in Figure 27.2.

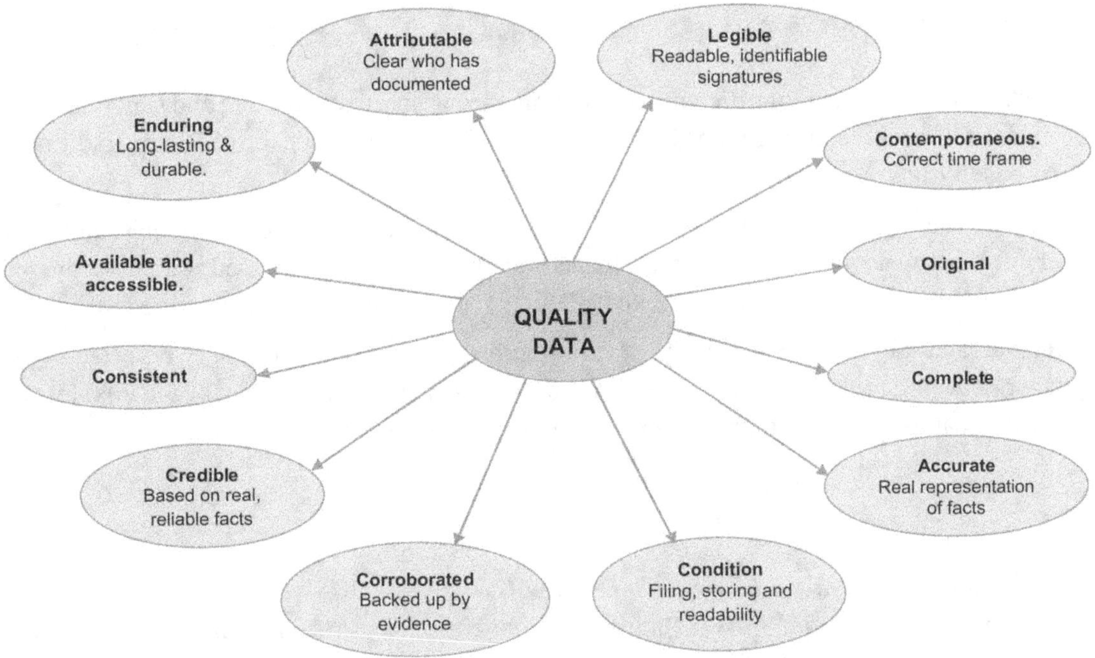

Figure 27.2 Attributes of a good quality data.

STRATEGIES TO ENHANCE THE QUALITY OF SOURCE DOCUMENTATION

- ✓ Regular and periodic trainings of personnel involved in clinical trial on GCP and GDP.
- ✓ Validation of medical data by Principal Investigator (PI) or co-investigators.
- ✓ PI should conduct frequent supervisions of study conduct and meetings with study staff.
- ✓ Establish and follow Standard Operative Procedures (SOPs) for good documentation.

DATA CAPTURE

"Data capture" refers to the compilation of data gathered in a clinical trial onto a database in a compatible and rational manner to enable its easy retrieval and search. Depending on the method employed for data capture in a particular clinical trial, they can be classified into:

- Traditional paper based trials
- Electronic Data Capture (EDC) based trials

ELECTRONIC DATA CAPTURE (EDC) OR REMOTE DATA CAPTURE (RDC)

It is a streamlined system for efficient compilation, cleaning, substantiation, and supervision of the data. EDC uses electronic records e.g. electronic CRF as against paper CRFs in traditional paper based trials

Electronic record: any amalgamation of data in the form of text, graphics, images, audio, or other information depicted in digital form that is generated, modified, retained, stored, recovered or distributed by a computer system. An eCRF is an example of an electronic record.

eCRF : an auditable electronic record of information which is conventionally reported to the sponsor pertaining to every trial subject, in accordance with a protocol. An eCRF enables the systematic capture, review, management, archival, analysis and reporting of clinical trial data.

METHODS OF DATA CAPTURE

1. ***Traditional methods in paper based trials***
   - *Single/Double Data Entry.* Data entry conventionally meant manual entry of data from a paper case record form (CRF) onto a central database through pre-set data entry screens, by trained specialist data entry operators utilizing a conventional keyboard. Data entry can be done at a single point of time (single entry) or successively (double entry), the latter with input by a second, separate data entry operator. Double data entry enhances accuracy by emphasizing differences between the two operators' versions of the data.
   - *Centralised vs Local Data Entry.* Data entry can be done in one centre (centralized) or at various individual investigator sites.
   - *Assimilation of data from an external database.* This involves specific data transfer in huge volumes to own database; for example, biochemical parameters from a central laboratory; thereby allowing less time consumption. However, measures need to be taken to maintain data integrity and safety while doing electronic transfer of data.
   - *Fax-based data capture.*

2. ***Methods in EDC based trials***
- *Manual entry of data on eCRF.*
- *Direct entry of data into the eCRF.*
- *Automatic transmission of data from devices or instruments directly to the eCRF.*
- *Transcription of data from paper or electronic sources to the eCRF.*
- *Direct transmission of data from the Electronic Health Record (EHR) to the eCRF.*
- *Transmission of data from Patient-Reported Outcome (PRO) instruments to the eCRF.*

TRADITIONAL PAPER-BASED TRIAL: DATA MANAGEMENT

Manual transcription/recording of data from source documents on paper case report forms (CRFs) by investigators at the investigational sites

⇓

Data verification (matching of data between CRF and source documents) by clinical monitors from sponsor pharmaceutical companies or from contract research organization (CRO) at the investigational sites

⇓

Collection of verified CRFs by monitor for further transmission to clinical data management (CDM) team

⇓

Resolution of any observed discrepancies within a predetermined time by CDM team with clinical monitors

⇓

Received CRFs marked as received in the clinical data management system (CDMS) to notify the data entry team for beginning data entry according to the established norms (double data entry-most preferred and most accurate).

⇓

Data validation and clean-up by authorized members in CDM team

⇓

In case of any queries, data clarification form (DCF) sent to investigational sites; resolved DCF sent back to CDM team

⇓

Database locked and analysis carried out followed by reporting

EDC BASED TRIAL: DATA MANAGEMENT

Data entry at investigational site by study personnel / investigator on electronic CRF (eCRF) via pre-set data entry screens

⇩

Addition, modification or deletion of data by the investigator in the EDC system subsequently at any time-point, until the eCRF pages are locked and no further addition or modification in the data is allowed.

⇩

Electronic signatures of investigator for all data entries, modifications or deletions to ensure the accuracy, credibility and completion of all data points.

(Data review/cleaning - a joint endeavor of site personnel / investigator, clinical monitor and CDM team in EDC based trial)

⇩

Database locked and analysis carried out followed by reporting

ADVANTAGES OF EDC OVER TRADITIONAL PAPER BASED METHOD

- Abbreviated paper utilization and paper amount.
- Speedy process of error management.
- Recognition of protocol violations and data outliers at the time of data entry itself.
- Reduction of load on clinical monitors.
- Reduced risk of loss/damage of CRFs and associated cost during transit of CRFs.
- Improved efficiency and accuracy of data.
- Reduced time to begin the study, database clean up and database lock.
- Data collation by EDC also plays important role in the conduct of adaptive clinical trials.

HURDLES/OBSTACLES FOR EDC

- EDC software must be as per the regulatory norms, sturdy, compelling and user-friendly.
- Investigational sites personnel / investigators may face difficulties in electronic data entry.
- Need of adequate training for EDC software, which is specific for a particular protocol.
- Increased costs in some regions; requires adequate information technology infrastructure and facilities.

DATA CODING

The data generated in a clinical trial needs to be coded in order to record and store data in a guarded, compatible and reproducible manner to retrieve and analyse the data.

Examples of various coding dictionaries used are;

- For adverse events:
  ✓ Medical Dictionary for Regulatory Activities (MedDRA).
  ✓ WHO-ART (Adverse Reaction Terminology).
  ✓ COSTART (Coding Symbols for Thesaurus of Adverse Reaction Terms).
- Systemised Nomenclature of Medicine (SNOMED) for medical terms.
- International Classification of Diseases –version 10 (ICD-10) for medical disorders.
- DSM-IV for psychiatric illnesses.
- Laboratory and clinical observation coding (LOINC).

Advantages of data coding. Coding facilitates various processes involved in data management like

- o Data recording and archival.
- o Searching and retrieving data.
- o Data manipulation and analysis.
- o Counting and tabulation.
- o Summarizing the data.
- o Presenting data in various different formats.
- o Reproducibility of data.
- o Data standardisation.

Problems with coding

- o Time-consuming and resource-intensive.
- o Codes need to be updated and validated.
- o Non-standardisation: communication problems.
- o Lumping: loss of specificity and original meaning.
- o Splitting: tedious data retrieval and aggregation.

DATA VALIDATION

The series of steps involved in turning the original or 'raw' data into the completed data, i.e. turning the data on CRF into a clean database. Validation must ensure data accuracy, consistency and as truly representing subject's profile.

The process of data validation begins at the trial site and finishes after issuance of final study report by the sponsor.

Data Validation steps performed by investigator, monitor and CDM team (Figure 27.3)

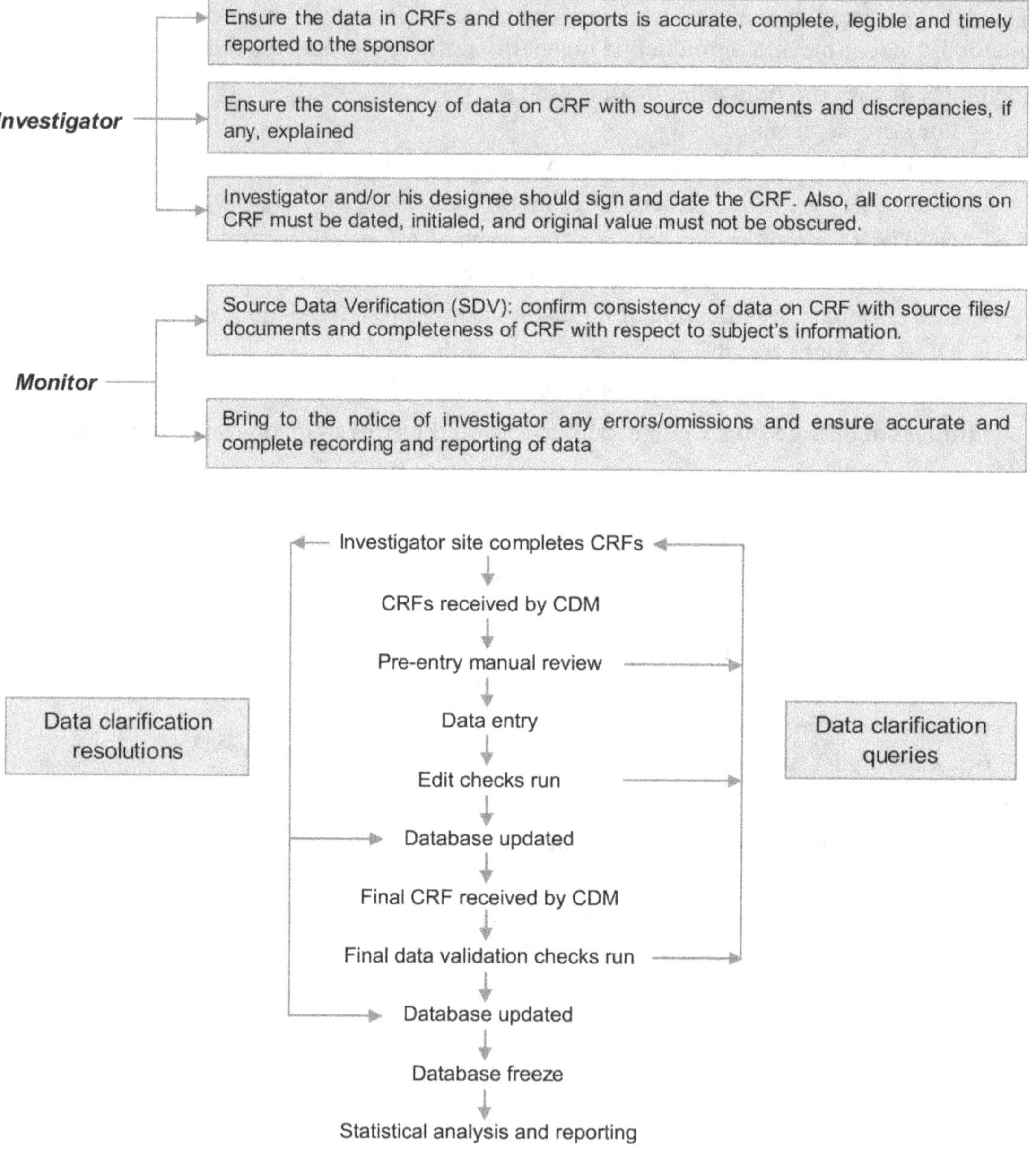

Figure 27.3 Data validation activities by investigator, monitor and CDM team.

DATA ARCHIVAL

CDM team and statisticians are responsible for archiving the electronic database, associated computer programmes, data monitoring conventions, audit trails and the final report. They also maintain all sponsor-specific essential documents as per the regulatory requirements.

REGULATORY GUIDANCE: GOOD DATA MANAGEMENT PRACTICE (GDMP)

INDIAN GCP AND ICH-GCP ON DATA HANDLING AND MANAGEMENT

- Proper documentation of all processes involved in data management should be done to facilitate stepwise retrospective evaluation of data quality and study conduct for the purpose of audit.
- All the information generated in clinical trial should be documented, managed, and archived in a manner to permit its accurate reporting, explanation and validation (ICH-GCP 2.10).
- Quality assurance and quality control systems with written SOPs should be implemented and maintained to ensure that trials are executed and data are obtained, documented and reported in accordance with the protocol, GCP and applicable regulatory requirement(s). (ICH-GCP 5.1.1).
- *Electronic data processing*
- ✓ Only authorized person should be permitted to enter or modify the data in computer and the system should have a recorded trail of the alterations and deletions made.
- ✓ There should be a security system to prevent unauthorised access to data.
- ✓ If any modification is done at the time of data processing, the same must be documented and the system validated.
- ✓ The designing of systems should facilitate documentation of any data modifications and ensure retention of data once entered.
- ✓ A list of authorized persons who are allowed to make changes in the computer system should be maintained.
- ✓ Data backup should be maintained adequately.
- *Validation of electronic data processing systems*. If data generated in the trial is entered directly into a computer, there should be a proper safeguard to ensure validation comprising of a signed and dated printout and backup records. Computerised systems – both hardware and software - should be validated and an updated record regarding their use should be maintained.

- *Language.* All written documents, information and other material used in the study should be in clearly understandable language.
- *Responsibilities of the sponsor and the monitor*
  - ✓ The sponsor should ensure that electronic data processing system adheres to certain essential requirements e.g. completeness, correctness, credibility and consistent planned performance or validation.
  - ✓ The sponsor should maintain SOPs for proper application of these systems.
  - ✓ If the computer system automatically adds any missing values – this should be clearly documented by the monitor.
  - ✓ Sponsor should ensure blinding, if any, during data entry and processing.
  - ✓ The subject identification code in use should be explicit to permit identification of all reported data for every subject.
  - ✓ Data ownership and any transfer should be documented and intimated to the concerned party(ies).

Case Report Form

INTRODUCTION

Definition. As defined in ICH-GCP guidelines, "case report form is a printed, optical or electronic document designed to record all of the protocol required information to be reported to the sponsor on each trial subject".

Aims of CRF. A CRF serves as a bridge between protocol, analysis and report. CRF aims

- to ensure that all data collected from the subjects reflects the objectives and rationale of the protocol.
- to ensure that the collected information is correct, complete and accurate and true reflection of the real facts.

TYPES OF CASE REPORT FORMS (CRFs)

- ◆ *Paper CRF.* It is the traditional method of data capture and mainly used for small studies with varying designs.
- ◆ *Electronic CRF (eCRF).* It is the improvised, validated version of CRFs, mainly used for large studies with similar designs.

Advantages of eCRF over paper CRF

- ✓ less time-consuming,
- ✓ ease of administration,
- ✓ facilitates conduct of large multicentric studies at the same time,

- ✓ zero/minimal errors,
- ✓ enhanced data quality,
- ✓ less chances of online discrepancies,
- ✓ facilitates an earlier database lock,
- ✓ good regulatory acceptance.

QUALITIES OF CRF

A CRF should be:

- ✓ designed as per the study protocol;
- ✓ robust in content;
- ✓ easy to enter and monitor data;
- ✓ representative of the essential contents of the study protocol;
- ✓ well-structured;
- ✓ easy to complete without much help.

DESIGNING OF CRF

Designing a CRF is a very crucial step as the data collected has a direct influence on the statistical outputs obtained. The responsibility of developing CRF lies with the clinical data manager, who takes the assistance of statistician, clinical operations team, the medical monitor, and the sponsor. The ideal timing of designing a CRF is after finalization of study protocol.

General considerations while designing CRF

- The design of CRF should be user-friendly i.e. address the requirements of all users like investigator, site coordinator, study monitor, data entry personnel, medical coder and statistician.
- Data in the CRF should be presented in a format facilitating and simplifying data analysis.
- For designing the CRF, standard operative procedures (SOPs) and recommended guidelines need to be considered.
- Duplication of data i.e. capturing same data at multiple points in CRF should be avoided
- Designing of CRF should be such that data is collected in sufficient detail without ambiguity and redundancies and avoids capture of unwanted details.
- There should be consistency in the format, font style and size used through the entire CRF document.

Ideally, any change in the CRF after the start of study should be avoided; however, in case a change is needed, the same has to be approved by ethics committee.

TYPES OF CRF FORMAT

- ♦ All visits on one page.
- ♦ Individual visits on separate pages.

STANDARD MODULES IN A CRF

CRF header. Identification of the study number, site number and subject identification number.

Patient Demography. Date of birth, age (years), gender, weight in kg, height (cms), informed consent.

Inclusion/ Exclusion criteria. Document at baseline if the subject meets inclusion/exclusion criteria for study participation. There should be positive response to all inclusion criteria and negative response to all exclusion criteria.

Medical history.

Physical examination. Vital signs and body system examination.

Laboratory data.

Efficacy endpoints. Diagnostic criteria, baseline and follow up visits (clinical symptoms, physical examination, scales, laboratory tests, radiology/imaging etc.).

Drugs. Study drug (compound name, dose, units, type, dispensing, packaging and regimen) and concomitant medication.

Safety. All adverse events with details like chronology, severity, action taken, seriousness, outcome, causality etc.

Patient reported outcomes (PROs). Information reported by a subject instead of being objectively assessed by study personnel e.g. symptoms, disability, emotional state, social functioning etc.

Reason for lost-to-follow up or withdrawal from therapy.

Information in case of death. Date and cause of death, causal relationship and if available, autopsy report.

Investigator signature.

REGULATORY GUIDANCE ON CRF: ICH-GCP (BOX 28.1)

Box 28.1 REGULATORY GUIDANCE ON CRF : ICH-GCP.

- • The investigator needs to make it certain that all the data entered in CRFs and other documents to be reported to the sponsor is accurate, complete, legible and well-timed.

Box 28.1 Contd...

- Data in CRF obtained from source documents has to be compatible with source documents and any inconsistencies need to be described.

- The records of any modifications and rectifications need to be retained by the investigator.

- Any modifications or rectifications in CRF have to be properly dated, described (if required) and initials added; and should not conceal the initial entry (i.e. audit trail should be sustained); this is applicable for both written and electronic modifications or rectifications. Sponsors need to furnish guidelines on incorporating any changes to investigators and/or their designated representatives.

- Sponsors must have written procedures to ensure that modifications or rectifications in CRFs are documented, inevitable and are countersigned by the investigator.

CLINICAL DATA ACQUISITION STANDARDS HARMONIZATION (CDASH) GUIDANCE ON DEVELOPING CRF

CDASH is part of the clinical data interchange standards consortium (CDISC) initiative, which is a global, multidisciplinary, non-profit organization which has developed standards to support the accession, interchange, acceptance and archival of clinical research data and metadata. CDASH provides guidance for developing case report form (CRF) with domains across wide therapeutic areas and applicable in most of the clinical trials.

CDASH version 1.0 was released by CDISC in October 2008. The latest available version 1.1 describes the contents of 16 standard domains e.g.

Interventions: exposure, drug accountability, prior and concomitant medications, substance use.

Events: adverse events, disposition, medical history.

Findings: lab results, vital signs, physical examination, eligibility, protocol deviations.

Special purpose: demographics, comments.

Advantages of using CDASH standard CRFs

- Consistent and standardized data collection.
- Lesser number of queries, thereby decreasing workload for data managers and site personnel.
- Captures only key data needed for statistical analysis; hence eliminates few unnecessary fields.
- Avoid duplicate data collection.
- CDASH domain CRFs can be used across studies, across the industry; thus minimizing time and effort wasted.

Quality Management in Clinical Research

INTRODUCTION

"Quality" is a measure of capacity of a product, process, or service to cater to proclaimed or inferred requirements satisfactorily. With respect to a clinical trial, quality may apply to

- ✓ data (e.g. data are accurate, legible, complete, consistent, reliable etc.) or
- ✓ processes (e.g. congruence with the study protocol and GCP; assuring informed consent; appropriate data handling and record-keeping, etc.).

In order to assure quality during a clinical trial, *standard operating procedures (SOPs)* need to be developed. SOPs are defined as "detailed, written instructions to attain uniformity of the performance of a specific function". SOPs along with close personal supervision of the trial's conduct by study investigator and careful monitoring by the sponsor helps to ensure consistent procedures and documentation.

A **quality system** is defined as an organizational structure, responsibilities, processes, methods and resources for the implementation of quality management. Within GCP, quality systems are executed through *quality management* which includes collaboration of activities by the sponsor, by the investigator(s) and site staff, by the IEC(s)/IRB(s) and by the regulatory bodies to manage their operations regarding quality.

QUALITY MANAGEMENT

This encompasses:
- ❖ Quality control.
- ❖ Quality Assurance
- ❖ Quality improvement.

Quality control (QC)

The operational methods and procedures undertaken within quality assurance system to ensure fulfillment of the quality requirements for all activities related to trial execution (ICH- GCP).

Quality Assurance (QA)

All the organized and programmed actions which are undertaken to assure that the clinical trial is conducted and the data are obtained, documented (recorded), and reported in accordance with GCP and the applicable regulatory requirement(s) (ICH- GCP).

Quality improvement

A systematic process for utilizing the knowledge obtained from quality assurance activities to modify systems and activities in order to enhance the ability to meet quality requirements.

QUALITY CONTROL VS. QUALITY ASSURANCE (TABLE 29.1)

Table 29.1 Comparison of quality control with quality assurance.

	Quality control	Quality Assurance
WHAT	QC encompasses steps taken during the clinical trial to assure that the trial conduct fulfils the protocol and methodological needs and is reproducible.	QA is an organized procedure to ensure that the quality control system is functioning and effective
FOCUS	Fulfilling quality requirements	Assuring that quality requirements are fulfilled
BY WHOM	Investigators; monitors	Auditors; Inspectors
HOW	Investigator supervision, Sponsor monitoring, and any ongoing review by regulatory authorities	Independent auditing by sponsors Inspection by regulatory bodies
WHEN	During clinical trial; at every step	Defined points (e.g. during the trial; upon completion)

COMPONENTS OF A QUALITY MANAGEMENT SYSTEM (FIGURE 29.1)

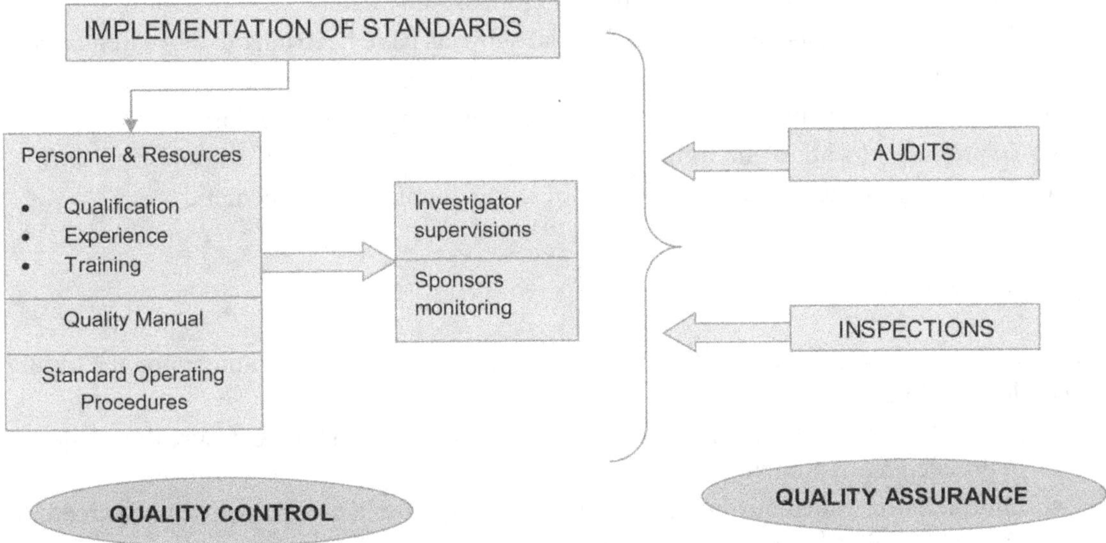

Figure 29.1 Components of a Quality Management System (QMS).

AUDIT

A systematized and independent evaluation of clinical trial related procedures and documents to ensure that evaluated trial related procedures were executed and the data were obtained, documented, analyzed and reported in accordance with the protocol, sponsor's SOP, GCP and the applicable regulatory requirement(s). Audit is generally conducted by the sponsor.

TYPES OF AUDIT

- *Internal audit:* carried out by sponsor's own personnel.
- *External audit:* carried out by a service contractor chosen by the sponsor.
- *In-house audit:* done at sponsor's company itself.
- *On-site audit:* done at investigator's facility.
- *Routine audit:* when the audit is systematic and done as routine.
- *For-cause audit:* when there is a doubt regarding data or process validity.
- *Systems audit (Horizontal audit):* Checks the quality of an operation through several of the sponsor's trials, conducted during a limited time period.
- *Clinical trial audit (Vertical audit):* Audit of a single clinical trial for study validation.

PURPOSE OF AUDIT

- To assure the integrity and credibility of clinical study data.
- To assure that rights and safety of the trial subjects have been adequately safeguarded.
- To prepare sites for a possible regulatory inspection.
- To ensure congruence with the protocol, GCP and applicable regulations.
- To provide education and training to study site staff and sponsor's monitoring staff.
- To obtain an independent assessment of study conduct across centers.

TIMING OF AUDIT

Audit can occur anytime during the study or after its completion. Depending upon the timing of conduct, audit can be:

- *Pretrial audit.* On-site examination by the sponsor and his team to ensure the adequacy of proceeding of clinical trial process.
- *Interim audit.* Taken during the course of trial e.g. after a certain number or percent of patients enrolled/ at a certain time point/ on a random basis.
- *Audit before analysis.* Done after data freezing for a final validation before statistical analysis.
- *Retrospective audit.* Done after the study report has been drafted.

QA PROCESS (FIGURE 29.2)

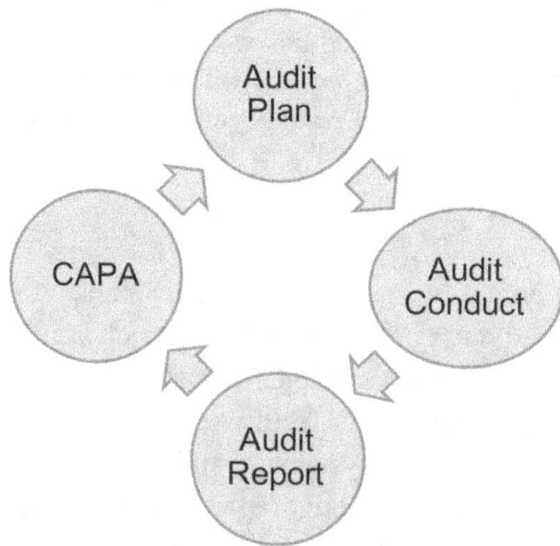

Figure 29.2 QA process (CAPA: Corrective Action and Preventive Action).

STEPS OF AN AUDIT

An audit is comprised of a series of steps.

State the Objectives of Audit

↓

Selection of site and investigators

↓

Inform the investigator

↓

Date of audit conduct decided

↓

Audit conducted

↓

Issuance of audit report and certificate

↓

Follow-up to assess recommended changes (CAPA)

AUDIT PLAN

An audit plan comprising of following is prepared in advance:
- Objectives and scope of audit.
- Identification of key personnel.
- Time period of audit.
- Identification of documents to be reviewed.

AUDIT CONDUCT

An audit usually is conducted over 1–2 days; the Principal Investigator (PI) is given an agenda and a list of documents required for review. The documents reviewed include:
- ✓ participant data/ case report forms,
- ✓ electronic data records,
- ✓ source documents,
- ✓ site study files,
- ✓ investigational product accountability records,
- ✓ regulatory documents e.g. IRB approval/ communications, signed consent forms.

Auditors also examine the study records to assure existence of an ***audit trail***. Audit trail refers to the ability to track the flow of data retrospectively as it is moved from the subject, via instruments or biological samples, to a laboratory, to a written report, to the sponsor, and through the steps of data management and analysis to a final report. This is especially vital when data are modified or rectified after initial entry at the investigator's site. Records must be maintained for all original and modified data along with an indication of who did the modifications and when the modifications were done.

AUDIT REPORT

This is generated upon completion of audit. The details generated during an audit are generally for internal use by the sponsor, and usually the site where audit is conducted is not provided a copy of the audit report. However, information regarding the overall results of audit and acceptability/ non-acceptability of trial data may be provided to the PI. An audit report includes

- ✓ Audit date and methodology;
- ✓ Documents examined and persons met;
- ✓ Percentage of data sampled and checked;
- ✓ Findings of non-compliance;
- ✓ Quality issues;
- ✓ Recommendations for improvement.

AUDIT CERTIFICATE

It is a declaration to confirm that audit has taken place. It describes the type of audit, date of audit, date of issue of audit report and the date when all the relevant corrective actions were taken by the relevant management.

INSPECTION

The act by a regulatory body to conduct an official review of the documents, facilities, resources, records and any other processes considered to be related to clinical trial and which may be present at the site of trial conduct, at the sponsor's and/or contract research organization's (CROs) or at other establishments.

PURPOSE OF INSPECTION

- To determine whether trial was executed in compliance with applicable laws and regulations.
- To ensure the safety and well being of human participants.

TYPES OF INSPECTIONS

❖ ***Study-directed inspections.*** These are carried out for trials which are required to apply for marketing authorization permissions of new drugs, biologicals or medical devices etc.

❖ ***Investigator-directed inspections.*** These may be initiated in situations like:

✓ sponsor's concerns about an investigator;

✓ complaint from a participant regarding issues like violation of subject's rights and safety;

✓ investigator's participation in many trials;

✓ very rapid and high recruitment;

✓ inconsistency in data at a site from other sites;

✓ atypically good safety/efficacy data;

✓ atypically consistent laboratory results.

This type of inspection is carried out much more meticulously than a study-directed inspection, reviews greater number of case reports, and may review multiple studies at a time.

NOTIFICATION TO THE PI.

After inspection, the inspector submits the *inspection report* to the regulatory authority which reviews it and sends a written notification to the investigator in the form of any of the following:

♦ *NAI (No Action Indicated):* No unacceptable processes or operations were identified during the inspection.

♦ *VAI (Voluntary Action Indicated):* Unacceptable processes or operations were identified but the regulatory authority is not ready to take or propose any administrative or regulatory action.

♦ *OAI (Official Action Indicated):* Regulatory and/or administrative actions are proposed. This may include issuance of a "warning letter" mentioning the deviations which require immediate action by the investigator. The study sponsor and site IRB may be informed of the insufficiencies. The sponsor may also be informed if any insufficiencies observed reflect inadequate monitoring by the sponsor.

COMMON OBSERVATIONS IN AUDITS AND INSPECTIONS

♦ *Principal investigator*
Inadequate management of clinical trial.
Improper assignment of tasks and responsibilities to study personnel.

♦ *Informed consent*
Use of stamped PI signature.

Missing signatures and/or dates.

Use of incorrect version of consent form.

Absence of important information in the consent form.

♦ *Protocol compliance*

Enrolment of subjects not as per the eligibility criteria.

Tests mentioned in protocol not conducted.

Use of disallowed medications.

♦ *IRB communications*

Missing approval of IRB for protocol amendment/s or revised consent form.

Absence of/ inadequate reporting to IRB.

♦ *Study data*

Improper data modifications.

Non availability of source documents.

Inconsistency between recorded data and source documents.

Biomarkers

OVERVIEW

INTRODUCTION

Biomarker (Biological marker). An attribute that is measured and assessed as an index of physiological or pathological processes or pharmacological outcomes of a therapeutic intervention.

Surrogate endpoint. It is a biomarker that serves as an alternative for a clinically meaningful endpoint and is supposed to estimate the response to a therapeutic intervention. Any modifications in the surrogate endpoint as a response to therapy are assumed to indicate effect on a clinically meaningful endpoint.

Clinical Endpoint. An attribute or variable that indicates the physical or mental state of a person.

HIERARCHY OF BIOMARKERS (FIGURE 30.1)

♦ **Type 0: Natural history marker**

It is a marker of disease severity reflecting underlying pathologic processes involved and speculates the clinical outcome irrespective of therapeutic intervention. It provides a biological plausibility for further being developed as a candidate marker. The frequency and extent of aberrance of a type 0 marker should be related to the stage or severity of disease.

Applications: (1) can be used as a stratification factor at baseline in trials to distinguish subjects at varying levels of risk for disease progression, and (2) act as landmarks of disease progression to monitor patients.

Validation: by demonstration of a strong correlation between the frequency and extent of marker aberrance at baseline and ultimate clinical outcome in a longitudinal study.

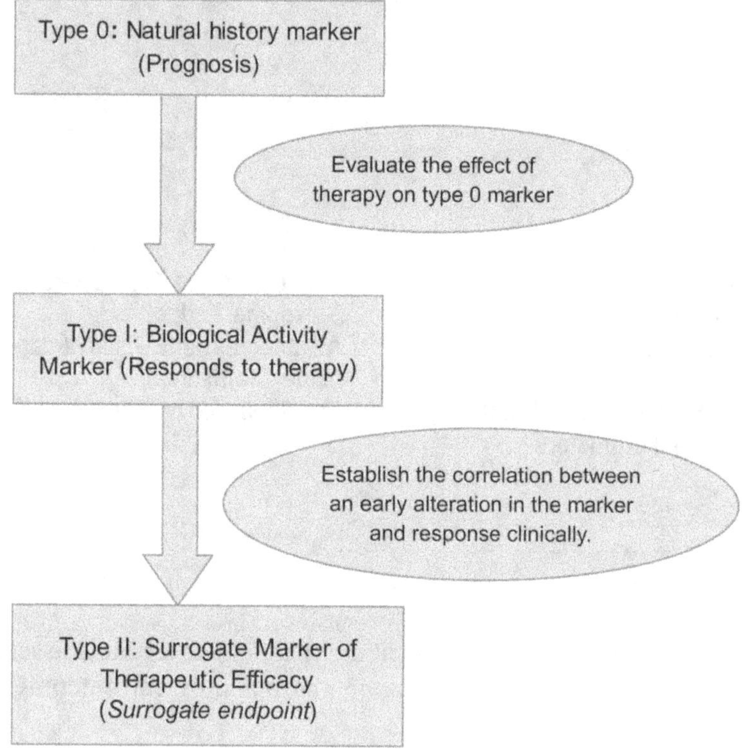

Figure 30.1 Hierarchy of biomarkers.

♦ **Type I: Biological activity marker**

It is defined as one that demonstrates response to a therapeutic intervention; the frequency and extent of the marker response should correspond with the magnitude of therapeutic effect.

Applications: In phase 1 /2 trials, where the primary aim of proof of concept studies is to determine the presence of effect of intervention on an appropriate marker. The magnitude of response of a type I marker can be used to predict an optimal dosing regimen.

Validation: In controlled phase 2 / 3 clinical trials, demonstrating a desirable effect on the marker with an active intervention, a diminished effect with a lower dose of active intervention or a less active agent, and absence of a significant effect with a placebo i.e. demonstration of a dose-response relationship.

♦ **Type II: Surrogate Marker of Therapeutic Efficacy**

A type II marker, either singly or as composite of various markers, is defined as one that completely explains the outcome of an intervention. A favorable effect on the marker denotes an ensuing desirable clinical outcome or, knowledge of the marker value imparts knowledge regarding prognosis irrespective of the treatment. Type II markers serve as "complete" surrogates of clinical outcome.

Validation: Positive outcome trials ideally phase 2 / 3; for example an early alteration in marker values can be reasonably elucidated to estimate or, indeed, mediate an ensuing therapeutic effect. Cross-study analyses are required for validation as (1) a marker may not be applicable at all different disease stages, (2) a marker may be used for one type of therapy but not another. Results observed consistently across studies are more reliable and ensure a greater confidence while using the respective biomarker as a surrogate endpoint for clinical outcome/s in efficacy trials.

CATEGORIES OF BIOMARKERS

- **Pharmacodynamic biomarkers**: these serve as indicators of the result of an interaction between a drug and its receptor/ target, comprising both efficacy and side effects.
- **Prognostic biomarkers**: markers that predict the possible outcome of a disorder irrespective of therapeutic intervention.
- **Predictive biomarkers**: markers which predict the population of patients likely to show response to a particular therapeutic intervention.

VALIDITY OF BIOMARKERS

The process of evaluating the validity of biomarkers is complex. Three aspects for measuring the validity of biomarkers have been suggested by "Schulte and Perera" as:

1. *Content validity*, which describes the extent to which a biomarker correlates with the biological phenomenon.
2. *Construct validity*, which describes the relation with other pertinent features of the disease e.g. other biomarkers or disease manifestations.
3. *Criterion validity*, which describes the degree to which the biomarker shows correlation with a particular disease.

CRITERIA FOR SURROGACY

Certain criteria for labeling a biomarker as surrogate endpoint have been defined (Figure 30.2).

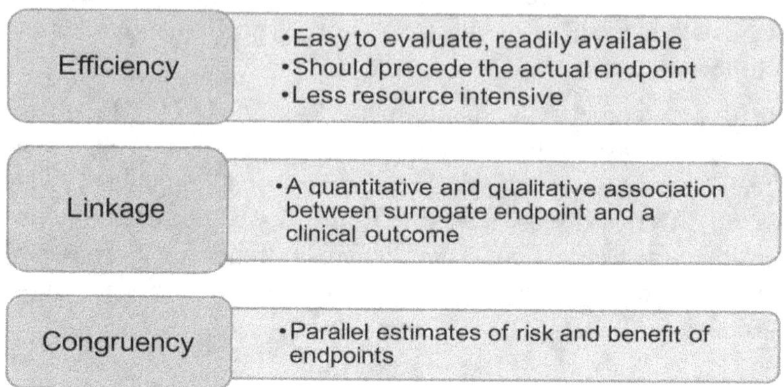

Figure 30.2 Boissel's clinical criteria for surrogacy.

Generally, a good level of stringency is needed when the response of a biomarker to drug treatment is recommended as a surrogate endpoint for a clinical outcome and is proposed to be utilized as the basis for regulatory approval to market a new drug.

BIOMARKERS AND SURROGATE END POINTS AS EFFICACY AND SAFETY PARAMETERS (TABLE 30.1 AND 30.2)

Table 30.1 Examples of biomarkers and surrogate endpoints as efficacy parameters.

Drug class	Biomarkers / Surrogate endpoints	Clinical outcome/ efficacy endpoint
Biochemical & other laboratory markers		
Antidiabetics	↓ Blood glucose, ↓HbA$_{1c}$	↓ Morbidity
Hypolipidemics	↓ Serum cholesterol	↓ Coronary artery disease
Antiretroviral drugs	↑ CD4 count, ↓HIV- RNA levels	↑ Survival
Drugs for osteoporosis	↑ Bone density	↓ Fracture rate
Antibiotics	Negative culture	Clinical cure
Drugs for prostate cancer	↓ Prostate specific antigen	Tumor response
Antiasthmatic drugs	Pulmonary function test	↓ Morbidity
Clinical markers		
Antihypertensive drugs	↓ Blood pressure	↓ Stroke
Drugs for glaucoma	↓ Intraocular pressure	Preservation of vision
Electrocardiographic markers		
Antiarrhythmics	↓ Arrhythmias	↑ Survival

In addition to their role in evaluating the efficacy of drugs, biomarkers have also been quite useful in safety monitoring.

Table 30.2 Examples of biomarkers and surrogate endpoints as safety parameters.

Drug class/ drugs	Biomarkers / Surrogate endpoints	Clinical safety endpoint
Anticancer drugs	Complete hemogram	Bone marrow suppression
Corticosteroids	Bone density, X rays	Osteoporosis
Statins	CPK-MB	Myopathy
Antitubercular drugs (INH, Rifampin)	Liver function tests	Hepatitis
Aminoglycosides	Renal function tests	Renal failure
Beta blockers	Electrocardiogram (PR interval)	Cardiac depression

CHARACTERISTICS OF AN IDEAL SURROGATE

- Reliability, reproducibility, ready availability, easy quantification, cost effectiveness and ability to demonstrate "dose-response" relationship.
- True indicator/ predictor of illness (or risk of illness).
- Existence of a biologically plausible explanation for association/ correlation between the disease of interest and surrogate end point.
- *Sensitive*- that is, a "positive" result for surrogate end point should be able to identify all or most subjects likely to experience efficacy/ adverse outcome.
- *Specific*-that is, a "negative" result should effectively exclude all or most subjects not likely to experience efficacy/ adverse outcome.
- There must be a clear cut off between within and outside normal range values.
- It should have good *positive predictive value*-that is, a "positive" result always or mostly indicates the subject's increased likelihood of experiencing efficacy or adverse outcome.
- It should have good *negative predictive value*-that is, a "negative" result always or mostly indicates the subject's decreased likelihood of experiencing efficacy or adverse outcome.
- Compliance with quality control monitoring.
- Any alteration/s in the surrogate end point should precisely and rapidly reflect the response to therapeutic intervention, especially there should be normalization of levels during states of remission or cure.

APPLICATIONS OF BIOMARKERS AND SURROGATE ENDPOINTS

Biomarkers and surrogate end points have useful applications during various phases of drug development and in clinical practice.

❖ ***Predevelopment studies of target illness***
- Correlation with disease diagnosis and prognosis.
- Explaining disease patho-physiology.

❖ ***Preclinical drug development***
- Confirm presence of anticipated pharmacological action *in vivo*.
- Probe concentration-response relationship in preclinical studies.
- Evaluate safety in animal models, e.g. toxicogenomics.

❖ ***Clinical drug development***
- Demonstrate pharmacological activity in humans.
- Evaluate optimal dosage and regimen to attain proposed pharmacologic effect.
- As safety markers in determining dose-response for toxicity.
- As a basis for stratification of subjects.
- Monitor compliance and adverse effects.
- Interim analysis of efficacy and safety.
- Determine role (if any) of differences in metabolism on efficacy and safety.
- To obtain conditional regulatory approval (please refer to box 30.1 for accelerated approval or subpart H approval).

❖ ***Post-marketing development***
- Studies aiming to evaluate newer indications for approved drugs.
- Basis for regulatory approval of new formulations and generics.

❖ ***Clinical practice***
- Confirmation of disease diagnosis and prognosis.
- Aid to select appropriate treatment.
- Monitor response to therapeutic intervention.

Box 30.1 Accelerated Approval or Subpart H Approval.

This strategy as described in NDA regulations of USFDA intends to make availability of favorable drugs for life threatening disorders in market based on some preliminary evidence prior to formal demonstration of efficacy in patient population. The marketing approval is granted based on studies evaluating a surrogate biomarker that is assumed to correlate with patient's response to therapy. Such an approval is considered a provisional approval with an obligation to conduct clinical studies formally demonstrating patient's response to therapy. Few examples of drugs receiving accelerated approval include *alemtuzumab*

Box 30.1 *Contd...*

> (in chronic lymphocytic leukemia patients treated with alkylating agents and showing failure to fludarabine therapy), *amifostine* (adjuvant therapy of postmenopausal women with hormone receptor positive early breast cancer) and *bortezomib* (multiple myeloma patients demonstrating disease progression despite being treated).

ADVANTAGES AND DISADVANTAGES OF USING BIOMARKERS

The applications of biomarkers are associated with certain advantages as well as disadvantages.

Advantages
- Objective evaluation.
- Accuracy in estimation.
- Reasonable reliability and validity.
- Less bias than other parameters like questionnaires.
- Disease processes often studied.
- Homogeneity of risk or disease.

Disadvantages
- Expensive (high analytical costs).
- Storage (issues like preservation of samples).
- Errors in laboratory measurements.
- Tedious to establish normal range in some cases.
- Confounding factors altering the measurement of biomarkers.
- Ethical issues when the source of biomarkers is critical and involves risk e.g. biopsy specimens, CSF.

THE DOWNSIDE OF BIOMARKERS / SURROGATE ENDPOINTS

Biomarkers/ surrogate endpoints may at times fail to truly reflect the clinical end points. There are examples of few large trials in the past where contrasting effects on validated surrogate biomarkers and clinical endpoints were observed with the therapeutic interventions.

- ❖ *CAST (Cardiac Arrhythmia Suppression Trial) trial.* This trial was designed to examine the hypothesis that prevention of premature ventricular complexes (PVC) with class I antiarrhythmic agents (encainide, flecainide, and morcizine) after a myocardial infarction would reduce mortality. It was found that the tested drugs increased mortality despite a successful reduction in the number of PVCs.

❖ ***ILLUMINATE trial.*** A significant improvement in serum lipid profile (HDL, LDL and triglycerides) was observed with torcetrapib compared to placebo when given in addition to atorvastatin in patients with coronary heart disease (CHD) or CHD risk equivalent. Torcetrapib arm, however, also demonstrated a significant increase in the risk of primary (composite of first major cardiovascular event) as well as secondary (all-cause mortality, hospitalization for unstable angina) end points.

❖ ***ACCORD (Action to Control Cardiovascular Risk in Diabetes) trial.*** In this trial, intensive glycemic treatment (targeted at HbA_{1C} less than 6.0%) was compared with standard treatment (targeted at HbA_{1C} less than 7.0–7.9%). An increased risk of primary outcome (composite of cardiovascular death, nonfatal myocardial infarction (MI), and nonfatal stroke) was associated with the intensive treatment strategy.

CHAPTER 31

Multicentric Clinical Trials

OVERVIEW

Introduction
Conduct of MCCTs
Ethical Review of Multicentric Research

Multinational/International Clinical Trials
Advantages of MCCT
Disadvantages of MCCT

INTRODUCTION

A multi-centric clinical trial (MCCT) is a clinical trial executed at the same time by multiple investigators working in different settings or organizations following the same protocol, identical techniques to pool the obtained data and analyzing them together. These are commonly undertaken in Phase III and Phase IV and less often in phase II clinical trials.

CONDUCT OF MCCTs

1. **Special requirements for MCCTs**

   Comparability of participating institutions
   - ✓ Equipment: All the equipments and methods including assay methods should be standardized. A central laboratory may be chosen to carry out the important tests or to check the results from each individual laboratory.
   - ✓ Staff personnel: The number, availability, experiences of staff personnel should ideally be similar across different centres.
   - ✓ Subject recruitment: The number of subjects enrolled in different centres should not be too different, nor should the subjects be too heterogenous.

   A common protocol. The protocol proposed to be used in MCCTs needs to be much more comprehensive as any variability in interpretation among different centres may lead to decreased homogeneity.

2. **Establishment of an Organizing Group.** An organizing group having the overall responsibility of organizing and overseeing all phases of trial should be established. This group consists of leaders from funding source (e.g. government agencies, private research organizations), and science (subject experts).

3. **Identification / Selection of trial sites.** The recruitment sites identified to be included in MCCT should have sufficient recruitment population; experienced, qualified and trained investigator group and adequate institutional support.

4. **Determine feasibility of study.** For trials with long duration and large sample size, it is desirable to instruct each center to conduct a feasibility pilot trial enrolling small number of patients.

5. **Coordinating the trial.** In all MCCTs, a *coordinating center* with appropriate secretarial facilities and data processing equipment should be established. This center plays vital roles in the design, management, conduct and analysis of trial; implementation of randomization scheme and ongoing communications with all centers. The *coordinating group* should include a clinician, a statistician, a person responsible for on-site trial monitoring, a pharmacologist (possibly) and one or more specialists in different fields. The members should meet frequently, direct and control the way the trial is conducted.

6. **Organizational structure.** An organizational structure for the clinical trial should be set up with clearly defined responsibilities and authorities.

✓ ***Data Monitoring committee***: works independently from the investigators and sponsor/s of the trial. This committee holds the responsibility of periodically monitoring study related data, evaluating center performance and reporting to either the organizing group or the study sponsor. The coordinating center also presents the data to the committee. The committee recommends to the organizers or to the sponsor of the trial on matters like premature termination of trial if there are serious safety concerns, more than predicted efficacy and high probability of indifferent observations.

✓ ***Steering committee/ executive committee:*** This committee oversees the trial at scientific and operational levels. It is comprised of a subset of investigators. For certain issues like compliance, quality control, categorization of response variables, publication policies etc. *focused subcommittees* can be constituted which ultimately report to the steering committee.

✓ ***Assembly of investigators:*** This is a representation of all the centres participating in the trial. Principal investigator from each centre is the voting member of the assembly. The purpose of this assembly is carrying out voting related to various issues, keeping the investigators conversant with trial progress and providing opportunities to train and educate staff personnel.

7. **Maintenance of highest quality standards.** Adequate training of all personnel involved and standardization of all procedures are keystones to enhance the quality of data generated in MCCTs. The staff at each center should be able to comprehend the protocol including the procedures to conduct various tests and maintain documents. The assistance of specialty centers may be taken in areas like laboratory testing, pathology or radiology reporting, ECG evaluation etc. to ensure unbiased assessment, decreased variability and quality control.

8. **Monitoring the progress of all centers.** A close monitoring of patient enrolment, quality of data obtained and documentation, quality of laboratory evaluations, and protocol compliance by subjects, investigators and other study personnel should be done regularly. The centers performing below average should be identified, and remedial measures and appropriate adjustments be implemented.

9. **Analysis of the results.** Several problems specific to MCCTs must be considered.

   The "center" factor. Inclusion of "center" factor into the analysis is useful in enhancing the power of study. This makes it possible to deduce the variability between centers from the residual variability and thus making detection of differences between treatments more sensitive. This method takes into account only those centers which contribute at least one case per treatment. Centers with very small recruitment are pooled into a big center.

   Interaction. It is important to verify if the difference between treatments vary outside random fluctuations across all centers. If major differences exist, the causes should be sought and test of interaction "treatment per center" be demonstrated to have significant result.

10. **Publication, presentation and authorship policies.** The dissemination issues should be planned essentially in advance as "credit" must be shared by all and to eliminate future misunderstanding. Usually sponsors are not a part of authorship. Investigators are allowed to publish their individual results of a MCCT, even when the statistical and clinical relevance of a single site's results would be highly questionable from a scientific perspective. However, in fairness to the pharmaceutical companies and other investigators, this may only be done a number of months (e.g., about 18 to 30) after the trial is completed in order to allow the sponsor time to analyze the data, prepare a manuscript, and have it published prior to an article being published on just one site's data from the trial that may not be representative of the overall data. Companies should show a summary of all results to each investigator at an early stage in the process so that the investigator is aware whether or not his or her results differ from the overall trial's results.

ETHICAL REVIEW OF MULTICENTRIC RESEARCH

❖ **Separate review by ECs of all the participating centers**

   Presently, in India, all the centers participating in multi-centric research need to obtain approval from their respective ECs whose responsibility is to consider the requirements of local populations and to safeguard the rights, safety and well being of trial participants. The ECs can also make suggestions on making amendments in study protocols and informed consent documents as per the site-specific needs. Such separate review may be especially needed in studies involving higher degree of risk, conditions when site/s have influence on trial conduct and other factors demanding closer review.

Separate review by all the concerned ECs, however, has concerns related to duplication of efforts, wastage of time and lack of communication among different ECs. Hence, in order to improve the feasibility and efficiency of such separate review, measures should be taken to establish communication between different ECs; also if approval is not granted by any EC, reasons for the same should be shared with other ECs and deliberated upon.

❖ **Common ethics review in multi-centric research**

Under common ethics review, EC of one participating center assumes the responsibility of conducting review of multi-centric research with mutual agreement of ECs of all the centers. Such EC is labeled as the ***Designated Ethics Committee (DEC)***. At all the participating centers, the ***Participating Center ECs (PECs)*** are located who are responsible for conducting detailed review of research proposals as per the local needs. A signed document in the form of letter of agreement (LOA) /letter of understanding (LOU) should be made to assign the roles and responsibilities of DEC and PECs.

The proposal of common ethics review in multi-centric research in India is currently under consideration.

Common ethics review of multi centre research

In 2019, ICMR has released draft guidelines for "Common ethics review of multi centre research" which provide details of the procedures involved in common ethics review (https://www.icmr.nic.in/sites/default/files/guidelines/Draft_ICMR_Guidelines.pdf as accessed on April 25, 2019).

❖ **Central IRB/ Central Ethics Committee for human research (CECHR)**

For FDA- regulated multi-centric studies of investigational drugs and biologics, there is the provision of centralized IRB review process. The central IRB is the IRB which conducts reviews on behalf of all those study sites which agree to participate in the centralized review process.

For sites at institutions having an IRB that ordinarily reviews research conducted at the institution, the central IRB should reach agreement with the institutions' IRBs about how to share the review responsibilities between local IRBs and the central IRB.

However, where a centralized IRB review process is used, the review should take into consideration the ethical issues pertaining to the local community and relevant local factors and adequate mechanisms should be in place to ensure consideration of such factors, for example:

✓ Central IRB should be provided with relevant local information by individuals or organizations versed with the local community, institution, and/or clinical research.

✓ Participation of consultants possessing pertinent expertise, or IRB members from the institution's own IRB, in the deliberations of the central IRB.

✓ Limited review of a central IRB-reviewed study by the institution's own IRB, with focus on issues that are of concern to the local community.

Centralized IRB review process in multicenter clinical trials

FDA Guidance: "Using a Centralized IRB Review Process in Multicenter Clinical Trials," issued in March, 2006 accessible at : http://www.fda.gov/cder/guidance/OC2005201fnl.pdf

---

MULTINATIONAL/INTERNATIONAL CLINICAL TRIALS

In cases where a large scale trial is being conducted in several countries, there may be additional complications owing to differences in many factors:

Differences in medical practice. Existence or prevalence of disease, classification of disease, genetic and ethnic background of individuals (metabolism and stature etc.), certain concepts related to disease and treatment, practice style of physicians.

Cultural differences. Language, ethical principles, dietary practices, customs and religions.

Regulatory differences. Placebo use, toxicology data requirements, import-export regulations.

Economic differences. Medical insurance, daily wagers etc.

Practical differences. Equipments used for investigations, central laboratories.

Problems in interpretation and extrapolation of data.

ADVANTAGES OF MCCT

- ❖ More rapid patient recruitment.
- ❖ Greater likelihood for a heterogeneous patient population to be enrolled.
- ❖ Helpful in studying a rarely occurring disorder or a restrictively – described subject population.
- ❖ Assure a more representative study or target population (e.g. in terms of geographical distribution, ethnicity, socioeconomic background, lifestyle etc.) which ensures a higher and more valid generalisability.
- ❖ More complex protocols may be conducted because of additional resources utilized for certain large trials.
- ❖ Less opportunity for one person's biases to influence the design or conduct of the clinical trial.
- ❖ Greater likelihood for data processing and analysis to be conducted at a high standard.

DISADVANTAGES OF MCCT

- ❖ Complex administrative arrangements and management details.
- ❖ Costly as compared to studying the same number of subjects in a single centre.
- ❖ Statistical data can be stronger from one or few centers than others.
- ❖ Some ethical committees/ IRBs may insist on changes that may be unacceptable to the sponsor and may delay the study start up or are unacceptable to other ethics committees.
- ❖ Individual investigators may receive little recognition during publication of results of large MC trials.

SECTION – H

CLINICAL DRUG DEVELOPMENT: PREMARKETING PHASES

CONTENTS

CHAPTER 32

Phase Zero Clinical Trials

OVERVIEW

Introduction
Objectives of Exploratory IND/Phase 0 Studies
Traditional Versus Exploratory IND Approach
Classification of Phase 0 Studies
Microdose Studies
   Relevance of Microdosing
   Conduct of Microdosing Studies

Non-Clinical Safety Data Requirements for Microdosing Studies
Correlation of Microdose with Therapeutic Dose
Current Status of Microdosing in India
Characteristics of an Ideal Drug Candidate for Microdosing
Advantages of Phase 0/Exploratory IND Studies
Limitations of Phase 0/Exploratory IND Studies

INTRODUCTION

Phase 0 trial (also called Exploratory IND/ Pre-Phase 1 study) is defined as a clinical trial that

- is carried out at an early period in phase 1,
- includes very less number of study subjects,
- does not have a therapeutic or diagnostic objective and
- is carried out prior to the conventional dose escalation studies assessing safety and tolerability of new compounds.

OBJECTIVES OF EXPLORATORY IND/PHASE 0 STUDIES

- ✓ Confirm the presence/absence of similar mechanism of action in humans as observed in preclinical studies (e.g. receptor binding property or modification of an enzyme).
- ✓ Furnish data on pharmacokinetics (PK) of new compounds.
- ✓ Helpful in choosing the most favorable lead compound from a group of molecules based on interaction with a potential therapeutic target in man, PK or pharmacodynamic (PD) properties.
- ✓ Elaboration of the bio-distribution profile of new compounds with the help of various imaging techniques.

TRADITIONAL VERSUS EXPLORATORY IND APPROACH

Exploratory IND approach involves administration of the drug product at sub-pharmacologic doses or doses assumed to have pharmacologic effect but producing no toxicity, hence, the probable risk of developing toxicity in human subjects is significantly less than in traditional IND approach. Also exploratory approach requires relatively less preclinical data than the traditional one. Table 32.1 lists important distinguishing features of traditional and exploratory IND approach.

Table 32.1	
Exploratory IND approach	**Traditional IND approach**
• Reduced preclinical data requirement	• Extensive preclinical data requirement
• ~ 3 – 6 months for preparing Exp IND	• ~9 – 18 months for preparing IND
• Could potentially reduce the failure rate	• >90% failure in clinical development
• <100 micrograms of drug required	• About 100 grams of drug required
• Cost of early phase of drug development:	
~US $0.3-0.5 million	~US $1.5-5 million

CLASSIFICATION OF PHASE 0 STUDIES

Phase 0 studies can be categorized into three different types depending upon the main study objectives (Figure 32.1):

❖ Phase 0 studies assessing pharmacokinetics / imaging studies (Microdose studies).

❖ Phase 0 studies aiming to determine pharmacologically relevant doses.

❖ Phase 0 studies exploring mechanism of action (MOA) related to efficacy/ Pharmacodynamic endpoint studies.

MICRODOSE STUDIES

These are the pharmacokinetic and mechanistic studies using a microdose. A *microdose* is described as less than 1/100th of the calculated dose of a test compound (on the basis of preclinical data) assumed to produce pharmacologic effect with a maximum dose of <100 micrograms. The maximum permissible dose for microdose studies involving protein products should not be more than 30 nanomoles due to relative dissimilarities in their molecular weights in contrast to chemical or synthetic products.

Human microdosing is based on the principle of safely administering sub-pharmacological amounts (microdoses) of NCEs to humans to attain useful information on PK, PD and metabolism at a much earlier stage.

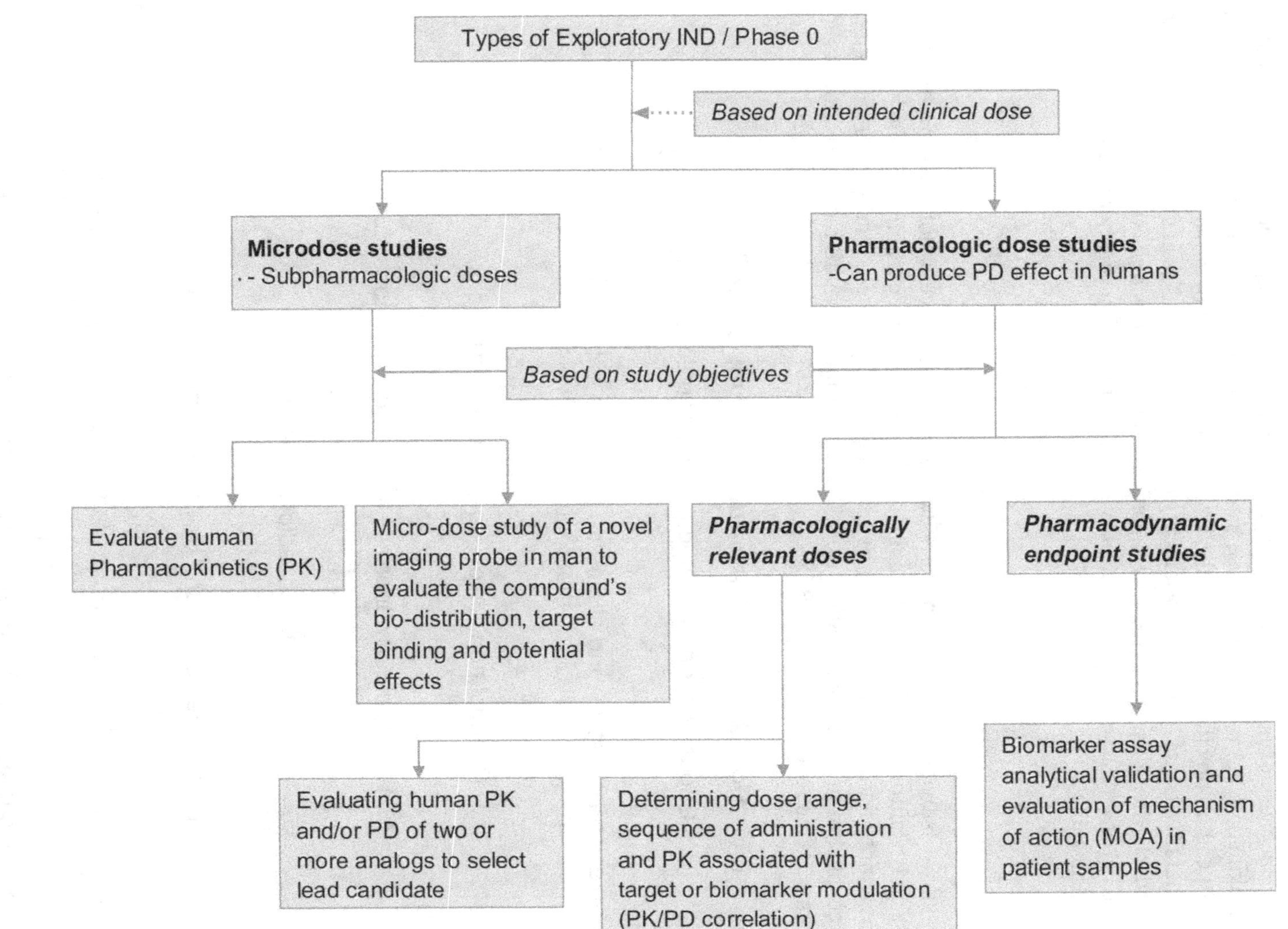

Figure 32.1 Types and objectives of Phase 0 studies.

RELEVANCE OF MICRODOSING

An important cause of failure of new drug candidates during development is non-favorable pharmacokinetic (PK) parameters. The existing methods to determine PK before clinical studies depend on preclinical models like animals, *in vitro* and *in silico*. There is always a concern that PK of drug might be substantially different in humans than predicted from these model studies. Microdosing studies, by evaluating human pharmacokinetics of new chemical entity (NCE) at a relatively early stage, provide key information in determining whether a NCE is 'druggable'.

CONDUCT OF MICRODOSING STUDIES

Highly ultrasensitive analytical 'big physics' technologies like accelerator mass spectrometry (AMS) and positron emission tomography (PET), which are capable of estimating the concentrations of drug/s and metabolites in the range of picograms to femtograms are central to the conduct of microdosing studies. Both these techniques require radioactive tracers to label drugs (^{14}C in AMS; ^{11}C or ^{18}F in PET).

Flow diagram of microdosing study procedures

Choose cohort of compounds for candidate selection.

⇩

Use animal PK study and allometric scaling to determine possible human therapeutic dose.

⇩

Conduct non clinical safety studies as required.

⇩

Obtain regulatory approval for human microdose study.

⇩

Obtain radiolabeled drug.

⇩

Standardize dosing and bioanalysis for microdose study.

⇩

Conduct human microdose study; Predict PK from microdose

⇩

Choose candidate to be taken through conventional development route.

NON-CLINICAL SAFETY DATA REQUIREMENTS FOR MICRODOSING STUDIES (TABLE 32.2)

Table 32.2 Non-clinical safety data requirements for micro dosing studies.	
US FDA guidelines (2006)	**EMEA guidelines (2004)**
Guidance: "Exploratory IND studies".	"Single dose pk study in humans using microdose."
Toxicity study: Extended (14-day) single dose toxicity study in single mammalian species (both genders), at multiple dose levels including one inducing minimal toxic effects	Similar to US-FDA
Route of administration: Single i.e. intended route	Both IV and intended routes of administration
Safety margin: 100x	1000x
Genotoxicity study: Not required	Required
Safety pharmacology: Not required	Required
Scope: Applies to all products, including therapeutic proteins and monoclonals.	Does not apply to biotechnology derived and anti-cancer drugs

CORRELATION OF MICRODOSE WITH THERAPEUTIC DOSE

The key concern with regard to the microdosing concept is whether the subpharmacological doses used in such studies are predictive of PK/PD at pharmacological doses. This aspect had been addressed in one of the pioneer microdosing studies - CREAM study (Consortium for Resourcing and Evaluating AMS Microdosing) in which 70% approximation between the pharmacokinetics at microdose and therapeutic dose was observed for 3 (midazolam, diazepam and ZK253) out of 5 drugs. The conclusion of the study was that microdosing can be adopted as a useful strategy to guide selection of drug compounds at an early developmental stage.

CURRENT STATUS OF MICRODOSING IN INDIA

Amendment to Section 2(6)(ii)(a) of Schedule Y (Human Pharmacology) states:

Very low dose pharmacokinetic studies (microdosing studies) may be conducted very early in development with the help of ultrasensitive equipment. The actual dose will depend on the potency of the investigational drug, but should not be more than 100 micro-grams in all cases. These single or multiple (maximum 7 days) microdose pre-phase I studies help in early appropriate drug candidate selection and reduce failure relating to pharmacokinetic parameters in early drug development. Microdosing studies are not appropriate for all new drug substances and have their own limitations which must be kept in mind when they are selected as an option in drug development.

In India, according to the New Drugs and Clinical Trials Rules, 2019, however, there is no concept of Phase 0 or Exploratory IND equivalent.

CHARACTERISTICS OF AN IDEAL DRUG CANDIDATE FOR MICRODOSING (BOX 32.1)

Box 32.1 Ideal drug candidates for microdosing.

- ✓ Compounds with linear pharmacokinetics.
- ✓ Small molecules with short half-lives.
- ✓ Compounds undergoing metabolism.
- ✓ Compounds having rapid dissociation from binding site on target.

ADVANTAGES OF PHASE 0/EXPLORATORY IND STUDIES

- ◆ Phase 0 studies by means of assessing human pharmacology including PK/PD profiles of new drug candidates help in earlier selection of potentially favorable compounds for further clinical development.
- ◆ Phase 0 clinical trials are welcomed in a big way in the field of oncology. The main objective of these studies in this field is to confirm the binding and further modulation of molecular targets in tumor cells by the drug candidate. In this way, they help in providing the basis for carrying the molecule for further development before exposing patients to potential toxic effects of new anti-cancer drugs.
- ◆ Phase 0 studies could be helpful in the discovery of endogenous biomarkers, which can be useful tools for quantitatively evaluating the in vivo effects of drugs.
- ◆ The cost of conducting an exploratory IND study is remarkably less, in comparison to a traditional IND/ full Phase I study.
- ◆ The requirements for preclinical toxicity data before carrying out phase 0 studies are very minimal, hence, number of animals tested and quantities of drug substance required are significantly less.

- Microdosing studies involve exposing human volunteers to sub-pharmacological dose of test compounds which is not intended to produce any pharmacological actions; hence the risk of adverse events is negligible.
- Using microdosing studies, pharmacokinetic data for determining initial dose is available within 4- 6 months, whereas in Phase I studies it takes 12-18 months.

LIMITATIONS OF PHASE 0/EXPLORATORY IND STUDIES

- A vital issue of concern is the predictive accuracy of microdosing. It is not clearly established that body's reaction to a compound given at microdoses is exactly similar to when therapeutic doses of the compound are administered.
- Microdosing studies may not be applicable to all new drug molecules, particularly drugs with complex pharmacokinetics (e.g. non-linear kinetics, high-affinity binding to their targets).
- Another limitation of microdosing is related to metabolism and stability of certain compounds. Some compounds show ready dissolution and good absorption characteristics at microdose; however, when administered at therapeutic doses, they exhibit limited solubility, and unfavorable absorption characteristics which cannot be anticipated at microdose levels. Also, many processes within the body involve the use of specialized transporters, enzymes and binding sites, which are saturable such that there is huge difference in pharmacokinetic profile at microdose from that at higher therapeutic dose.
- Microdosing studies utilize advanced technologies like AMS and PET which demand huge investments. Besides cost, these techniques employ radiotracer assays which carry inherent limitations like short half-life of tracers and compromised specificity (metabolites may also be included in assays).
- Another limitation relates to the absence of therapeutic objective in Phase 0 trials. Also, patients may be subjected to serial tissue biopsies, invasive procedures or multiple pharmacokinetic samplings. These issues pose huge challenge in recruiting subjects thus hampering successful conduct of Phase 0 trials.
- Although the participation of subjects in Phase 0 studies is short lasting, usually not more than 1 week, but the mere fact that they are being enrolled in phase 0 study might delay or exclude their participation in other clinical trials which may offer some therapeutic advantage to subjects.
- Another limitation is related to their application in the field of oncology. In this field though their main objective is to assess the anti-cancer potential of new drugs but lack of availability of validated biomarkers and assays limit their utility in this area.

Phase 1 Clinical Trials

INTRODUCTION

Clinical trials of an investigational medicinal product (IMP) that are not assumed to render any benefit to subjects, whether they are healthy subjects or patients, are called phase 1 or non-therapeutic trials. Conventionally, this is the phase when new drug is administered to the human beings for the first time hence also known as First in human (FIH) or First time in human (FTIH) trials.

OBJECTIVES OF A PHASE I TRIAL

PRIMARY OBJECTIVES

- Define safety and tolerability of the new compound i.e. determine the maximum tolerated dose (MTD).
- Identify dose-limiting toxicities (DLTs) and the recommended phase 2 dose (RPTD).

SECONDARY OBJECTIVES

- Describe the toxicity profile of the new treatment in the schedule being evaluated.
- Assess pharmacokinetics (PK).
- Assess pharmacodynamic effects (PD).
- Document any preliminary evidence of objective drug activity.

FEW DEFINITIONS RELEVANT TO PHASE 1 TRIALS

- ♦ ***Maximum tolerated dose (MTD):*** Dose level prior to the dose level where the adverse effects lead to stopping further dose escalation or reaching stopping criteria.
- ♦ ***Dose-limiting toxicity (DLT):*** Toxicity which is considered unacceptable (due to being severe and/or irreversible in nature) and limits further dose increment. DLT is specifically defined for a protocol and in advance prior to trial initiation. It is defined according to some standard method e.g. common terminology criteria for adverse events (CTCAE).
- ♦ ***Recommended phase 2 dose (RP2D or RD):*** Dose at which DLT appears in a pre-defined proportion of subjects (usually ranges from 20-40%) – this is the dose which would be used subsequently in phase II trials.

TYPES OF PHASE 1 TRIALS

Phase 1 trials are usually carried out in two stages viz. early and late phase studies.

EARLY PHASE 1 STUDIES

These include single ascending dose and multiple ascending dose studies.

Single ascending dose (SAD) studies

Small groups of subjects are administered small doses of the drug to be tested and observed for a defined duration. If no side effects appear during the period of observation, a higher dosage of the same drug is administered to a new group of individuals. This process continues until intolerable side effects of the drug appear.

Study design:
- ♦ Fasting, randomized, double blind, placebo controlled, parallel group studies.
- ♦ SAD cohort- Generally, at each dose level, eight volunteers are tested: 6 receiving test drug and 2 placebo (6+2).
- ♦ Safety monitoring – clinical examination, 12-lead ECG, ambulatory BP, holter monitoring, clinical laboratory tests, monitoring of vitals and adverse event monitoring.

- Pharmacokinetics evaluation – Blood samples at baseline, pre and post drug administration at various intervals according to the kinetic properties of drug. Simultaneous collection of urine for drug analysis over stipulated intervals is also done.
- Follow –up: The investigator must follow up:
  - o All subjects after their last dose of IND, for a period depending on the IND and the trial.
  - o Subjects with adverse events, including clinically relevant abnormal laboratory results, until being resolved or resolving.
  - o Subjects who withdraw from a trial.

Multiple Ascending Dose (MAD) studies

Only when single dose administration is completed can multiple dose studies begin. The participants receive various doses of the drug ranging from the lowest dose upto a predetermined level. Samples of blood and other body fluids are taken each time the dose of the drug is raised and it is analyzed in order to evaluate tolerability to drug.

Study design:
- Randomized, double blind, placebo controlled, parallel group studies.
- Duration- till steady state levels reached/ 1-2 weeks.
- MAD cohort- 8-12 volunteers at each dose level (6+2); 4-6 dose levels tested.
- Safety/tolerability assessment.
- Kinetic data (Cmax, Tmax, AUC, $t_{1/2}$, CL, Vd) – blood and urine samples after first and last doses of the trial at the times described in SAD study. Additionally, information about accumulation and attainment of steady-state blood concentrations is obtained by taking blood samples each day immediately before drug administration.
- Follow-up.

LATE PHASE 1 STUDIES

These comprise the additional studies which can be carried out during Phase 1 for example:
- ❖ Drug drug interaction studies.
- ❖ Fed state studies.
- ❖ Special populations- elderly, pediatrics etc.
- ❖ Special clinical conditions – renal/ hepatic disease.
- ❖ New formulation studies.
- ❖ Definitive PK/ PD studies.
- ❖ Bioavailability studies.

CONDUCT OF PHASE 1 TRIALS

INFORMATION REQUIRED BEFORE BEGINNING A PHASE 1 TRIAL (BOX 33.1)

> **Box 33.1** Information required before beginning a Phase 1 trial.
>
> 1. ***General Pharmacology***: in order to indicate the main pharmacological actions of the drug and to provide a background information for the development of the compound as Phase 1.
> 2. ***Non-clinical toxicity studies*** (as per the New Drugs and Clinical Trials Rules, 2019):
> - Systemic toxicity studies:
>   - Single dose toxicity studies.
>   - Dose ranging studies.
>   - Repeat dose systemic toxicity studies of adequate duration supporting the anticipated human exposure.
> - Male fertility studies.
> - In-vitro genotoxicity tests.
> - Relevant local toxicity studies with proposed route of application (duration based on proposed period of exposure clinically).
> - Allergenicity / Hypersensitivity tests (in cases having a cause for concern, parenteral drugs, including dermal application).
> - Photoallergy or dermal phototoxicity tests (if the drug or a metabolite belong to a group of agents known to be associated with photosensitivity or the nature of action indicates such a potential).
> 3. ***Animal pharmacokinetic studies:*** preferably in the species used for toxicity studies.
> 4. ***Chemical and pharmaceutical data***

RISK MANAGEMENT PLAN AND STRATEGY

A proper risk management plan and strategy is essential before starting a Phase 1 clinical trial in order to ensure a minimal risk throughout the trial. The factors to be considered for risk management strategies for phase 1 trials include:

- Study subjects
- Starting dose/First human dose
- Dose escalation protocols
- Dose administration and route
- Facilities and staff

I. STUDY SUBJECTS

In Phase 1 trial, the usual practice is to recruit healthy volunteers/ normal subjects who
- are males,
- aged 18-35 years,
- not currently on any medication/s,
- do not abuse alcohol or any other drugs,
- have no clinically significant hematological or chemical pathological abnormality, and
- have no serological evidence of past or present hepatitis and HIV infection.

Definition of normal subjects as per USFDA (Box 33.2)

Box 33.2 FDA definition of healthy volunteers.

With increasing number of studies in apparently healthy volunteers, it is becoming clear that clinical observations hitherto been regarded as indicators of disease may occur in normal subjects. Recognizing this problem, FDA has defined "healthy volunteers" as *"the individuals who do not suffer from any disorder or abnormality which is expected to interfere with results of the experiment or which can increase the susceptibility of subject to toxic effects of the drug"*. Thus, individuals with mild and stable illness like hypertension, arthritis could be considered for phase 1 trials.

Reasons for selection of healthy volunteers
- *Methodological*: It is easier to establish a causal relationship between drug and adverse event in healthy volunteers due to their lesser susceptibility to adverse events in contrast to patient population.
- *Ethical*: In early stages of drug testing, it is ethically more desirable to involve healthy volunteers than patients.
- *Logistical*: It is relatively simpler and faster to recruit healthy volunteers than patients. Also, healthy subjects are better at completing long and complex trials.

Certain issues of concern regarding selection of study subjects in Phase 1 trials (Box 33.3)

Box 33.3 Issues of concern regarding subject selection criteria in Phase 1 trials.

Appropriate age for inclusion. For drugs mainly consumed by elderly patients e.g. drugs for Alzheimer's disease, the exclusion of volunteers aged over 35 years will fail to elicit essential data about tolerance and pharmacokinetics of drug in later life.

Box 33.3 Contd...

Female subjects in Phase 1. Female subjects of child-bearing potential are usually not enrolled in phase 1 trials, presumably because of the possibility of permanent damage to their germ cells which could lead to congenital malformations in subsequent pregnancies. However, the risk of potential gonadal damage and teratogenicity cannot be completely ruled out for drugs given to males. In fact, some drugs given to males may result in unwanted effects in offspring, also, any male germ cell damaged by a drug is most unlikely to be able to succeed to fertilize the ovum *in vivo*.

Females may show differences from males both in drug kinetics and pharmacodynamics, may have a greater tendency to drug-induced immune reactions and tend to report subjective adverse reactions to drugs more frequently than men. Hence, underrepresentation of females in new drug trials may do women a disservice. In fact, the risk of unfavorable outcome of a hypothetical pregnancy may be easily offset by the greater risks to women due to inadequate pharmacological data for new drugs.

Issues with subjects abusing drugs. Subjects taking other medications or abusing alcohol or drugs of dependency must be excluded from phase 1 studies. It is ideal to carry out a toxicological screen on urine (for salicylates, alcohol, barbiturates, amphetamine, phenothiazine, tricyclic antidepressants, opiates, cocaine, cannabinoids etc.) prior to entry to the trial. The inclusion of nicotine addicts, however, remains a matter of debate. In many studies, they are included and even allowed to smoke on the grounds that the physiological and psychological disturbances produced by withdrawal are more disruptive to the conduct of research than are the actions of nicotine. However, the possible effects of smoking on drug disposition and cardiovascular parameters must also be taken into consideration during subject recruitment and interpretation of results, and it is desirable to balance smokers and non-smokers as far as possible within the study.

IMP potentially toxic or dangerous to healthy volunteers. e.g. anticancer and anti-HIV drugs, gene therapy trials. In such cases, patients with respective disease are invited to participate in phase 1 studies.

II. STARTING DOSE/FIRST HUMAN DOSE

The selection of starting dose for phase 1 studies is a very critical issue. Too low a starting dose may not yield desired information and may necessitate expenditure of extra time and resources to reach to a conclusion, while too high starting dose may pose a threat to subject safety and overlook clinical significance of lower doses.

The choice of method for determination of starting dose in phase 1 studies depends on the nature of the IMP as shown in figure 33.1.

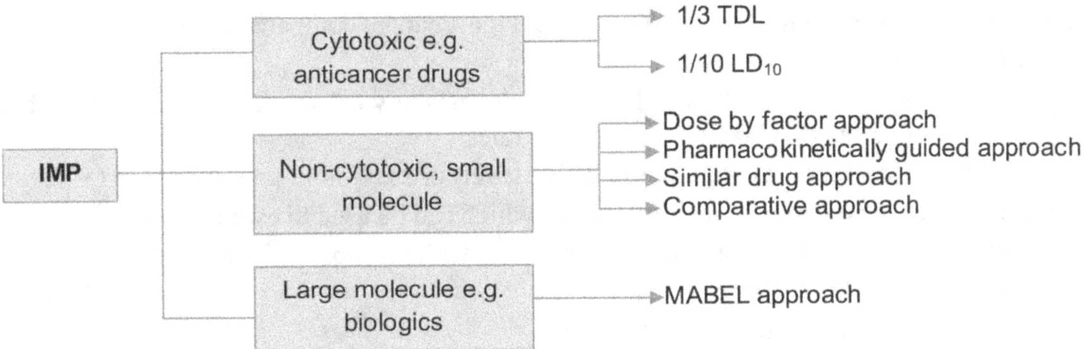

Figure 33.1 Decision tree to calculate starting dose in Phase 1 studies.

A. Cytotoxic compounds

Calculation of the starting dose for cytotoxic compounds is usually done on the basis of a dose and dosage schedule that have elicited some toxicity in animals rather than on a dose identified as totally safe in preclinical studies.

- ***One-third of the toxic dose level (1/3 TDL) in a large animal species.*** Starting dose is calculated as one-third of the toxic dose level (TDL; expressed as mg/m^2) in a large animal species (either dog or monkey). TDL is defined as the lowest dose producing drug-induced pathological changes in hematological, chemical, clinical, or morphological parameters and which, when doubled, produces no lethality. The TDL is estimated on two basic schedules, single dose and daily for 5 days.

- ***One-tenth of the lethal dose in mice.*** The starting dose is calculated as one tenth of a dose producing lethality in 10% of non-tumor bearing mice (LD$_{10}$; expressed in mg/m^2) during a specified duration of observation. LD$_{10}$ is estimated on two basic schedules (single dose and daily for 5 days) including groups of ten mice at each dose level.

B. Non-cytotoxic, small molecule compounds

For such compounds, the starting dose to be used in phase 1 studies can be calculated using different approaches like

- Dose by factor approach (on the basis of allometric scaling of dose).
- Pharmacokinetically guided approach (based on allometric scaling of drug clearance).
- Similar drug approach.
- Comparative approach.

(i) 'Dose by factor' approach.

This is the commonest approach followed for starting dose calculation in phase 1 studies. FDA guidance entitled "*Estimating the Maximum Safe Starting Dose in Initial Clinical Trials for Therapeutics in Adult Healthy Volunteers*" has outlined a 5 step approach to determination of maximum recommended starting dose (MRSD) for first-in-human clinical trials.

Step 1. No Observed Adverse Effect Level (NOAEL) determination. NOAEL is defined as the highest dose level that does not lead to a significant increase in biologically significant adverse events (even in the absence of statistical significance) compared to the control group. NOAEL is different from:

- ♦ no observed effect level (NOEL), which denotes any effect, not only adverse effect, even though the two may be identical at times.
- ♦ LOAEL (lowest observed adverse effect level) or maximum tolerated dose (MTD)

Observations in nonclinical toxicology studies which can be used to estimate NOAEL:

1. manifest toxicity (e.g. clinical signs, gross and microscopic lesions);
2. surrogate markers of toxicity; and
3. exaggerated pharmacodynamic effects.

> In general, definition of NOAEL from pre/non clinical toxicity studies should be done on the basis of an adverse effect that would be considered as unacceptable if produced by the starting dose of drug in a Phase 1 trial in adult healthy volunteers.

Step 2. Human Equivalent Dose (HED) calculation

❖ ***Conversion on the basis of body surface area***

The basis of this conversion is an assumption that doses scale 1:1 between species on normalization to body surface area.

The body surface area normalization and the extrapolation of the animal dose to human dose should be carried out in one step by the multiplication of NOAEL determined in each animal species with appropriate body surface area conversion factor (BSA-CF). This conversion factor is a unit less number which converts mg/kg dose for each animal species to the mg/kg dose in humans, which is equivalent to the animal's NOAEL on a mg/m^2 basis.

HED= NOAEL x BSA-CF

BSA-CF = k_m of animal/ k_m of human

where k_m = $100/K \times Weight^{0.33}$; where K is a value unique to each species;

The k_m value does not remain constant for any species, but increases with increase in body weight.

Alternatively, BSA-CF = (Weight of animal in kg / Weight of human in kg)$^{1-b}$

where b = exponent for body surface area; value of b = 0.67

The conversion factors and divisors (as given in FDA guidance) are recommended to be used as standard values for interspecies dose conversions for NOAELs.

> The approach to convert NOAEL doses to an HED based on body surface area correction factors should ideally be preferred for starting dose calculations in phase 1 studies due to the fact that correction done for body surface area leads to the estimation of more conservative starting dose eventually increasing the chances of safety.

❖ *Calculation on the basis of mg/kg conversions*

Under certain circumstances, it is preferable to do scaling on the basis of body weight i.e. HED (mg/kg) = NOAEL (mg/kg) provided the available data demonstrates similar NOAEL in mg/kg dose across species.

> It is to be noted that HED calculated from *mg/kg scaling* is twelve-, six-, and twofold higher than *mg/m² approach* for mice, rats, and dogs, respectively.

❖ *Other exceptions to mg/m² scaling between species*
- Drugs administered by *alternative routes* (e.g. topical, intranasal, subcutaneous, intramuscular) when local toxicities determine the dose. Such drugs should be normalized to concentration (e.g. mg/area) or amount of drug (mg) at the application site.
- Drugs administered into *anatomical compartments* (e.g. intrathecal, intravesical, intraocular etc.) and mainly limited within the compartment. In these cases, between species normalization should be done according to compartmental volumes and drug concentrations.
- *Proteins with M. wt > 100,000 daltons administered intravascularly.* Normalization should be done to mg/kg.

Step 3. Selecting the most appropriate species

The species generating lowest HED is known as the most sensitive species. However, the species considered more relevant for assessing human risk is generally the most appropriate species. In case the data on species relevance is not available, the most sensitive species is taken as most appropriate species to derive the MRSD.

Step 4: Applying the safety factor

Once HED is calculated in the most appropriate/sensitive species, a safety factor should be applied to yield a safety margin to ensure protection of human subjects who would receive the starting dose. This safety factor adjusts for any variability in dose extrapolation from animals to humans arising due to:
- ✓ uncertainties because of increased susceptibility to pharmacologic effect in humans compared to animals;
- ✓ practical issues in identifying certain adverse effects in animals (e.g. headache, mental state changes);
- ✓ differences in receptor characteristics e.g. density or affinity;
- ✓ unanticipated adverse events; and
- ✓ differences in drug pharmacokinetics between species.

One strategy to accommodate such variabilities is to lower the human starting dose from the calculated HED.

The default safety factor generally used is 10. However, in certain instances, safety factor may be modified as mentioned below.

Increasing the safety factor (>10):
- ✓ Steep dose response curve.
- ✓ Toxicities- severe/non-recordable/ irreversible/ have no premonitory signs.
- ✓ Issues with bioavailability.
- ✓ Undescribed lethalities.
- ✓ Huge variations in drug doses or plasma levels producing effect.
- ✓ Nonlinear pharmacokinetics.
- ✓ Insufficient dose-response data.
- ✓ Novel therapeutic targets.
- ✓ Animal models having doubtful applications.

Decreasing the Safety Factor (< 10):
- ✓ Therapeutics belonging to a well characterized class; administered by same route, dosage regimen and duration; identical bioavailability; similar metabolic and toxicity profiles across all tested species including humans.
- ✓ NOAEL determination on the basis of longer duration toxicity studies compared to the proposed duration in healthy subjects.
- ✓ Toxicity can be readily monitored, reversed, predicted and demonstrates a moderate-to-shallow dose-response relationship.
- ✓ Relatively consistent toxicities across the species tested.
- ✓ Toxicities are cumulative, not associated with peak drug concentrations.
- ✓ No toxicities observed earlier in the repeated dose study.

Step 5: Considering the pharmacologically active dose (PAD)

After calculating the MRSD, it is compared to the PAD derived from suitable pharmacodynamic models. If PAD is lower than MRSD, it may be preferable to decrease the starting dose.

Advantages of 'Dose by factor' approach.
- ✓ Conservative, hence good safety record.
- ✓ Simplicity; easy and practical to apply.

Disadvantages
- ✓ Assumes that drug has similar pharmacokinetics and pharmacodynamics in both species. (In case these presumptions are not sustainable, there are chances of underestimating the effective dose which in turn needs numerous dose escalations to derive therapeutic range).
- ✓ Mechanical (i.e. strict algorithm based).
- ✓ The main focus is on toxicity with relatively lesser incorporation of pharmacology
- ✓ Not applicable to endogenous hormones and proteins (i.e. recombinant clotting factors). used at physiological concentrations or prophylactic vaccines.
- ✓ Not applicable to locally administered drugs.
- ✓ Gives no directions on dose escalation or maximum allowable doses.

(ii) 'Pharmacokinetically guided' approach

In this approach, *systemic exposure* rather than dose is used for extrapolating human dose from animals (Figure 33.2).

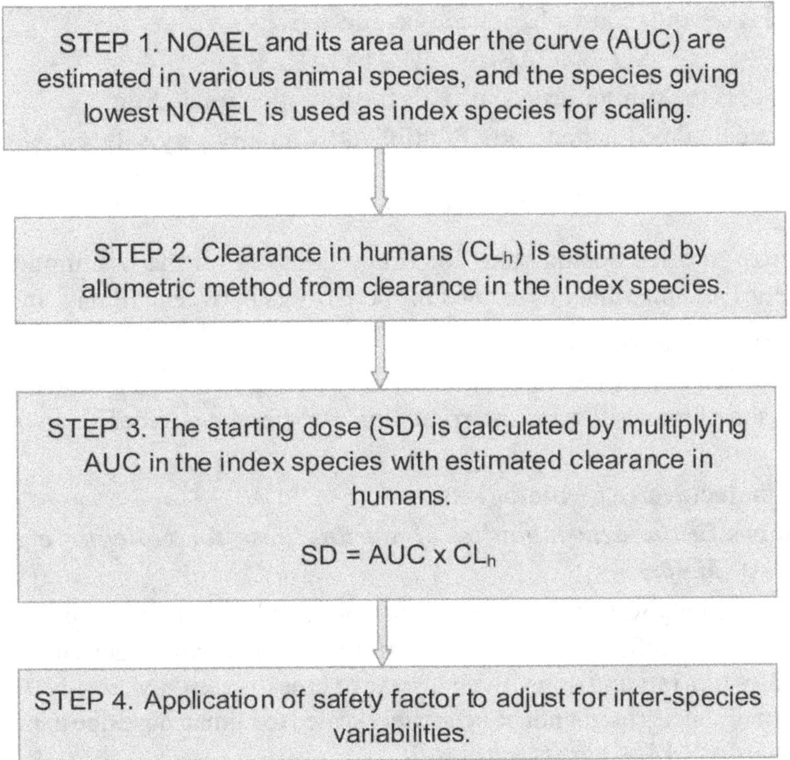

Figure 33.2 Steps in 'Pharmacokinetically guided' approach.

Advantages of 'Pharmacokinetically guided' approach

- ✓ Safe
- ✓ Takes into account preclinical pharmacokinetic data.

Disadvantages

- ✓ Not applicable to drugs following non linear kinetics and drugs having active metabolites.
- ✓ Does not adjust for inter-species differences in drug potency (adjusted by applying safety factor).
- ✓ Uncertainty in prediction of CL(h) using allometric scaling.

(iii) Similar drug approach

This approach is utilized when safety data in humans is available for a drug similar to the investigational drug and can be used as a reference to calculate the starting dose. The "similar drug" is generally of the same chemical class, having similar or related chemical structure and is already approved.

This method relies on the presumption that ratio of the optimal starting dose (SD) of the similar drug to its NOAEL is equal to the ratio of the starting dose of the investigational drug to its NOAEL (optimal starting dose is one which is not associated with any drug-related adverse events or laboratory abnormalities after single dose administration in man and is devoid of any pharmacodynamic activity).

$$SD_s / NOAEL_s = SD_i / NOAEL_i$$

where "s" is the similar drug and "i" is the investigational drug.

The dose calculated is generally multiplied by an arbitrary safety factor to adjust for any uncertainities.

Limitation:

Applying a cross-species dosing ratio for drugs is based on the assumption of identical pharmacokinetics and pharmacodynamics for both drugs between animals and humans.

(iv) Comparative approach

This approach comprises calculation of the starting dose using at least two methods, comparison of the results and interpretation of differences to derive an optimal starting dose.

C. Large molecules (e.g. biologics)

Challenges in the determination of starting dose for biologics e.g. monoclonal antibodies (MAbs)

❖ Adequate toxicity testing may not be possibly conducted in preclinical *in vivo* models due to human specificity of many MAbs and absence of cross-reactivity among different test species like rats and dogs. Even in case of cross-reactive MAbs, NOAEL estimated from animal species might not be accurately scaled to human dose due to pharmacological differences of MAbs across species.

❖ The toxicity of biologics is usually the result of exaggerated pharmacological effects. Hence, characterization of the pharmacological response in preclinical studies is vital to understand the safety implications of these compounds when used clinically.

❖ The prediction of pharmacological effect in humans from preclinical studies is a challenging task due to the different mechanisms of interaction of MAbs with their targets, as compared to small molecules.

❖ Selection of very low starting dose of biologics may demand their administration for longer duration in clinical studies to yield useful information. Further, due to their long half-lives, toxicity with biologics in humans is assumed to sustain for longer periods. Therefore, rational determination of starting doses is of added significance for MAbs.

Taking into consideration the risks involved with biologics and the fact that none of the above methods for starting dose determination is easily applicable to them; an additional method to calculate starting dose needs to be followed.

One recommended approach utilizes the '**Minimal Anticipated Biological Effect Level**' (**MABEL**) which is defined as the dose level anticipated to produce a minimal biological effect in humans. The determination of MABEL incorporates the pharmacokinetic/ pharmacodynamic information from all *in vitro* and *in vivo* models, for example:

- ✓ *in vitro* studies assessing target binding and receptor occupancy in human and animal target cells,
- ✓ *in vitro* assessment of concentration-response relationships in human and animal target cells,
- ✓ *in vivo* dose/exposure-response relationship in relevant preclinical animal models,
- ✓ assessment of exposure at pharmacological doses in preclinical studies.

The data thus obtained should ideally be integrated in a PK/PD model for the estimation of MABEL.

Further, to limit the toxicity in humans, a ***safety factor*** may be applied after taking into consideration various risk criteria e.g. novelty of the molecule, its biological potency and mechanism of action, degree of species specificity, characteristics of dose-response curve and degree of uncertainty in the calculation of MABEL.

When the estimated starting dose in humans determined from various approaches (e.g. NOAEL, MABEL) is different, it is wise to choose the lowest values, unless specified.

III. DOSE ESCALATION PROTOCOLS

The main principle for dose escalation in phase I trials is to implement gradual increments in dose levels to avoid unnecessary exposure of sub-therapeutic doses of an investigational drug to subjects while preserving safety simultaneously. Dose escalation methods for phase I clinical trials can broadly be classified into two categories: the rule-based designs and the model-based designs (Figure 33.3).

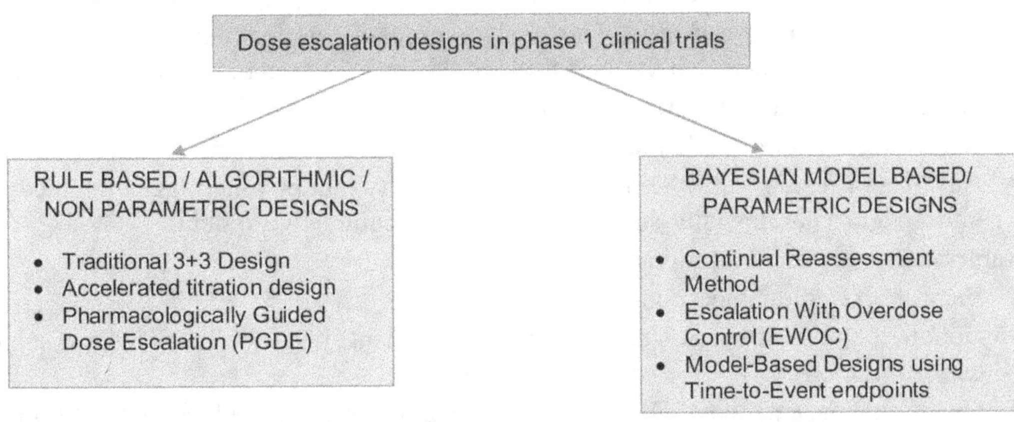

Figure 33.3 Various dose escalation designs used in phase 1 clinical trials

RULE BASED DESIGNS. These methods administer the dose levels to subjects according to pre-defined rules on the basis of actual observations of target events (e.g. the dose-limiting toxicity). These designs are comprised of "up-and-down" designs because they permit dose escalation as well as de-escalation.

1. **Traditional 3+3 Design.** This design proceeds with cohorts of three subjects as follows: 3 subjects are administered dose K.

   ♦ If no subject experiences DLT, escalate to dose K+1.
   ♦ If 2 or more subjects experience DLT, de-escalate to level K-1.
   ♦ If 1 subject experiences DLT, administer dose K to 3 more subjects.
   - If 1 of 6 experiences DLT, escalate to dose level K+1.
   - If 2 or more of 6 experiences DLT, de-escalate to level K-1.

   Dose increments: Conventionally, the dose is doubled at each increment and this practice is justified by a log-linear dose-response curve.

   In phase 1 trial of anticancer drugs, ***Modified Fibonacci sequence*** is followed in which dose increments become smaller with increases in dose (e.g. the dose first increases by 100% of the previous dose, and thereafter by 67%, 50%, 40%, and 30% – 35% of the respective previous doses).

Merits:

   ✓ Simple to implement.
   ✓ Safe.
   ✓ Provides additional information on inter-subject pharmacokinetic variability due to inclusion of 3 subjects at each dose level.

Demerits:

   ✓ Many subjects are administered sub-therapeutic doses.
   ✓ Dose escalation is done quite gradually.
   ✓ Uncertainty about the RP2D.
   ✓ The dose to be administered to a subject is determined by findings from the dose given just before; information on other doses is not considered.

2. **Accelerated titration design.** This design combines the features of traditional 3+3 design and its variants and the model-based designs. The major characteristics are:

   - Escalation done rapidly during initial phase.
   - Within-subject dose escalation.
   - Analysis of results with the help of a dose-toxicity model which takes into account information regarding inter-subject variability and cumulative toxicity.

Example of an accelerated titration design:

   ♦ Begin with single subject cohorts.
   ♦ Double the dose at every step (i.e., 100% increment) per dose level (within-subject dose escalation).
   ♦ On the first appearance of DLT or the second appearance of moderate toxicity (in any course), the cohort for the current dose level is expanded to three subjects.
   ♦ At this point, the trial resumes the traditional 3+3 design for further cohorts with dose increments done by 40%.

   The *model* suggested to be used includes parameters for cumulative toxicity and inter-subject variability. However, in practice, at the end of trial, traditional 3+3 escalation rule is used to determine MTD without incorporation of models. Hence, the original model based accelerated titration designs have been modified mainly as rule-based designs.

Merits:

- ✓ Dose escalation done quite rapidly.
- ✓ Relatively larger number of subjects may be exposed to higher dose levels.
- ✓ The data from all subjects, cumulative toxicities and inter-subject variability may be applied in a model to establish RP2D.

Demerits:

If model fitting is not executed (as generally done in practice):

- ✓ Within-subject dose escalation may conceal the cumulative or delayed toxicities.
- ✓ Tedious elucidation of results with within-subject dose escalations.

3. **Pharmacologically Guided Dose Escalation (PGDE).** This approach is based on the principle that dose-limiting toxicities can be anticipated from plasma drug concentrations and this relationship can be accurately studied in preclinical models. This method is done in two stages.

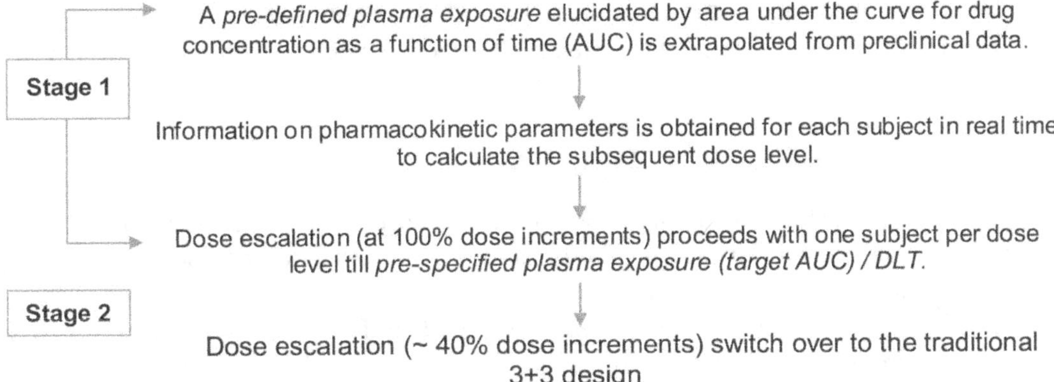

Merits:

- ✓ Dose escalation done more rapidly.
- ✓ Provides information on inter-subject variability in PK data

Demerits:

- ✓ Requirement of real-time PK information.
- ✓ Inter-subject variability may affect further dose escalation.

MODEL BASED DESIGNS

These designs employ statistical models which aim to precisely compute dose–toxicity curve and to determine the dose level producing a pre-defined likelihood of dose-limiting toxicity based on toxicity data from all enrolled subjects.

The Bayesian methods employed in these designs require a prior assumption or distribution of θ, which characterizes the shape of the dose–toxicity curve. Any manifestation of toxicity in enrolled subjects at any dose level imparts added information for the statistical model leading to an adjustment of θ; i.e. posterior distribution of θ according to Bayes' theorem. The posterior distribution is then examined to identify the dose level closely associated with target toxicity, and this dose is used in further subjects and to determine the recommended dose for phase II trials.

Merits

- ✓ Clear definition of target toxicity level.
- ✓ Dose escalation done rapidly.
- ✓ Relevant information from all subjects used to estimate dose.
- ✓ Determination of the RP2D with a confidence interval.
- ✓ Late-onset toxicities are taken into consideration (time-to-event continual reassessment method).
- ✓ Both toxicity and efficacy are duly considered.

Demerits

- ✓ Need to have a prior estimate of RP2D.
- ✓ Computations needed after each subject or cohort of subjects.
- ✓ Biostatistical support needed for making decisions on dose escalation (may also be an advantage).

IV. DOSE ADMINISTRATION AND ROUTE

- ◆ For a low risk IMP to be administered orally, cohorts of subjects can be dosed during same session at short intervals of 5-10 minutes. At least 2 subjects should be used on each dose.
- ◆ If the route of administration is intravenous, it should be given by slow infusion over several hours rather than rapid injection.
- ◆ For a high risk IMP, initially only one subject should be administered the active drug. Following this, *"staggered dosing within a cohort"* can be done with increasing doses as shown in Figure 33.4.

	Dose administration Time = t (time of dose administration)	Dose administration Time = t + 3 hours
First day	Subject 1	Subject 2
Second day	Subjects 3-8	

Figure 33.4 Staggered dosing within a cohort.

V. FACILITIES AND STAFF

Phase 1 trials are conducted at specialized sites – Phase 1 unit/ Clinical Pharmacology Unit (CPU). A phase 1 unit should:
- ✓ be purpose-built or modified as per the purpose;
- ✓ in line with local planning, health and safety requirements;
- ✓ having ready access to the emergency services;
- ✓ be close to or on site of a hospital having acute medical services;
- ✓ have adequate utility services, including emergency lighting and a back-up power supply, and collection of hazardous and clinical waste.

There should be adequate medical, nursing, scientific, technical and support staff for the types and number of trials that are conducted in the unit. All staff should be adequately qualified, trained and experienced.

PHASE 1 STOP RULES

- Poor tolerability: unacceptable serious ADR's.
- Poor/ inadequate bioavailability.
- Saturable clearance : change to steep DRC
- Too short $t_{1/2}$: need for high frequency of dosing.
- Multiple active metabolites, not covered in preclinical toxicity studies.
- Active metabolites with very long $t_{1/2}$
- Development of major organ toxicity in man.

RISKS INVOLVED IN PHASE 1 TRIALS

The overall safety profile of phase 1 trials is good. The incidence of serious adverse events related to IMP has been reported as 0.02%. However, few healthy subjects died during phase 1 trials. A man died due to cardiac arrest after taking an IMP in Ireland in 1984. At the time of screening for the trial, he did not inform that he had recently received a depot injection of an anti-psychotic medicine. A woman died after receiving a high dose of lidocaine to prevent discomfort from endoscopy in a trial in USA in 1996. Another woman with mild asthma died of lung damage after inhaling hexamethonium in a trial in the USA in 2001 (Box 33.4).

> **Box 33.4** Parexel tragedy: the disaster.
>
> This dreadful tragedy occurred during phase 1 trial of ***TGN1412***, a recombinant humanized monoclonal antibody, a CD28 superagonist. The trial was sponsored by TeGenero, Germany and conducted at Parexel Clinical Pharmacology Research Unit, U.K (Northwick Park Hospital in North London). For the trial, 8 healthy young men were enrolled (6 - TGN1412; 2 - Placebo). All the six subjects suffered from "cytokine release syndrome" and life threatening multi-organ failure. The starting dose administered to subjects was 0.1 mg/kg (calculated by dose by factor approach, FDA guidance), which on product analysis was stipulated to be close to the maximum immuno-stimulatory dose. The MABEL method gave a much lower starting dose (5 µg/kg).

PAYMENT FOR PARTICIPATION IN PHASE 1 TRIALS

- Many trials have challenging issues for the subject and involve long duration of stay, multiple visits to the trial site, urine collections, and multiple blood tests and other procedures associated with discomfort, as well as lifestyle restrictions. So payment of subjects, whether healthy volunteers or patients, more than just any expenses they bear is justified.
- The *amount* should be proportionate to the duration of stay in the unit, frequency and length of visits, lifestyle restrictions, and the nature and intensity of inconvenience and discomfort associated. As a rule, payments should be on the basis of minimum hourly wage and should be increased proportionately for procedures demanding extra care.
- *Payment* should not be determined by the risk involved. For subjects withdrawing themselves or being withdrawn for medical reasons, the amount of payment may be decided by the investigator depending on circumstances.
- Payment may be reduced if a subject fails to comply with the protocol, or may be increased if any protocol amendment is made to add extra tests or visits.
- Payment should be appropriately made to reserve or 'stand by' subjects.
- The policy on payment of trial subjects and the amount must be mentioned in the subject information sheet and be approved by the Ethics Committee.

CHAPTER 34

Phase 2 and 3 Clinical Trials

OVERVIEW

PHASE II CLINICAL TRIALS (THERAPEUTIC EXPLORATORY TRIALS)

INTRODUCTION

Phase II clinical trials are controlled clinical studies undertaken early during clinical phase of drug development with an aim to gain preliminary knowledge on efficacy of drug for the proposed indication in patient population. These trials are helpful in determining frequent short-term adverse effects and risks associated with drug use in patients. Phase II studies may also be conducted as pilot (or feasibility) studies to predict probability of success in subsequent phase III trials.

OBJECTIVES OF PHASE II CLINICAL TRIALS

- To prove drug activity on specific pharmacodynamic outcomes.
- To determine dose range and dosage regimen for subsequent phase (phase 3) clinical trials.
- To obtain safety and tolerability data on drug use in patient population.

TYPES OF PHASE II TRIALS

Phase II trials are often called "***Therapeutic Exploratory trials***" and are further comprised of two phases:

Phase IIa. Proof of Concept (PoC) or Proof of Principle studies

Phase IIb. Dose selection or dose ranging or dose finding studies

PHASE IIA (PROOF OF CONCEPT)

These clinical experiments are based on the principle that binding of a drug to a specific target/ receptor is associated with meaningful change in a clinical/surrogate end-point. Their main objective is to confirm the fundamental biological and pharmaco-dynamic concepts associated with the mechanism of action of a new drug. Hence, they are especially useful when the compound under investigation is an innovative one.

These trials are usually small, complex and of great strategic significance as failure to prove the concept warrants termination of drug development program.

Features of PoC studies

- ✓ Homogenous study population.
- ✓ Early efficacy indicator (mechanistic efficacy) and therefore early dose selection for phase 3.
- ✓ Focused target population (ideally genetically defined).
- ✓ Focused safety (predicted).
- ✓ Small sample size (N = 20 -100; few sites) and small duration.
- ✓ Validated pharmacodynamic model.
- ✓ Novel, innovative approach (e.g. challenge agent paradigm, use of novel biomarker such as PET imaging).
- ✓ Novel designs.

PHASE IIB (DOSE FINDING OR DOSE RANGING)

These are the studies done for establishing the dose/s and dosing frequencies for further studies. In addition, useful data on pharmaco-dynamic and therapeutic profile of the drug can be obtained from these studies. They also serve as proof of concept studies in the absence of Phase IIa studies.

Dose-ranging trials in humans are often conducted to characterize responses obtained at specific doses and to identify specific doses (e.g., minimum effective dose, maximum effective dose, maximum tolerable dose, optimal dose, minimum toxic dose). Information on the therapeutic index also is sought in most dose-ranging trials. In a pilot clinical trial where dose ranging is conducted, the purpose may be to identify a range of effective doses.

A major goal of dose-ranging trials is to identify the optimal dose or dose range appropriate for a specific indication in terms of both safety and efficacy for a specific population of patients. This involves determining the:

- Amount of drug to be taken in each dose.
- Number of doses to be taken each day.
- When during the day (or night) each dose is to be taken.
- Conditions under which each dose is to be taken (e.g., with food, amount of water).

As the dose given to each patient or group of patients increases in a clinical trial, the response of each patient may also increase (i.e. a greater effect may be observed). In addition, more people may respond to treatment; this is more likely to occur if clinical responses are not graded but, instead, are all-or-none.

Characteristically, these are open-label or double-blind pilot trials that are specifically designed to evaluate the safety and/or preliminary efficacy of a number of doses. Usually two or more doses of a drug are tested to seek efficacious effects.

Designs used in dose ranging studies:

Fixed-dose parallel group trial: equal number of patients receive each dose.

Titrated-dose trial: individuals are titrated to their most effective and safe dose.

In Phase 2, the lowest dose tested for efficacy is the one that led to the plasma concentration in Phase 1 predicted to be effective based on animal studies. An even lower dose, which is anticipated to be sub-therapeutic, may also be tested in Phase 2, or a higher dose may be tested. If clinical efficacy is not observed at any of the doses studied in early Phase 2 trials or an insufficient response is observed, it is generally decided to repeat a Phase 1 trial studying higher doses and then to evaluate efficacy of those doses in Phase 2 dose-ranging trials.

TYPES OF DESIGNS USED IN PHASE II TRIALS

- ❖ **Single-arm study.** This is the most uncomplicated design in which all subjects receive the study intervention. Its advantage is being less resource intensive. Some studies are designed to impart information on the number of subjects required to respond to the new intervention to justify further clinical development.

- ❖ **Single-arm two-stage study (Design of Gehan).** In this, small number of participants are first administered the intervention and evaluated. A 'stopping rule' is defined according to which if a specified proportion of subjects show response at the end of first stage, the trial is continued with further recruitment of second group of participants; otherwise the trial is terminated This design is particularly useful when the outcome is based on binary data e.g. counting the subjects. Such two-stage designs are particularly applicable when the new intervention is expected to produce serious adverse effects or is expensive, because of very limited exposure to study intervention which may well be devoid of any clinical benefit.

❖ **Randomized phase II trial with control arm.** The trial comprises two intervention groups viz. new intervention group and a control (standard treatment or placebo) group. The results in two groups form basis for designing the corresponding treatment groups in a phase III trial, especially to calculate sample size. Additional information gained with this design includes estimate of recruitment rates, subjects' willingness to get enrolled in a randomized trial, possible logistical issues, etc. which may prove quite helpful in designing future trials.

❖ **Randomized phase II trial with multiple intervention groups.** Two or more new interventions can be evaluated simultaneously in this design. Each treatment group is designed as a single-arm study, and subjects are randomized to all different groups. The primary objective of this design is not comparison of results between different groups/ arms but to identify the intervention (one or more) having potential for further investigation as is done in single-arm phase II study. The study may also be designed to include standard treatment or placebo in one of the treatment arms.

❖ **Randomized phase II trial with multiple intervention groups: two-stage design.** This is an extension of the single-arm two-stage design. During the first stage, few subjects (as defined in the sample size calculation) are randomized to all the new intervention groups. Efficacy is assessed at the end of first stage and the interventions showing promising results are proceeded to second stage.

PHASE III CLINICAL TRIALS (THERAPEUTIC CONFIRMATORY TRIALS)

INTRODUCTION

The primary objective of Phase III trials is to demonstrate or confirm therapeutic benefits(s). Studies in Phase III are planned with an objective to substantiate the preliminary evidence generated in phase II regarding safety and efficacy of the intervention in the proposed indication and patient population.

These studies also intend to provide sufficient evidence for marketing authorization of new intervention.

Phase III trials may also be conducted to explore
- dose-response relationships (relationships between drug dosage, concentration in plasma/ target site and clinical response),
- drug usage in broader populations with different stages of disease, or
- safety/ efficacy profile of the drug when administered with other drug(s).

For drugs expected to be administered for long durations, trials comprising of extended exposure to the drug are generally carried out in phase III, though they may be started in phase II. Such phase III trials provide sufficient data to complete the drug's prescribing information.

Phase III trials have broad inclusion/exclusion criteria making the study population more heterogenous. This strategy is helpful in getting results which are more generalizable, thereby, increasing the external validity of these trials.

FACTORS DETERMINING ENTRY INTO A PHASE III TRIAL: A CONCEPTUAL DECISION MODEL (FIGURE 34.1)

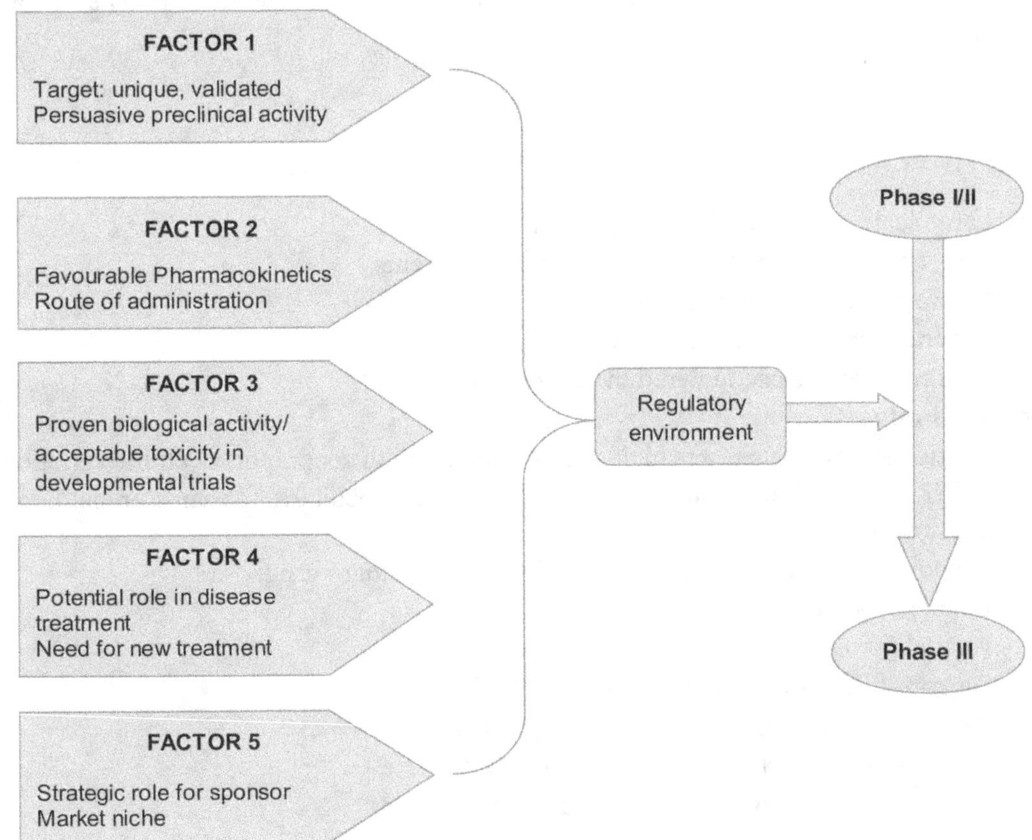

Figure 34.1 Phase III decision model: Critical deciding factors for advancing from developmental trials (Phase I/II) to Phase III.

TYPES OF PHASE III CLINICAL TRIALS

Phase III A clinical trials

These comprise the clinical trials conducted up to NDA submission.

End of Phase III A studies must include special patient populations and pharmacoeconomic data collection.

Phase III B clinical trials

- ✓ Ongoing trials at time of NDA submission.
- ✓ Undertaken after NDA submission but before NCE is marketed.
- ✓ New indications may be included.
- ✓ New patient populations may be included.
- ✓ Special features explored e.g. drug interactions.
- ✓ Multicenter trials, superiority trials, non-inferiority trials, combination trials, bridging studies, vaccine clinical trials.

CHARACTERISTIC FEATURES OF PHASE III TRIALS

- Large scale, randomised, controlled trials.
- Target population: hundreds to thousands of patients.
- Heterogenous study population.
- Generally executed by clinicians in the hospital.
- Minimises errors encountered in phases I and II.
- **Methods**
  - Multicentric which ensures inclusion of subjects with geographic & ethnic variations.
  - Different patient subgroups may be included e.g. pediatric, geriatric, renal/hepatic impaired.
  - Randomised assignment of test drug /placebo/ standard drug.
  - Double blinded.
  - Parallel / cross over designs used commonly.
  - Superiority/ non-inferiority/ equivalence trials.
  - Cautious monitoring of all adverse drug reactions.
  - Meticulous statistical analysis of all clinical data.
- Usually long duration studies: up to 5 years.
- Variable success rates.

For new drugs approved outside India, Phase III trials should mainly be conducted to gather evidence on efficacy and safety of the drug in Indian population when used as suggested in the prescribing information. Before conducting Phase III trials in Indian subjects, regulatory authority may demand conduct of pharmacokinetic studies to verify the concordance of data obtained in Indian population with that generated abroad.

CLINICAL DRUG DEVELOPMENT: POSTMARKETING PHASES

CONTENTS

CHAPTER 35

Phase 4 Research

OVERVIEW

Introduction
Phase 4: Meeting the Unmet Needs
Objectives of Studies Conducted
during Phase 4

Categories of Phase 4 Research
FDA- Mandated/Negotiated Studies
Non- FDA Mandated Phase 4 Studies
Post Marketing Evaluation of New Drugs

INTRODUCTION

Postmarketing (Phase 4) research is a general term which denotes all studies carried out on a drug product after being granted approval by the regulatory authority. The main purpose of Post-marketing or Phase 4 studies (apart from routine surveillance studies) is to optimize the use of newly approved drug in approved indication/s.

PHASE 4: MEETING THE UNMET NEEDS

The need of Phase 4 studies arises due to the existing drawbacks of clinical trials conducted during the premarketing phase (Phases 1, 2 and 3) of drug development like:

- ✓ Failure to identify adverse events which are infrequent/ rare or present after a long latent period.
- ✓ Failure to reflect the real-world use of drugs due to:
- Narrow inclusion criteria to recruit patients.
- "Short" study period; short duration of drug use.
- Small user population.
- Include intensive medical supervision which is not practically feasible in standard clinical practice.
- Narrow set of indications.
- Limited comparison groups, most often limited to placebo.
- ✓ Commonly employ surrogate endpoints as measures of efficacy.
- ✓ Limited generalizability of results to routine clinical practice.
- ✓ Inherent bias during the conduct of clinical trials.

OBJECTIVES OF STUDIES CONDUCTED DURING PHASE 4

- Gain a better medical and scientific *understanding of adverse events* so patients can be more effectively treated.
- Gain more insight into the *real-world use of the drug* in order to produce better product information for healthcare professionals and patients. Hence, these studies are also known as "Real-world data" studies.
- Adhere to *regulatory* requirements and agreements made as part of the drug's approval.
- Demonstrate that any *potential or real safety issues* are being assiduously investigated, which would help to protect the company from liability suits that might result from the issue being studied.
- Learn more about benefits of the drug that may *expand the indication* (e.g., to a less ill or more severely ill group of patients).
- Learn more about *dosing regimens or combinations with other drugs* that may provide greater convenience or enhanced benefits.
- Expand the knowledge base for *specific patient groups* or circumstances that may not have been included in the development program or were only minimally represented, such as the elderly, different racial and ethnic groups, those with organ impairment, and long-term treatment.
- Discover *new indications* (occurring through serendipity or informal tests) that are then explored and developed in Phases 2 and 3.

CATEGORIES OF PHASE 4 RESEARCH (FIGURE 35.1)

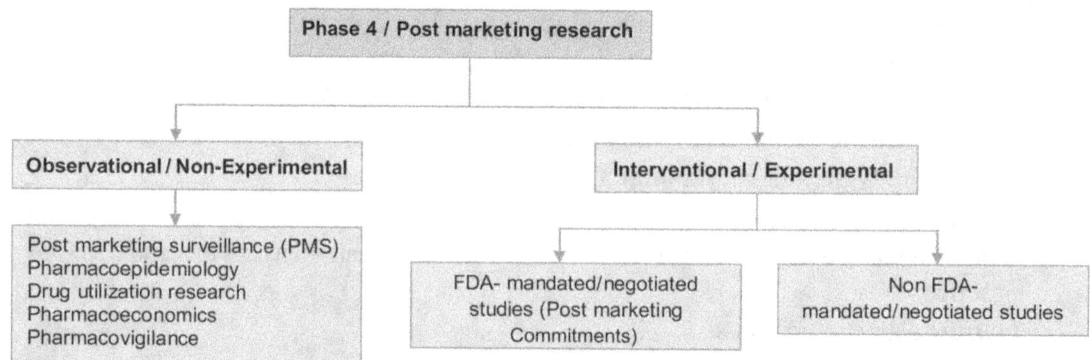

Figure 35.1 Types of research conducted during Phase 4.

FDA-MANDATED/NEGOTIATED STUDIES

These are the studies required by FDA after the approval of new drugs, and are labeled as Phase IV Post Marketing Commitment studies (PMCs). These are particularly indicated when the new drug has received approval through US-FDA expedited program for NDAs e.g. fast track or accelerated approval.

Types of study designs

- Standard RCTs.
- Drug interaction studies.
- Studies in special group of patients e.g. pediatric, geriatric, pregnant, lactating etc.
- Formulation advancement studies.
- Special safety studies.
- *Exploratory special population studies.* These aim to assess the effect and/or adverse effect profile of a drug in special subset of patients such as neonatal abstinence syndrome.
- *Phase V trials.* Supplementary scientifically exhaustive studies carried out during post marketing period, especially if they are RCTs, are sometimes labeled as 'phase V' trials.

NON- FDA MANDATED PHASE 4 STUDIES

These are of various types like:
- RCTs aiming to evaluate *superiority/ equivalence/ non-inferiority* of study treatment compared to control treatment.
- *Large Simple Trial.* These large trials are based on the assumption that the drug effects are identical among various participants, hence the subject eligibility criteria can be broadened, simplified techniques can be utilized for data management, thereby reducing the cost involved. Such types of trials are however feasible with easily administered intervention/s and conveniently determined outcome/s. An advantage of large simple trials is reasonably fair probability of detecting rare ADRs.
- *Prospective, Randomized, Open-Label, Blinded Endpoint (PROBE) Design.* The advantages of open label design are feasibility of study conduct when comparing interventions with different routes of administration and physical characteristics, drugs producing some obvious symptom or sign like discoloration of secretions, and in studies involving clinical titration of drugs. However, in such open label studies, the personnel involved in assessing outcomes are generally blinded to avoid assessment bias.
- *Practice Based Clinical Experience Studies/ Physician Experience Studies (PES).* These are usually commenced by the sponsor but may be required by the FDA at times. Generally, PES are not designed as a randomized controlled trial, hence their scientific rigor is an issue of concern. Another disadvantage is a lot of missing data in these studies. However, they are helpful to provide experience to physicians on the use

of new drugs, in addition to gathering 'real world' evidence regarding the benefit-risk profile of the drugs by exposing huge population to the newly launched drugs.

- ***Marketing-oriented studies/ Seeding studies.*** These are uncontrolled cohort studies that appear to be planned more for marketing advantage rather than the detection of new ADRs. They mainly aim to alter the physician prescribing and as this is not mentioned in the protocol they are inherently dishonest and bring discredit to the industry and doctors involved. Features suggestive of seeding studies include:

✓ No comparator group.

✓ Poor statistical power.

✓ Large number of doctors with small number of patients each.

✓ Involvement of medical representatives.

✓ Invalid or inappropriate outcomes.

✓ Short duration study with a drug intended to be used for long duration.

✓ Directly sponsored by manufacturing company.

POSTMARKETING EVALUATION OF NEW DRUGS (BOX 35.1)

Box 35.1 The New Drugs and Clinical Trials Rules, 2019, India.

Post market evaluation of new drugs can be conducted through:

❖ ***Phase IV (Post marketing) trial.***

- These may include drug interaction studies, dose response or safety studies, mortality or morbidity studies etc.

- Such trial should be carried out after obtaining approval from CLA with the new drug under approved conditions of its use.

- Fees to be deposited with application for permission to conduct Phase IV trial is Rs. 2,00,000. *(Earlier, no fees was defined for Phase IV studies).*

- In these trials, study drug may be given free of cost to the trial subjects unless there is some specific concern to the satisfaction of CLA or EC.

❖ ***Post marketing surveillance study / observational or non-interventional study for active surveillance.***

- Such studies need prior approval from CLA.

- Subject inclusion criteria are determined by the recommended use of drug/s according to the prescribing information or approved package insert.

- Regulatory guidelines applicable for clinical trial of a new drug do not apply in these cases as drugs are already approved for marketing.

❖ ***Post marketing surveillance through periodic safety update reports***

(For details, please refer to Chapter 36).

Post Marketing Surveillance

OVERVIEW

Introduction
PMS: Methods
  Spontaneous/Voluntary/Targeted Reporting
  Prescription Event Monitoring (PEM)
  Record Linkage

Periodic Safety Update Reports (PSURs) /
Periodic Benefit-Risk Evaluation Reports
(PBRERs)
Detection of Adverse Effects of Drugs

INTRODUCTION

Post Marketing Surveillance (PMS) has traditionally been defined as "the systematic detection and evaluation of adverse experience/s occurring in association with drugs or biologics under customary conditions of use in ordinary medical practice".

PMS: METHODS

1. Spontaneous/ voluntary/ targeted reporting (Figure 36.1)

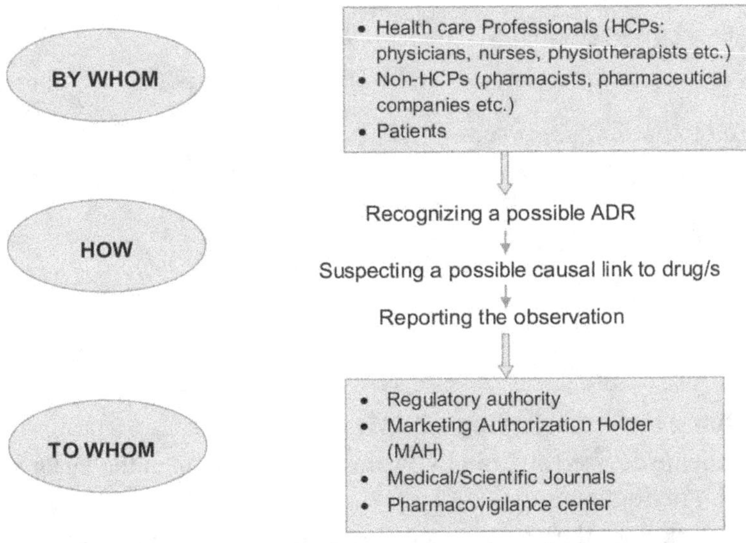

Figure 36.1 The process of spontaneous/ voluntary reporting of adverse events.

Merits

- Very good for generating new ADR hypotheses, especially rare ADRs.
- Wide scope: available immediately after a new drug is marketed, continues indefinitely, involves all doctors and covers the entire population receiving the drug.
- Also detect and characterize common reactions.
- Helps in confirming the suspicions aroused during clinical trials.

Demerits

- Under reporting (Table 36.1).
- Reporting influenced by various factors (volume of sales, how long the drug has been in the market, type and severity of ADR, publicity about the drug and reaction etc.).
- Do not confirm the ADR hypothesis.
- Incidence rate of ADR can't be determined; only reporting rate can be calculated.

Table 36.1 ADR Under-reporting: Reasons.

Reasons related to HCPs

- Guilt-ridden feeling.
- Fear of prosecution.
- Busy schedule.
- Lack of interest.
- Lack of risk perception with regard to new drugs.
- Reservedness.
- Poorly trained in ADR identification.
- Insufficient knowledge on reporting process.
- Inability to precisely correlate ADR with biochemical or pathologic observation/s.

Reasons related to patients/subjects

- Lack of ADR recognition.
- Failure to associate ADR with drug.
- Inadequate knowlegde about PV program.
- Poor inclination.
- Mindset and expectations.

2. Prescription event monitoring (PEM)

PEM is a scheme devised and run by Professor Bill Inman at the Drug Safety Research Unit (DSRU) in Southampton, UK.

Figure 36.2 describes the various steps involved in the PEM process.

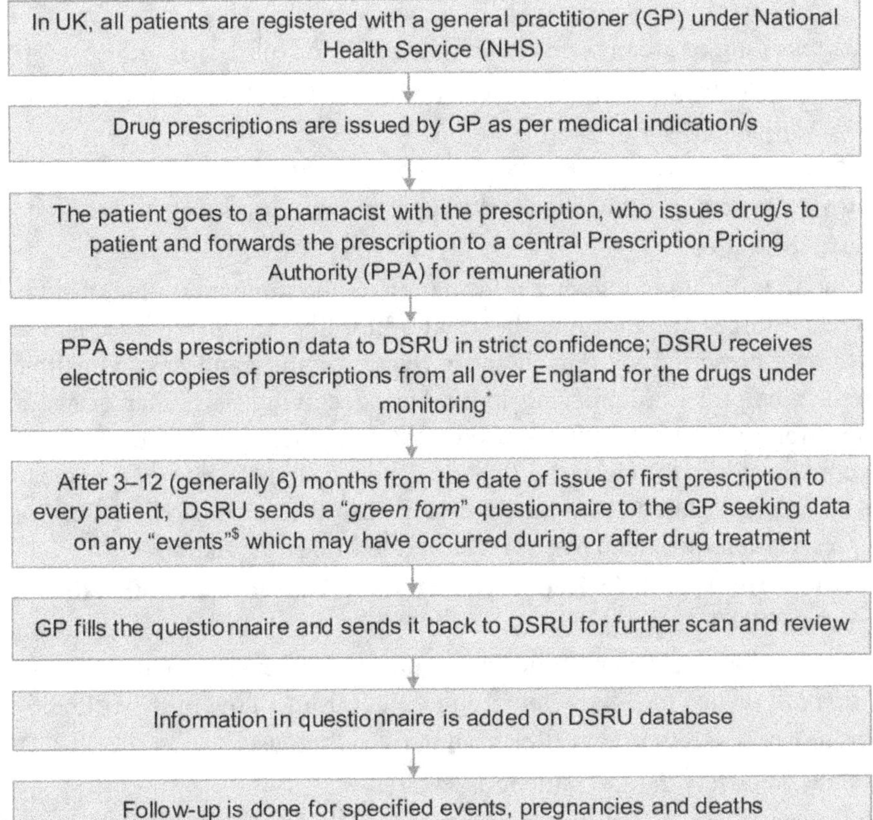

*Drugs monitored by PEM are generally new drugs assumed to be commonly prescribed by GPs or already existing products prescribed for a new indication or new group of patients

$Criteria for event definition:
- diagnosis of a previously non-existing condition,
- any condition demanding consultation or hospital admission,
- an unpredicted worsening (or betterment) in a coexisting disorder,
- any known reaction to drug administration,
- any clinically significant derangement in laboratory parameters or
- any other reported symptom or sign entered in the patient's notes.

Figure 36.2 The PEM Process

Merits

- Non-interventional; does not influence prescribing decisions.
- Monitors prescriptions that have actually been dispensed.
- Supplies "real-world" data on drug use.
- Helps in the identification of unexpected adverse events.
- Patients in the cohort can be enrolled in future studies like nested case–control studies or pharmacogenetic studies to identify risk factors.

Demerits

- Under reporting of green forms leading to selection bias.
- Dependent on the quality of GPs record keeping as well as completeness and accuracy of information in green forms.
- Compliance of dispensed prescriptions is not measured
- Limited to general practice; hence does not monitor drugs used in hospital settings.

3. **Record linkage**

   This involves bringing together information on the same individual from two or more different sources for example, hospital admission and discharge data and general practitioner prescriptions. This helps in relating significant remote health events. The system is helpful in identifying individuals receiving particular drugs and select a comparator group, it can hence be used to test hypotheses and quantify risk. An example of record linkage in the UK is the Tayside system called MEMO (MEdicinesMOnitoring Unit) which uses patients' unique community health numbers to link data from hospitals and prescriptions provided by the Prescription Pricing Division.

4. **Periodic Safety Update Reports (PSURs) / Periodic Benefit-Risk Evaluation Reports (PBRERs)**

   PSUR is a document containing a regular and extensive evaluation of the safety information related to a marketed drug product from all over the world. PSUR aims to

✓ report any new safety information arising from drug use;

✓ correlate the safety data to patient exposure;

✓ outline the worldwide marketing authorization status including any significant differences due to safety aspects;

✓ provide regular update of the overall safety assessment;

✓ indicate the need to make any modifications in product information to ensure optimal drug use.

As per the New Drugs and Clinical Trials Rules, 2019 (Box 36.1),

✓ PSURs need to be submitted to regulatory authority six monthly for the first two years after drug approval and annually for next two years.

✓ The total period for submitting PSUR can be increased by licensing authority if deemed essential in public interest.

✓ PSURs for a defined period have to be submitted to licensing authority within 30 calendar days of the last day of the reporting period. However, all serious unpredicted adverse reactions need to be reported within 15 days of receipt of their initial information by the applicant.

✓ In case of delayed marketing of new drug after grant of approval, data has to be delivered on deferred basis from marketing of new drug.

Box 36.1 The New Drugs and Clinical Trials Rules, 2019, India.

Changes in the format of PSUR compared to that in Schedule Y:

- ✓ More elaborate format of PSUR.
- ✓ Inclusion of information on risk management plan (not included earlier).
- ✓ Need to enclose copy of marketing authorization in India, which was not required previously.

Structure of PSUR (as per the New Drugs and Clinical Trials Rules, 2019, India)

- ✓ Title page.
- ✓ Introduction.
- ✓ Current worldwide marketing authorization status.
- ✓ Any safety related regulatory actions taken during reporting interval.
- ✓ Modifications, if any, to reference safety information.
- ✓ Estimated patient exposure (Data on cumulative and interval subject exposure in clinical trial, cumulative and interval patient exposure from marketing experience in India and from rest of the world).
- ✓ Inclusion of individual case histories.
- ✓ Studies.
- ✓ Other information including risk management plan.
- ✓ Overall safety evaluation.
- ✓ Conclusion (details on the safety profile of drug and any actions taken by the licence holder with regard to safety).
- ✓ Appendix: including the copy of marketing authorisation in India, copy of prescribing information, line listings with narrative of Individual Case Safety Reports (ICSR).

PBRER. Compared to PSUR, the scope of PBRER extends to include benefit as well as safety, hence it gives a comprehensive and clear assessment of benefit-risk profile of the medicinal product.

DETECTION OF ADVERSE EFFECTS OF DRUGS

Various factors which determine the potential of a surveillance method to identify adverse effects associated with drugs include:

- Time lapse between administration of drug and appearance of adverse effect (the latency period).

- Sample size studied.
- Background frequency of the condition.
- Additional frequency due to drug.
- Size of the control group, if background incidence is unknown.

The probability of detecting a drug effect in a particular study is determined by the study's sample size and background frequency of drug effect. For instance, in a cohort study, if the background frequency of drug induced ADR is 1 percent, the probability of finding one or more ADRs in a sample of 100 people would be 63 percent. As the sample studied is increased, the probability of detecting ADR will increase (Table 36.2).

Table 36.2 Probability of observing an ADR (95% probability).

Number of patients in ADR study	Frequency of ADR		
	1/100	1/1000	1/10,000
100	0.63	0.10	0.01
200	0.86	0.18	0.02
500	0.99	0.39	0.05
1000	0.99	0.63	0.10
2000	0.99	0.86	0.18
5000	0.99	0.99	0.39
10,000	0.99	0.99	0.63

In other words, how many users need to be observed to have 95 percent certainty of finding at least 1 case of ADR when the background incidence (frequency) of ADR is known? The *'rule of three'* indicates if an event occurs in 1 of every 5000 exposed persons, 3x5000 (i.e. 15000) people would be needed in a sample to be 95% certain that the sample includes one case (Table 36.3).

Table 36.3 Number of subjects needed to detect one, two, or three ADRs when background frequency of ADR is not known (95% probability).

Expected incidence of adverse reaction	Required number of ADRs		
	1 ADR	2 ADRs	3 ADRs
1 in 100	300	480	650
1 in 200	600	960	1,300
1 in 1,000	3,000	4,800	6,500

The size of sample required to detect a drug's effect increases as the expected incidence of an event decreases and as the incidence of the drug's additional contribution to the event increases.

In cases where there is no background information regarding the incidence of drug induced adverse event and has to be determined by observing control groups, the smaller the size of control group, the larger the sample size of drug users should be to attain same level of confidence in the observations.

Pharmacovigilance

OVERVIEW

INTRODUCTION

The definition of Pharmacovigilance (PV) given by World Health Organization (WHO) is: "The science and activities relating to the detection, assessment, understanding and prevention of adverse effects or any other possible drug related problems". Pharmacovigilance (PV), one of the drug safety surveillance activities in the post marketing phase, has a crucial function of assuring safe use of drugs.

In 1968, WHO set up its "Programme for International Drug Monitoring" aiming at an organized gathering of data on serious ADRs through the developmental phases of new drugs especially after their availability for communal use. Since 1978 this programme is being operated by Uppsala Monitoring Centre (UMC) in Sweden.

IMPORTANT DEFINITIONS RELATED TO PHARMACOVIGILANCE (BOX 37.1)

Box 37.1 Important Definitions Related to Pharmacovigilance.

Adverse Event (AE): any undesired and unfavorable medical event occurring in a patient or clinical trial participant which may not essentially have a causal relationship with the administered medicine/ intervention.

Box 37.1 *Contd...*

Adverse Drug Reaction (ADR): defined by WHO as "a response to a drug that is noxious and unintended and occurs at doses normally used in man for prophylaxis, diagnosis and therapy of disease or for the modification of the physiological function".

Serious Adverse Event (SAE): an undesired medical event observed during a clinical trial that is associated with

- death,

- in-patient hospitalization (if the trial involved out-patients),

- prolongation of hospitalization (if the trial involved in-patients),

- persistent or significant disability or incapacity,

- congenital anomaly or birth defect or is

- life threatening

Suspected Unexpected Serious Adverse Reaction (SUSAR): an adverse reaction that is:

- Suspected i.e. presence of a reasonable likelihood of a causal association with the drug;

- Unexpected i.e. not congrous with the current product information e.g. USPI (United States Product Information), EU-SmPC (Summary of Product Characteristics); and

- Serious in nature.

Treatment Emergent Adverse Event (TEAE): defined as an ·

- undesirable event that was not existing before the administration of medical treatment; or

- an already existing event which shows deterioration with respect to severity or frequency after administration of treatment.

Signal: is the recorded description of an adverse event with a drug, the association between the two being plausible; the drug-event association is so far being not specified or insufficiently described in literature. The generation of signal is usually conditional on more than one report of drug-event combination, seriousness of event and attributes of the report.

SIGNAL PROCESSING IN PHARMACOVIGILANCE

An important issue of concern in PV is the identification of unspecified and unpredicted associations between exposure to pharmacological interventions (medicines) and untoward or undesirable events.

The process of signal identification and development includes a sequence of steps as:

- Identifying a drug-adverse event combination of potential concern.
- An initial examination of the evidence of association in literature.
- Working through the process of signal development.

Figure 37.1 depicts the sequence of steps involved in the signal processing.

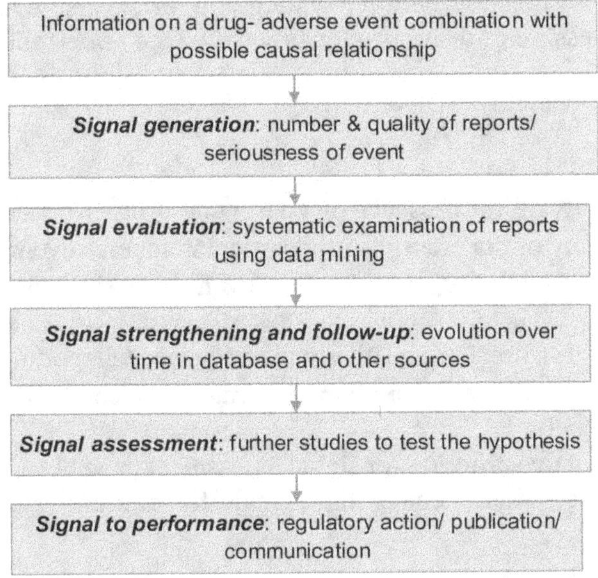

Figure 37.1 Signal processing in Pharmacovigilance: from suspicion to an explained phenomenon.

❖ **Signal generation and evaluation**

Once there is a report on a possible causal association between a drug and an adverse event, a signal is generated depending upon the quantity and attributes of reports and seriousness of the event. This is followed by evaluation of signal which involves a methodological and detailed evaluation of the adverse event reports by means of statistical or mathematical techniques; this procedure is called "data mining". Data mining is based on highlighting the drug-event combinations which are significantly larger in number and need further review.

The techniques used in data mining are:

1. Point estimate.

   This involves the calculation of odds ratio (case/ non-case analysis).

Suspected drugs	Reported suspected ADRs	
	Event of interest	Other events
Exposure of interest	P	Q
Other exposures	R	S

Odds ratio = (P/R) / (Q/S)

2. Bayesian logic.

At WHO–UMC, automated quantitative signal generation- Bayesian confidence propagation neural network (BCPNN)-based technique is routinely applied. Using this network, the individual reports in UMC database are counted to obtain - all reports with a particular drug (A), all reports with a particular event (B) and all reports having both A and B i.e. particular drug-event combination.

The degree of association between a drug and an adverse event is calculated by a logarithmic measure of disproportionality called the *information component (IC)*.

$$IC = \log_2 \frac{p(x, y)}{p(x)p(y)}$$

where:

p (x) = probability of the presence of a particular drug 'x' in a report.

p (y) = probability of the presence of a particular adverse event 'y' in a report.

p (x, y) = probability that a particular drug-event 'x' and 'y', appear in a report.

Hence, a positive value of IC implies that a particular drug- event combination is reported more frequently than predicted relative to the frequency of reporting of the drug and event. This process is thus utilized to spotlight the drug- event combinations having likelihood of becoming signals.

Once the quantitative criterion for signal assessment have been met using data mining approach, further assessment of the signals for qualitative criteria is carried out (Table 37.1).

Table 37.1 Determinants for signal evaluation in Pharmacovigilance.	
Determinant	**Explanation**
Quantitative	
Strength of the association	The number of case reports (related to drug exposure), statistical disproportionality and significance
Qualitative	
Data consistency	General occurrence of a particular attribute, and rare occurrence of reverse findings.
Exposure-response relationship	Time relation, site of involvement, relationship with dose, reversible/ irreversible nature
Biological credibility of the hypothesis	Pharmacological and pathological processes involved
Experimental observations	Rechallenge, drug-specific antibodies, plasma or tissue drug concentrations, metabolites, diagnostic markers
Analogy	Past incident/s with related drugs, event recognized to be commonly drug-induced
Features and attributes of data	Distinctive features and objectivity of the event, authenticity and legitimacy of documentation, case causality evaluation

❖ **Signal strengthening and review**

After a signal has been recognized and evaluated, review of the database needs to be done to see the evolution of signal over time with respect to number of reports with and without particular drug, consistency in reporting pattern and characteristic features, and statistical parameters (Table 37.2).

Table 37.2 Signal review.
Identical database
Evolution of data with respect to quantity and consistency.
Signal reinforcement.
Evaluation of individual cases.
Country (source) comparisons.
Targeted comparisons.
Nested case-control studies.
Other databases and sources
Presence of an identical relationship.
Supplementary clinical findings (e.g. literature, spontaneous reporting).
Experimental observations (e.g. pharmacological, immunological).

❖ **Signal assessment**

Signal identified through spontaneous adverse event reporting is mainly helpful in generation of a new hypothesis which however demands further testing to provide the basis for any decision making by regulatory authorities. Such signal assessment is generally carried out by means of follow-up pharmacoepidemiological studies.

❖ **Signal to performance**

Figure 37.2 depicts various outcomes which can happen after a signal is generated.

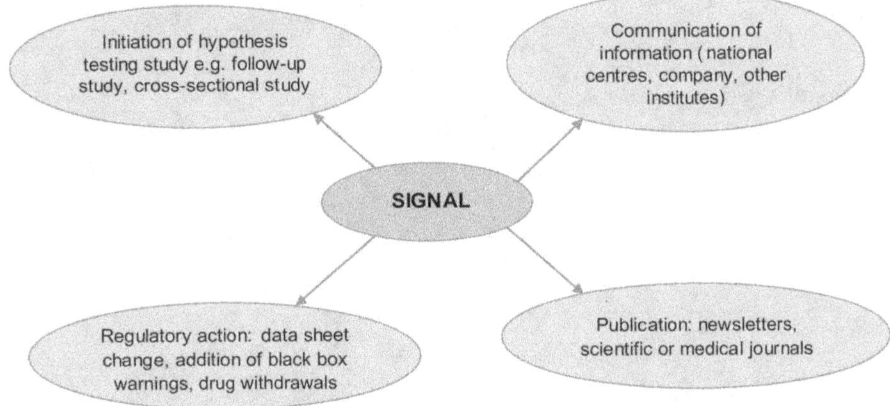

Figure 37.2 Various outcomes of signal generation.

SIGNAL DETECTION PROCESS AT UMC (FIGURE 37.3)

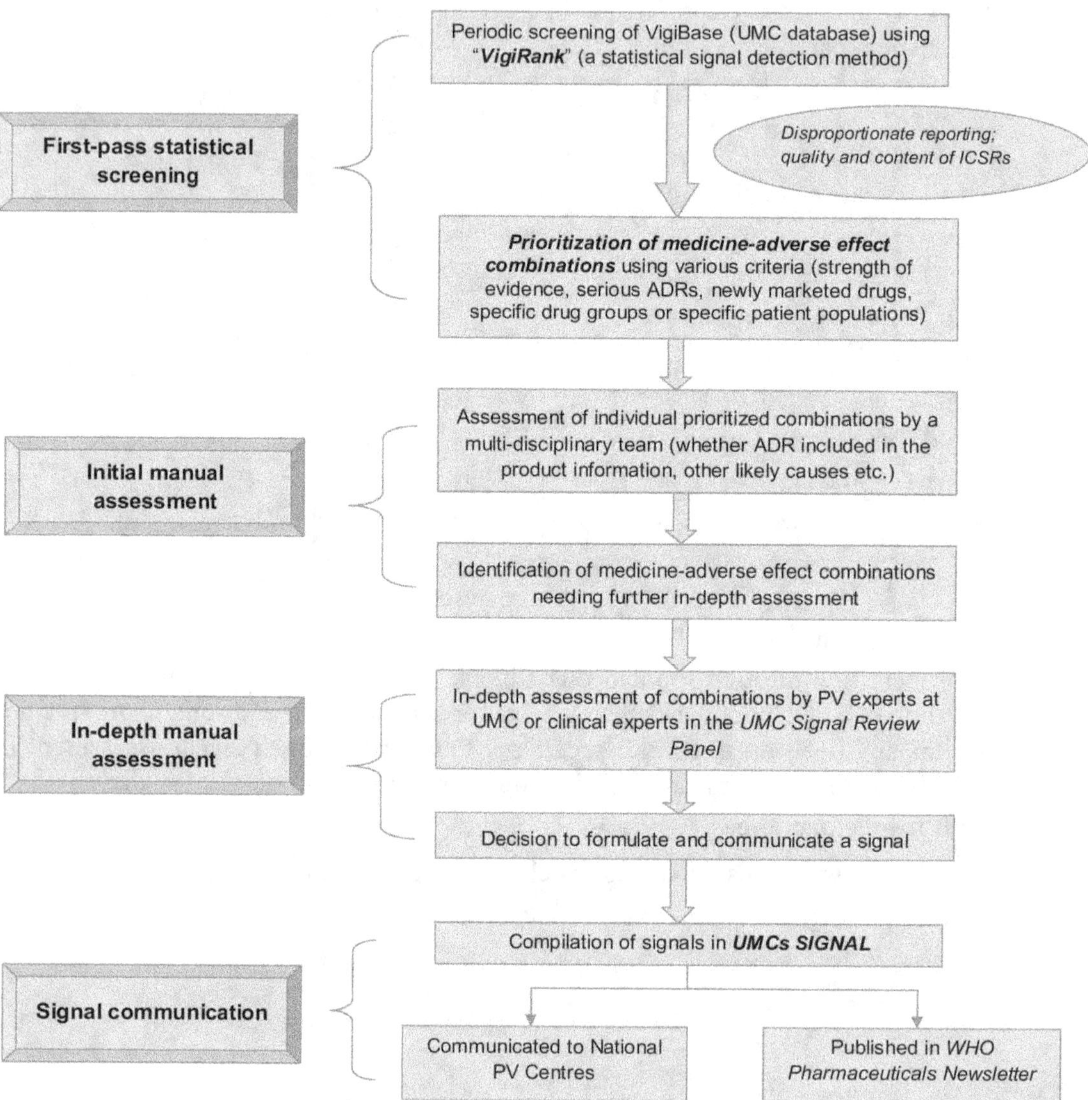

Figure 37.3 Signal detection process at UMC.

PHARMACOVIGILANCE IN INDIA

EVOLUTION OF PV IN INDIA

Figure 37.4 depicts various stages through the evolution of PV in India.

1982: first formal ADR monitoring program by Dr. Molly Thomas at Christian Medical College, Vellore.

1986: formal establishment of PV in India by DCGI (12 main centers) .

Failed: illiteracy, strong influence of traditional medicine, over-the-counter drug. availability, inadequate numbers of trained personnel and costs.

1997: India joined the WHO ADR Monitoring Programme based in Uppsala, Sweden.

3 centers: Department of Pharmacology, AIIMS New Delhi as National. Pharmacovigilance Centre; KEM Hospital (Mumbai) and JLN Hospital, Aligarh Muslim University (Aligarh).

Failed: lack of knowledge and awareness among prescribers and poor funding from government.

2005: **National Pharmacovigilance Programme (NPVP) for India**, (WHO sponsored and World Bank funded) under CDSCO.

2 zonal centres (the *South-West zonal centre* - Department of Clinical Pharmacology, Seth GS Medical College and KEM Hospital, Mumbai and the *North-East zonal centre*. - Department of Pharmacology, AIIMS, New Delhi); 5 regional and 24 peripheral centers.

2010: NPVP reformulated as **PvPI (Pharmacovigilance Programme of India)**; operational since mid July 2010.

National Coordination Centre (NCC): Department of Pharmacology at AIIMS, New Delhi later shifted to Indian Pharmacopoeia Commission (IPC), Ghaziabad.

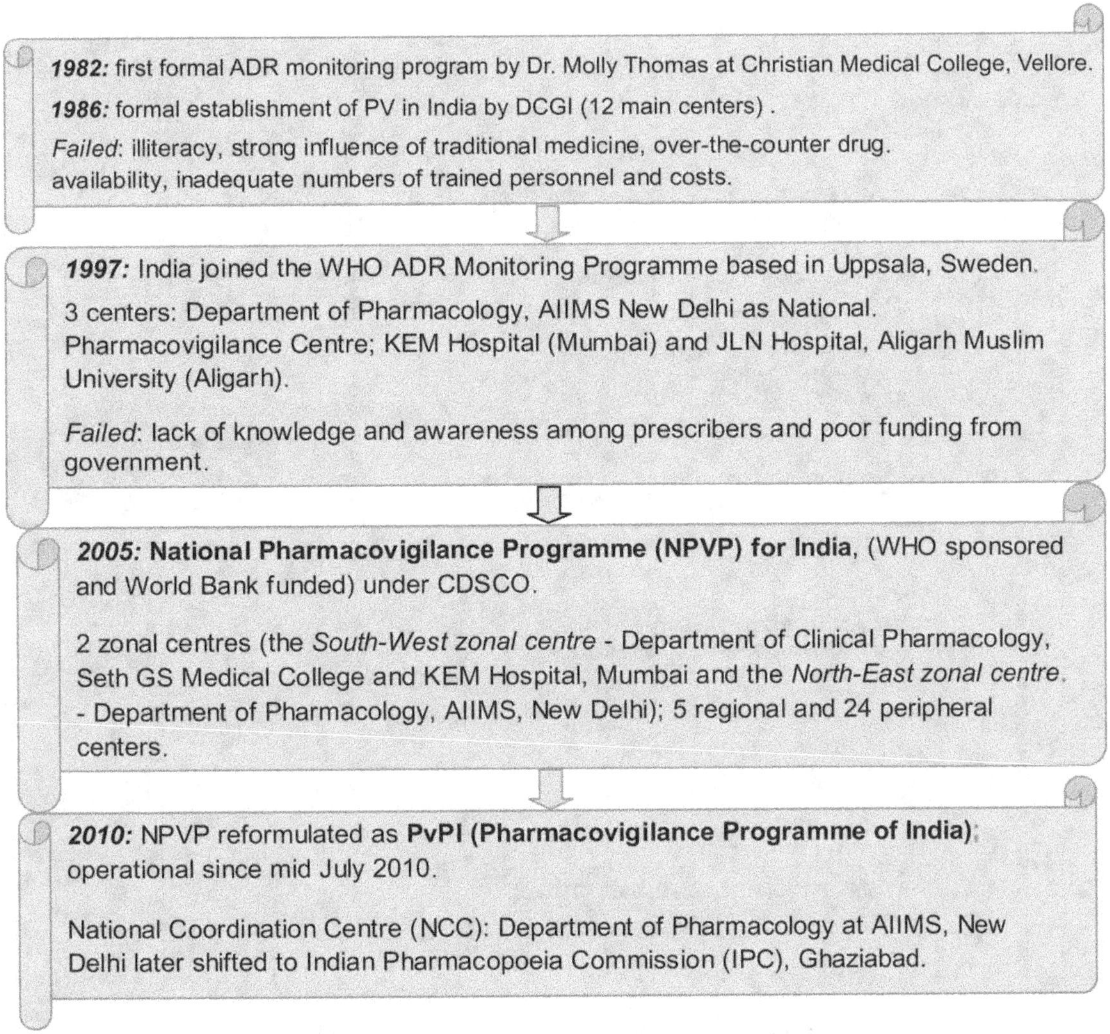

Figure 37.4 Evolution of PV in India.

ORGANIZATION AND WORKING OF PVPI (FIGURE 37.5).

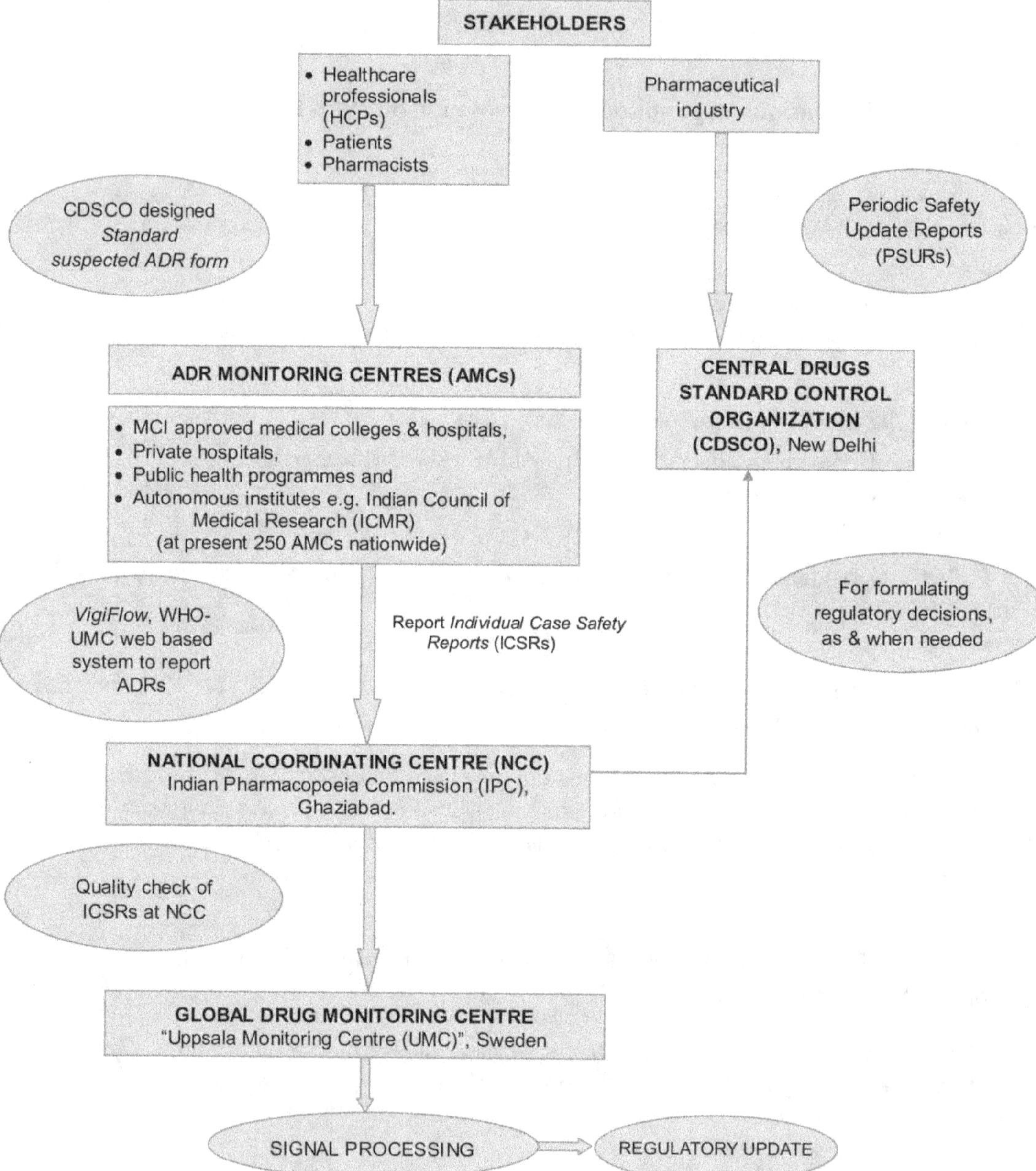

Figure 37.5 Diagram representing organization and working of PvPI.

CHALLENGES FOR PV IN INDIA (TABLE 37.3)

Table 37.3 Challenges for PV in India.

- Underreporting of ADRs (entirely relies on spontaneous/voluntary reporting).
- Lacunae in existing teaching curriculum (lack of training to medical/paramedical students)
- Lack of adequate funding sources.
- Traditionalist infrastructure.
- Wide time lags between guidelines and their implementation.
- Conservative beliefs on new drug research.
- Non-existent inspections pertaining to PV.

STRATEGIES TO STRENGTHEN PV IN INDIA

- ✓ Enhancing awareness among HCPs and patients/consumers/ society about PV by means of conducting regular trainings, workshops and medical education programmes.
- ✓ Reminders to HCPs for reporting ADRs telephonically, or by sending mails or message alerts periodically or SMS alerts.
- ✓ Provision of incentives to physicians for example publications from ADR data.
- ✓ Reassuring physicians with regard to no legal consequences of reporting ADRs.
- ✓ Mandatory incorporation of PV in the teaching curriculum by Medical Council of India.
- ✓ Post marketing surveillance and ADR reporting to be made legally compulsory.
- ✓ Active monitoring systems and registries for new medicines and vaccines.
- ✓ Improved funding by means of separate budgeting.
- ✓ Motivation of consumers/civil society groups through public health programmes and active campaigns.
- ✓ ADR form should be simple, clear, include non-complex terms, easily accessible; and available in local languages.

CONTRIBUTION OF PVPI IN CONTAINMENT OF ANTIMICROBIAL RESISTANCE (AMR)

AMR is an emerging public health threat globally. According to a CDC (Centre for disease control and prevention) report in 2013, around 2 million persons attain an antibiotic resistant infection annually out of which 23,000 die. In the 2017 scoping report on AMR, India has been identified as having the highest rates of antimicrobial resistance among bacteria causing many communal and nosocomial infections; the factors identified as responsible in this report include rampant use of broad-spectrum antibiotics, injudicious consumption of antibiotic fixed-dose combinations, self-medication, gaps in knowledge and awareness among healthcare professionals regarding optimal use of antimicrobials and AMR etc. To embark upon this issue, Government of India (GOI) adopted many strategies like:

- ✓ National program on containment of antimicrobial resistance launched by GOI in 12th five year plan, 2012-17.

✓ Implementation of Schedule H1; rendering the availability of 24 antibiotics (previously under OTC sale) under restricted sale, on providing a valid prescription only.

Further, in this direction, PvPI, a flagship programme of MoHFW, has taken many initiatives to curb the menace of AMR in India. These include:

❖ Providing regular updates on situation of AMR to IPC. Due to the alarming trends observed in collated data, an appendix has been included in latest (5th) edition of National Formulary of India stating the mechanisms involved in AMR and strategies to control AMR in health care settings.

❖ Expansion of scope of PvPI to monitor AMR. PvPI has included AMR in the updated training modules and skill development programs.

❖ Collaboration with Department of Microbiology, Nizam Institute of Medical Sciences, Hyderabad, and National Institute for Research in Tuberculosis, Chennai with an aim to generate database on AMR and plan measures for its containment in an effective manner.

❖ Collaboration with public health programmes like Revised National TB Control Program (RNTCP), National AIDS Control Organization (NACO), Adverse Event Following Immunization (AEFI), and National Vector Borne Disease Control Program (NVBDCP) to identify the cause of resistance to antimicrobials used in these programmes.

❖ Collaboration with NABH to promote monitoring and reporting of ADRs by NABH accredited hospitals and provide training-cum-workshops on AMR to staff in such hospitals.

❖ Expanding the scope of PvPI to district level hospitals with an objective to raise awareness on safe drug use among rural masses and health care professionals with special emphasis on appropriate antimicrobial use and adherence to antimicrobial therapy.

VACCINE PHARMACOVIGILANCE

According to the CIOMS/WHO Working Group, vaccine pharmacovigilance is defined as "the science and activities relating to the detection, assessment, understanding and communication of adverse events following immunization (AEFI) and other vaccine or immunization-related issues, and to the prevention of untoward effects of the vaccine or immunization".

In 2013, PvPI collaborated with Adverse Events Following Immunization (AEFI) Programme for the monitoring of ADRs from vaccines.

General principles / objectives of AEFI surveillance
✓ Identification, rectification and avoidance of immunization fallacies.
✓ Recognition of potential concerns with particular vaccine lots.

- ✓ Ensuring a constant faith in vigilance by timely reacting to patient / community matters.
- ✓ Signal recognition for unexpected adverse events and generation of hypothesis which can be later validated by controlled studies.
- ✓ Determination of rates of AEFI within local communities.
- ✓ Strategies to enhance awareness about vaccine PV among HCPs and patients in particular and society as a whole.

HAEMOVIGILANCE

A conjugation of various surveillance strategies aimed to gather and evaluate information on unpredicted or untoward events occurring by the use of blood or blood products for therapeutic purposes and to take measures to avoid their occurrence in near or distant future. This strategy covers the entire chain of steps in transfusion process from collecting blood and its components from donor/s to occurence of any consequences in recipients. Haemovigilance Programme of India (HvPI) was launched by IPC in collaboration with National Institute of Biologicals in 2012 under PvPI with following terms of reference:
- ✓ To keep a record of adverse events/ reactions occurring as a result of therapeutic use of blood and blood products (haemovigilance).
- ✓ To assist in detecting any trends, advocating best strategies and methods for improving patient safety, while decreasing expense of medical care system.

"Haemo-vigil" is the software developed to collect and analyse data regarding haemovigilance from across the country.

Objectives of HvPI:
- Keep a track of adverse events associated with transfusions.
- Sensitize the healthcare professionals.
- Advocate recommendations on the basis of evidence.
- Provide advice to regulatory authority for health related decisions.
- Disseminate the results to major stakeholders.
- Create national as well as international linkages.

The number of centres covered under HvPI till 2016 were 206. The HvPI has become the member of International Haemovigilance Network.

BIOVIGILANCE

The National Institute of biologicals (NIB) in alliance with IPC introduced the Biovigilance Programme of India (BvPI) in 2013 with the main aim to monitor adverse reactions and incidences related to biologicals as well as tissue, organ and cell therapy transplantation.

MATERIOVIGILANCE

In order to track the safety aspects of medical devices in the country, Materiovigilance Programme of India (MvPI) was launched on 06th July 2015 at IPC, Ghaziabad by DCG(I). The Indian Pharmacopoeia Commission functions as National Coordination Centre for MvPI and Sree Chitra Tirunal Institute of Medical Sciences & Technology (SCTIMST) functions as National Collaborating Centre. National Health Systems Resource Centre (NHSRC) under MoHFW, Govt. of India is the technical support and resource centre.

HERBAVIGILANCE
(PHARMACOVIGILANCE OF HERBAL MEDICATIONS)

Herbs/ herbal supplements are commonly preferred and used as alternatives or as adjunct to the prescribed treatment because they are natural and believed to be 'safer' and having 'lesser side effects' than synthetic drugs. However, since they contain a number of active ingredients with potential to alter the physiological system, they may produce side effects as well. Hence, there is a rising awareness of the requirement to promote pharmacovigilance practices for herbal drugs.

Numerous challenges come in the way of herbavigilance due to peculiar characteristics of herbal products (unknown composition, presence of multiple ingredients, lack of standardization for the dose of active ingredient, insufficient knowledge regarding the mechanism of action of active ingredients, inappropriate dosing, improper labeling, herb-drug interactions etc.).

Few strategies proposed to be implemented in the field of herbavigilance include:
- ✓ The use of herbal anatomic-therapeutic-chemical (HATC) classification for the therapeutic classification of herbal products. HATC is being incorporated within the WHO-DD structure as part of the global WHO database. Also, using a system checklist for citing botanical and vernacular names used as names of ingredients can be promoted.
- ✓ Use of proper scientific binomial names for medicinal herbs to ensure consistency in the naming of herbs in adverse reaction reports.
- ✓ Training of herbal experts in the science of Pharmacovigilance and their involvement not only in reporting but also analyzing ADRs.

WHO has prepared guidelines for tracking the safety aspects of herbal drugs in Pharmacovigilance systems. In India, CDSCO and Department of AYUSH, Ministry of Health and Family welfare, Government of India monitor ADRs related to herbal medicines.

NUTRAVIGILANCE

Nutravigilance is defined as "the science and activities relating to the detection, assessment, understanding and prevention of adverse effects related to the use of a food, dietary supplement, or medical food". The need of nutravigilance arises due to insufficient information regarding preclinical and clinical profile and product characteristics for dietary products e.g. stability, shelf life etc. and unawareness among health care professionals about the side effects of nutraceuticals.

In USA, dietary supplements are regulated by FDA under the Dietary Supplement Health and Education Act of 1994 (DSHEA). In European Union, food supplements are regulated by the European Food Safety Authority (EFSA) while in Canada, they are regulated by Food and Drug Regulations (FDRs). In India, Food Safety and Standards Authority of India (FSSAI) regulates nutraceuticals under the Food Safety Act, 2006.

ECOPHARMACOVIGILANCE

The scientific discipline that is based on various activities related to identification, assessment, knowledge and prevention of harmful effects of drugs/ pharmaceuticals in the environment, which in turn adversely impact humans and other animal species.

Various drugs used in humans have been detected in the environment in recent times. The routes of environmental entry of pharmaceuticals may be:
- excretion of drug/ metabolites through drainage system;
- release of drug from hospitals or place of manufacture into waste water;
- disposal of drug via toilets/ sinks.

Consequences of contamination of environment with pharmaceuticals
- Substantial decline in the number of vultures secondary to indirect exposure to diclofenac; it was observed that vultures when fed on the corpses of livestock who had received high doses of diclofenac prior to their deaths, eventually died of kidney failure. As a result of this, veterinary use of diclofenac was banned in India.
- Adverse effect of ethinylestradiol on the growth of sexual characteristics in male fish.
- Presence of traces of oral contraceptive pills in water lead to sterility in frogs.

Environmental Risk Assessment of Pharmaceuticals

Environmental Risk Assessment (ERA) of Pharmaceuticals is mandatory before applying for marketing authorization in Europe (Box 37.2).

> **Box 37.2** Evaluating Environmental Risk Assessment (ERA) of Pharmaceuticals.
>
> ERA of pharmaceuticals is done by calculating risk quotient.
>
> *Risk Quotient (RQ) = PEC / PNEC*
>
> PEC: Predicted Environmental Concentration i.e. maximum concentration of pharmaceutical predicted in environment based on use and elimination in waste water.
>
> PNEC: Predicted No-Effect Concentration, calculated from ecotoxicological tests employing algae, daphnids and fish (representing three trophic levels).
>
> Interpretation of risk quotient (RQ):
>
> Value of RQ
>
> <1 : no further information needed.
>
> >1 : needs further testing and risk management strategies.

Nowadays, measures like environmental risk management plans (ERMPs) are emerging which aim to identify drugs which are potentially hazardous to the environment during early phases of development and help in timely decision making.

CAUSALITY ASSESSMENT OF ADVERSE EVENTS

Causality assessment of adverse events (AEs) is the systematic and elaborate evaluation of individual case safety reports for the possibility of causal relationship between the suspected drug/s and the particular AE. Establishing a cause-and-effect association between a drug and a particular adverse event is quite challenging due to the presence of various confounding factors like associated co-morbidities, concomitant medications, non-drug variables etc.

Numerous strategies have been developed to evaluate causality of an adverse event with a drug treatment. Broadly, these are classified into:

❖ Expert judgement/ Global introspection.

❖ Probabilistic methods.

❖ Operational algorithms.

1. **Expert judgement/ Global introspection.** This approach includes judgement made by an expert on the possible causal association of the particular drug with the adverse event after taking into consideration the relevant information in the given case. However, due to subjectivity and lack of standardization, this method is associated with poor reproducibility and intra and inter-rater disagreements. Based on this approach, few methods have been described like WHO-GI (global introspection), Wilholm, Miremont et al, Arimone et al etc.

2. **Probabilistic/Bayesian methods.** These are based on Bayes' theorem, which in the context of causality assessment, express the relationship between the probability that a drug caused an event before (prior) and after (posterior) the acquisition of supplementary criteria (e.g. time relationship, patient attributes, clinical findings). The prior probability is estimated from epidemiological data while posterior probability is estimated by combining prior probability and the pertinent evidential information in the considered case.

   Posterior odds = Likelihood ratio x Prior odds

   These methods are not feasible for routine use due to the usual lack of required information for calculating the estimate of causation. Moreover, the prior probability might not be identical in different settings and populations. The calculation of likelihood ratio is complicated due to usual nonavailability of data and the fact that the variables used may not be independent. Thus, the calculations may result in quasi-accurate probabilities. A computerized system- Bayesian Adverse Reactions Diagnostic Instrument (BARDI) is utilized for complex calculations.

3. **Algorithms /scales.** These estimate the probability of a causal-effect relationship on the basis of scores obtained in respective questionnaires. These are most commonly employed to assess causality due to their simplicity and higher intra and inter-rater agreements. Various algorithms available for this purpose are Naranjo, Kramer, Karch and Lasagna, Jones, Liverpool etc.

   Out of the various methods available, WHO GI method and Naranjo adverse drug reaction (ADR) Probability Scale are the two most commonly applied and agreed causality assessment methods in clinical as well as experimental scenario. Both these methods are generic and their relevance in various settings has been time tested.

   ♦ ***WHO-GI method:*** This method was proposed by Uppsala Monitoring Centre, the World Health Organization Collaborating Centre for International Drug Monitoring (WHO–UMC). The WHO method takes into consideration various factors like clinical and pharmacological details in the report, attributes of the documentation with a relatively less information on prior knowledge and statistical probability.

   Depending on various criteria taken into consideration while assigning causality (e.g. recognised pharmacological phenomenon, time relationship to drug intake, presence of other disease, drugs co-administered, dechallenge and rechallenge), there are six causality categories defined in this method:

   - Certain.
   - Probable/likely.
   - Possible.
   - Unlikely.
   - Conditional/ unclassified.
   - Unassessable / unclassifiable.

   ♦ ***Naranjo's algorithm:*** This algorithm involves checking each individual case against a set of 10 questions which take into consideration factors like:

- Presence of any earlier definitive report on adverse reaction in literature,
- Time relation of adverse event with drug administration,
- Dechallenge; also any improvement of adverse event on administration of specific antagonist,
- Presence of alternative explanation/s,
- Rechallenge; any reappearance of adverse event on placebo administration,
- Concentration (if toxic) of suspected drug/s in blood/ body fluids,
- Any change in adverse event severity on dose modifications,
- Past history of any similar reaction,
- Objective evidence of adverse event

Each 'positive', 'negative' or 'missing' information is allotted a score which is then summed up and interpreted as: 9=highly probable/definite, 5-8=probable, 1-4=possible and 0=doubtful.

MOdified NARanjo Causality Scale for ICSRs (MONARCSi) (Box 37.3).

Box 37.3 MOdified NARanjo Causality Scale for ICSRs (MONARCSi).

This, a novel decision support tool, is based on aspects of Naranjo algorithm to evaluate the causality of drug-event pairs. In this method, an "aggregate score" is calculated after taking into consideration various aspects of drug-event relationship which is then logistically transformed to yield a binary measure for the presence or absence of 'relatedness' of a drug-event pair.

Features

Nine features are taken into consideration and noted as present, absent or unknown/ applicable. The features include significant safety event, previous association, temporality, mechanism of action, de-challenge, re-challenge, dose response, experimental data and confounding factors.

Process flow to determine causality using MONARCSi

Input to the tool: On the basis of information regarding molecule and specific ICSR, and utilizing aspects of Naranjo's algorithm, Bradford-Hill criteria and additional attributes highly suggestive of causal relationship

↓

Processing: Information entered is combined with a weighting vector to derive an "aggregate score" which is mapped to a probability logistic function

↓

Output: a binary classifier to determine if the drug-event pair is "related" or "not related"

ISCR-MRCT Investigational Drug Adverse Event Causality Assessment Tool

A comprehensive framework for causality assessment of adverse events from the perspective of clinical trials has been developed by the Indian Society for Clinical Research (ISCR) in collaboration with Harvard Multi-Regional Clinical Trials (MRCT) Center. In this, factors considered in determining causality of adverse event include:

- Investigational product.
- Clinical trial procedures.
- Clinical procedures for care of patient.
- Underlying disease procedures.
- unrelated causes to clinical trial enrolment.

This tool is an expansion of WHO-UMC system and is composed of:
- ✓ Table 1 (22 listed items; information to be collated to analyze each adverse event),
- ✓ Table 2 (29 listed items; binary response causality assessment questionnaire) and
- ✓ Table 3 (interpretation of responses).

Details of this tool can be accessed at http://iscrmrctcausalityassessment.org/login.php

CAUSALITY ASSESSMENT OF ADVERSE EVENTS FOLLOWING IMMUNIZATION (AEFI)

An adverse event following immunization (AEFI) is defined as any untoward/ undesirable medical event that occurs following an immunization and may not essentially have causal association with the administration of vaccine.

Determining causation is especially demanding in the case of vaccines due to reasons like:
1. Lack of complete information on dechallenge and rechallenge.
2. Administration of vaccines mainly to the country's birth cohort at an age when the chances of concomitant illnesses are very high.
3. Administration of multiple vaccines in routine at the same immunization visit.
4. The possibility of immunization errors must be considered. Vaccine storage, management, transportation and administration should strictly abide by specified conditions. Any of these, if not followed properly, may cause an adverse event.

Elements in causality assessment of AEFI
- ❖ Determining the *eligibility* of AEFI for causality assessment:
- ✓ *AEFI case*. Ensure the completeness of AEFI investigation and availability of all case details.
- ✓ *Identify vaccine(s)*. Identify one vaccine (implicated) administered prior to event occurrence.

✓ *Valid diagnosis.* Determine the undesirable or unpredicted medical occurence, deranged laboratory parameter/s, or any other sign whose causality is to be checked.

✓ *Case definition.* Brighton Collaboration definition, standard literature definition, national definition or other approved definition.

❖ ***Considerations*** for causality assessment:
- Temporal relation. Association (time, place).
- Biological plausibility.
- Previous knowledge.
- Clinical characteristics and laboratory findings.
- Quality of data. Accuracy, reproducibility and consistency.
- Probability/ rejection of other causes.
- Precision and robustness of association.

Classification of causality categories for AEFI (Figure 37.6)

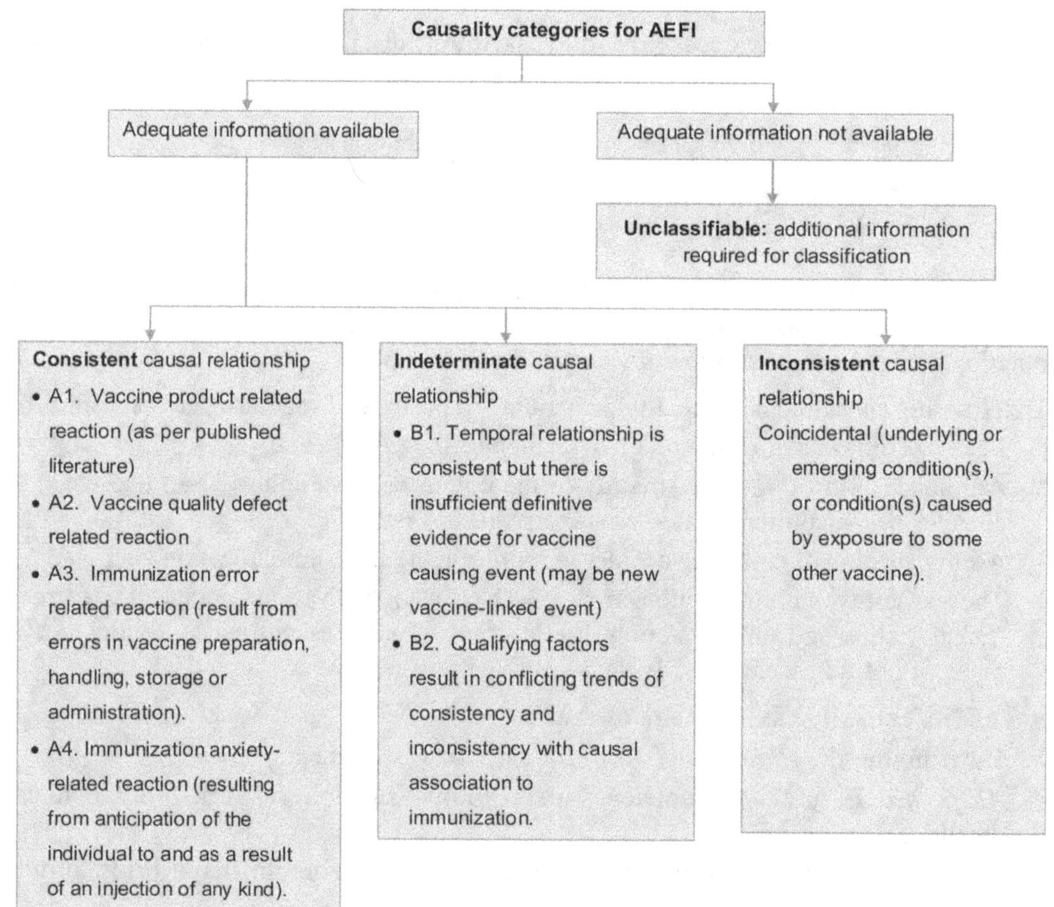

Figure 37.6 Causality categories for AEFI.

SIGNIFICANCE OF CAUSALITY ASSESSMENT

- Causality assessment of AEs is extremely important as the revealing of association of a drug with an adverse event, particularly serious or severe one, may lead to regulatory actions like black box warnings, ban or withdrawal of the drug.
- Standardized case-causality assessment helps in decreasing ambiguity of data and preventing erroneous conclusions.
- The basic knowledge of causality assessment is indispensable for healthcare professionals as uncertainty of the potential causal relationship between drug and AE remains one of the major reasons of under reporting in pharmacovigilance.

PRACTICAL ISSUES WITH CAUSALITY ASSESSMENT

- The methods for causality assessment are semi-quantitative in nature as they do not exactly measure the likelihood of a relationship. An explicit outcome (unrelated or certain) is given in a minority of cases.
- There is a high threshold in assigning a 'definite/ certain' ADR which is of paramount importance from public safety and regulatory point of view.
- The knowledge of dechallenge and rechallenge holds a high importance when assigning causality by both WHO and Naranjo methods. However, few peculiar issues pertaining to these concepts exist e.g. the concept of dechallenge may not be applicable where the drug is a one dose treatment (e.g. vaccine), reaction resulted in death and reaction occurred after the drug was discontinued. Also, in certain cases the evaluation may be tedious like irreversible or long lasting reaction e.g. congenital anomaly, hepatotoxicity, bone marrow suppression with cytotoxic drugs. Moreover, dechallenge cannot be addressed in cases of adverse reactions showing spontaneous recovery despite continuation of therapy. A rechallenge may range from a similar episode in the past to a true planned prospective re-exposure. Due to ethical and medical concerns, a true rechallenge is a rarity particularly in serious reactions. Also, in a subjective reaction, more than one rechallenge may be required to achieve a convincing result. Moreover, the situation during rechallenge (dose or duration of treatment) may not be exactly identical to the original episode.
- None of the methods addresses the issue of lack of efficacy/ unexpected therapeutic failure, which is also categorised as an ADR (type F).

IMPORTANT LINKS

1. The use of the WHO-UMC system for standardised case causality assessment. https://www.who.int/medicines/areas/quality_safety/safety_efficacy/WHOcausality_assessment.pdf

2. Forms for reporting to FDA.
   https://www.fda.gov/safety/medwatch/howtoreport/downloadforms/default.htm

3. Reporting forms.
   https://yellowcard.mhra.gov.uk/downloadable-information/reporting-forms/

4. Suspected adverse drug reaction reporting form. http://www.ipgmer.gov.in/PharmacovigilanceCommittee/ADR_Reporting_formVersion1.3.pdf

5. Medicines side effect reporting form (for consumers). https://www.mkcgmch.org/admin/MenuDocument/DownloadForms_171.pdf

6. Reporting form for adverse events following immunization (AEFI) https://www.who.int/vaccine_safety/AEFI_reporting_form_EN_Jan2016.pdf

7. Transfusion Reaction Reporting Form (TRRF) For Blood & Blood Components & Plasma Products.
   http://nib.gov.in/Haemovigilance/TRRF_Form.pdf

8. Medical device adverse event reporting form. https://ipc.gov.in/images/MEDICAL_DEVICE_ADVERSE_EVENT_REPORTING_FORM.pdf

9. Scoping Report on Antimicrobial Resistance in India. November 2017. Available at https://cddep.org/wp-content/uploads/2017/11/AMR-INDIA-SCOPING-REPORT.pdf. (Last accessed on 2019 August 2)

Drug Utilisation Research

INTRODUCTION

Drug utilization research (DUR) is defined as "the marketing, distribution, prescription, and use of drugs in a society, with special emphasis on the resulting medical, social and economic consequences" (WHO, 1977). It has also been defined as "an authorized, structured and continuing program that reviews, analyses and interprets patterns of drug use against predetermined standards".

Aims of DUR

- To quantify present usage and estimate future demands.
- To measure the effects of informational, educational and regulatory activities.
- To promote the rational utilization of drugs in population.

ROLE OF DUR IN CLINICAL PRACTICE

DUR holds a crucial place in clinical practice as it forms the basis for making amendments in the drug dispensing policies at local and national levels. DUR contributes to rational use of drugs in many important ways as described below:

1. ***Description of drug use patterns.*** DUR increases our understanding of how drugs are being used by providing information on:

   ✓ Number of patients who received the drugs being studied in a given period.
   ✓ The magnitude of drug use at a certain point of time and/or in a particular setting.
   ✓ The extent of drug use whether adequate, over-use or under-use.
   ✓ The extent to which alternative drugs are being used to treat particular conditions.

2. ***Early indicators of irrational drug use.*** DUR helps in identifying the indicators of irrational drug use by:

✓ Comparing the patterns of drug utilization between different settings or at different times.

✓ Comparing the observed patterns of drug use for treating a particular disease with current recommendations or guidelines.

3. ***Interventions to improve drug use.***

✓ Monitoring and evaluation of the results of strategies adopted to curtail undesirable drug use patterns.

✓ Assessing the impact of regulatory policies or modifications in insurance or reimbursement systems.

✓ Assessing the extent to which strategies like drug promotional campaigns by pharmaceutical industry influence the drug utilization patterns.

4. ***Quality control of drug use.*** DUR forms a framework for continuous quality improvement. Making comparisons on data from drug utilization patterns or research from varied settings or regions can prove to be helpful in detecting the deficiencies which need further assessment, ultimately leading to identification and encouragement of best practice.

SOURCES OF DATA IN DRUG UTILIZATION RESEARCH (TABLE 38.1).

Table 38.1 Sources of data in drug utilization.

1. Large databases
2. Data from drug regulatory agencies
   - *Drug registration; drug importation*
3. Supplier (distribution) data
   - *Drug importation; local manufacture; customs service*
4. Practice setting data
   - *Prescribing data*
   - *Dispensing data*
   - *Aggregate data*
   - *Over-the-counter and pharmacist-prescribed drugs*
   - *Telephone and Internet prescribing*
5. Community setting data
   - *Household survey; compliance*
6. Drug use evaluation
   - *Drugs and therapeutic committee*
   - *Prospective evaluation (e.g. indications, drug selected, doses, route and dosage form, costs, duration of therapy, quantity dispensed, contraindications, therapeutic outcome, adverse drug reactions, drug interactions)*
   - *Retrospective evaluation (e.g. evaluation of indications, monitoring use of high-cost medicines, comparison of prescribing between physicians, cost to patient, adverse drug reactions, drug interactions)*

TYPES OF DUR

Descriptive research - describe patterns of drug use and identify the issues demanding further detailed evaluation.

Analytical research – relate data on drug utilization research to morbidity, impact of therapeutic interventions and quality of life, evaluating rationality of drug therapy.

WHO/INRUD DRUG USE INDICATORS (FIGURE 38.1)

These indicators measure the various aspects of behavior of health care providers at primary health care facilities, irrespective of the data collector. These have been extensively field-tested and are quite reliable in providing information related to drug use, prescribing patterns and different facets of health care.

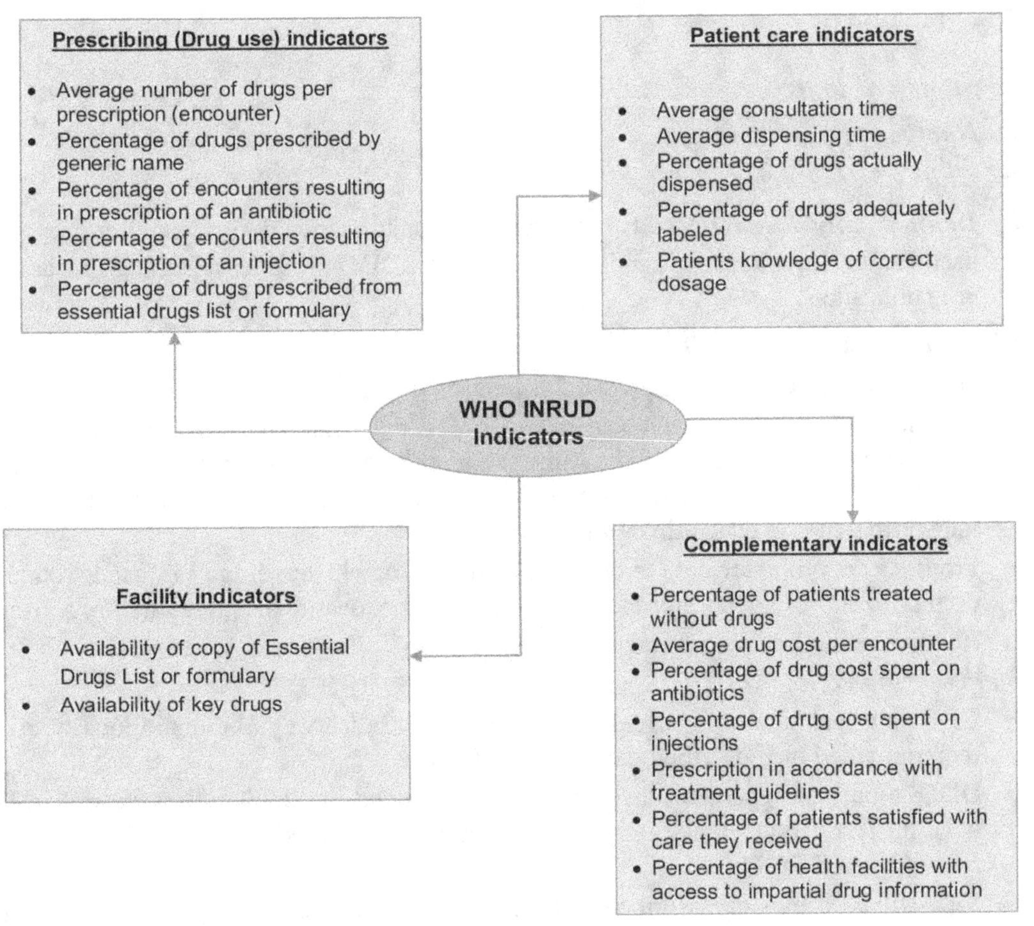

Figure 38.1 WHO INRUD (International Networks of Rational Use of Drugs) Indicators 1993.

CODING SYSTEM IN DUR

The reference standard for drug utilization is WHO ATC/DDD (Anatomical Therapeutic Chemical / Defined daily dose) methodology. The main objective of ATC/DDD system is serving as a tool to demonstrate drug utilization statistics to improve drug use patterns. This system is widely in use in drug utilization studies since early 1970s and has been found to be quite suitable for:

✓ Comparing drug utilization patterns at national and international levels,
✓ Examining long lasting trends in drug use,
✓ Evaluating the influence of certain measures on drug usage
✓ Contributing denominator data in experiments of drug safety (trends in frequency of ADR reports examined against drug exposure: Ratio: ADR/DDDs).

DRUG UTILIZATION METRICS

❖ *Monetary units.*

❖ *Number of prescriptions.*

❖ *Units of drug dispensed.*

❖ *Defined daily dose (DDD).* It is the average maintenance daily dose of a drug when used for its major approved indication in adults. DDD provides a standard measure of drug utilization.

Merits of the concept of DDD.
- Used to describe and compare drug utilization patterns.
- As a standardized unit of measurement, DDD serves as a means to compare the usage patterns of different drugs in the same therapeutic group, different systems providing health care facilities or different geographical regions, and evaluation of short term or long term trends in drug utilization.
- Provides denominator data to conduct epidemiological screening for issues related to drug utilization, and monitor the impact of various educational and regulatory activities.
- Relatively uncomplicated and economical to use.

Demerits of the concept of DDD.
- DDD is a technical unit of calculation and may not always be analogous with the recommended or prescribed daily dose (PDD).
- DDD is only assigned for drugs which are included in ATC/DDD methodology and have an ATC code. Hence, the concept cannot be applied to drugs which have not been assigned DDD.
- Pediatric uses are usually not considered in any calculations.

- Problems can arise when doses vary widely or there is more than one major indication for a drug e.g. aspirin.
- DDDs are not based on equipotency data.
- DDDs are independent of quality of treatment, side effects and outcomes.

Drug utilization figures are represented as:

- *Number of DDDs per inhabitant per year*. It is a measure of the average number of days in a year during which all inhabitants receive treatment.
- *Numbers of DDDs per 1000 inhabitants per day*. It is a measure of the proportion of study population who receive the drug or group of drugs being evaluated on daily basis. This is especially applicable for drugs used to treat chronic disorders which usually demonstrate a good correspondence between DDD and average prescribed daily dose.
- *Number of DDDs per 100 bed-days*. This measure is utilized when the research involves drug usage by inpatients.
- ***Prescribed daily dose (PDD).*** This is the mean per day dose of a drug which is truly prescribed and is calculated from an illustrative specimens of prescriptions.

  Caution needs to be exercised when there is difference in the recommended dosage of drug prescribed for different indications to another (e.g. antipsychotics), severe versus mild disease (e.g. antibiotics) and where PDDs may be different for varied populations (e.g., different PDDs depending on gender, age, or geographic region).

  In situations where there is a significant discrepancy between DDD and PDD, this fact needs to be taken into consideration while analyzing and defining drug utilization measures, particularly in terms of morbidity.

  PDD may not always be a true reflection of actual drug utilization. This may be due to the fact that sometimes medications prescribed may not actually be dispensed, and the patients may not necessarily always take all the dispensed medications. A proposed strategy to address this issue is assessment of parameters like actual drug intake by the patient i.e. ***consumed daily dose*** in special studies incorporating certain designs like patient interviews.

CHAPTER 39

Pharmacoepidemiology

OVERVIEW

Introduction
Aims of PE
Applications of PE
Measurement of Outcomes in PE
  Outcome Measures
  Risk Measures
Types of Study Designs in Pharmacoepidemiologic Research
  Descriptive Designs/Studies
    Case Reports
    Case Series
    Cross Sectional Study
    Ecologic Studies
  Analytical Studies
    Case-Control Study
    Cohort Study
    Hybrid Studies
Advantages of Pharmacoepidemiological Methods
Disadvantages of Pharmacoepidemiological Methods
Biases in Pharmacoepidemiology

INTRODUCTION

Pharmacoepidemiology (PE) is the branch of science that deals with the study of incidence and proportion of disease conditions in human populations occurring as an outcome of harmful and favorable effects of pharmacological interventions. It can also be described as the implementation of pharmacological knowledge in the field of epidemiology, various epidemiologic techniques and judgement to study the effects of drug use (useful and harmful) in human populations (Table 39.1).

Table 39.1 Focus of Pharmacoepidemiology and related areas of study.

Discipline	Focus	Indicator of drug exposure	Result studied
Clinical Pharmacology	Individual patient	Clinical effect	Drug effectiveness
		Adverse reaction	Drug toxicity
Drug utilization research	Groups	Utilization patterns	Excessive or inadequate use
		Appropriateness of use	Quality of care
		Correlation with outcome	Drug safety, possible relationships
Pharmacoepidemiology	Populations (defined)	Exposure-outcome relationship	Causality
		Comparative effectiveness	Quantification of benefit
		Comparative toxicity	Quantification of risk

AIMS OF PE

- **Signal generation:** for recognition of new adverse drug reactions (ADRs) and identification of new applications of medicines.
- **Risk / benefit quantification:** quantification of risks i.e. adverse consequences as well as benefits accrued from drug use in humans. Such risk/ benefit quantification often requires large population studies.

Study sample size required to detect adverse events depending on their background frequency

Incidence of adverse events (%)	Sample size	Type of study
1	1,000	Clinical trial
0.1	10,000	Large clinical trial
0.01	100,000	Postmarketing surveillance
0.001	1,000,000	Long term survey

- **Hypothesis testing:** this requires the use of comparison groups to determine whether there are differences in variables of interest.

APPLICATIONS OF PE

- ✓ Estimation of risks of drug use:
- • Quantify benefit : risk ratio.
- • Identify risk situations.
- ✓ Patient counselling.
- ✓ Formulation of public health policy decisions:
- • Withdrawal of drugs.
- • Measures to be taken if high rates of improper prescribing detected.
- ✓ Formulation of therapeutic guidelines.
- ✓ Discovery of new indications.
- ✓ Facilitation of pharmacoeconomic analysis.
- ✓ Finding new areas worth investigating.

MEASUREMENT OF OUTCOMES IN PE

These can be studied as outcome measures, drug use measures and risk measures. Drug use measures are discussed in detail under drug utilization research.

❖ **Outcome measures**

♦ *Morbidity Measures*
  - Morbidity: No. of cases of disease or event per unit population (per 1000) or per unit time (per year) or both (events per 1000 inhabitants per year).
  - No. of hospitalizations due to or prevented by drug use.
  - Days of hospitalization.
  - Days of hospitalization prevented by drug use.
  - Deaths due to or prevented by drug use.

♦ *Prevalence:* Proportion of people affected with a disease or exposed to a particular drug in a population at a given time. It is a cross sectional measure usually determined by surveying the population of interest. It is generally expressed as percentage e.g. 1%.

♦ *Cumulative incidence:* The number of new cases of a disorder or outcome that occur in a population during a specified amount of time divided by the initial population size i.e. count of persons in population at beginning. It is a longitudinal measure; and reflects the average risk of the individual developing the outcome in a specified time interval. It is expressed as percentage or cases per 1000.

♦ *Incidence rate:* Ratio of new cases to the person-time at risk. The denominator is sum of all exposures multiplied by the length of these exposures. It is expressed as number of cases per person-year (or any other time unit) of exposure.

❖ **Risk measures**

Risk is the probability of developing an outcome regardless of severity. CIOMS (Council for International Organization of Medical Sciences) has suggested a scale of risk level terms as given below:

Very common	≥ 1 in 10 exposures
Common	< 1 in 10 but ≥ 1 in 100
Uncommon	< 1 in 100 but ≥ 1 in 1000
Rare	< 1 in 1000 but ≥ 1 in 10000
Very rare	< 1 in 10000 exposures

♦ *Attributable risk (AR):* is an estimate of the risk in excess that can be considered to be associated with intervention, over and further away from other causes. This can be expressed as below:

Factor Status	Outcome		Total
	With AE	**Without AE**	
Exposed	A	B	e1
Not exposed	C	D	e2
Total	c1	c2	

In this example, $AR = \dfrac{(A/A+B) - (C/C+D)}{A/A+B}$

- ◆ ***Relative risk (RR) or risk ratio:*** Probability of experiencing an outcome in a group of exposed persons relative to the baseline risk. RR is expressed along with confidence interval.

$$RR = \{A/A+B\} / \{C/C+D\}$$

- • A RR of 1: the two groups exhibit similar risk of experiencing outcome.
- • A RR of <1: the risk of having outcome in experimental group is less than the control group.
- • A RR of >1: the risk of having outcome in experimental group is greater than the control group.

RR associated with particular exposure is relevant to the clinician while AR forms basis for public health policy decisions.

- ◆ ***Odds ratio (OR):*** The OR is a measure to compare the chances/ probability of a certain event in two groups; OR of 1 denotes equal likelihood of occurrence of event in two groups. The odds of occurrence of an event is denoted as a ratio i.e. the presence of occurrence of the event divided by the absence of its occurrence. OR is an estimate of RR and is applied in case control studies as a substitute of RR.

  In the above example, the odds of having adverse event (AE) in the exposed group is A/B; and the odds of having AE in not exposed group is C/D hence, the odds of AE is (A/B) / (C/D) i.e. AD/BC.

- ◆ ***Relative Risk Reduction (RRR):*** is the measure of difference in rates of event occurrence between two groups (e.g. a treatment and control group).

$$RRR= (1-RR) \times 100$$

- ◆ ***Absolute Risk Reduction (ARR):*** is just expressed as the difference in incidence rates between two groups.

$$ARR= (A/A+B) - (C/C+D)$$

- ◆ ***Number needed to treat (NNT):*** number of people required to be treated to produce 1 or more case of the outcome. It is the reciprocal of ARR.

$$NNT = 1/ARR.$$

- ◆ ***Number needed to harm (NNH):*** is calculated by subtracting the adverse event rates in the treatment and control group.

$$NNH= 1/ \text{(adverse event rate in exposed- adverse event rate in not exposed)}$$

Table 39.2 gives a list of formulae to calculate various measures of risk.

Table 39.2 Formulae for various measures of risk.

Measures of risk	Formula
Attributable risk	(Rate of event occurrence in treatment group – Rate of event occurrence in control group) / Rate of event occurrence in control group
Relative risk	Rate of event occurrence in treatment group / rate of event occurrence in control group
Odds ratio	Odds of event occurrence in treatment group / Odds of event occurrence in control group
Relative risk reduction	(1- Relative Risk) × 100
Absolute risk reduction	Event rate in treatment group – Event rate in control group
Number needed to treat	1/ Absolute risk reduction
Number needed to harm	1 / difference in adverse event rate between treatment and control groups

TYPES OF STUDY DESIGNS IN PHARMACOEPIDEMIOLOGIC RESEARCH (FIGURE 39.1)

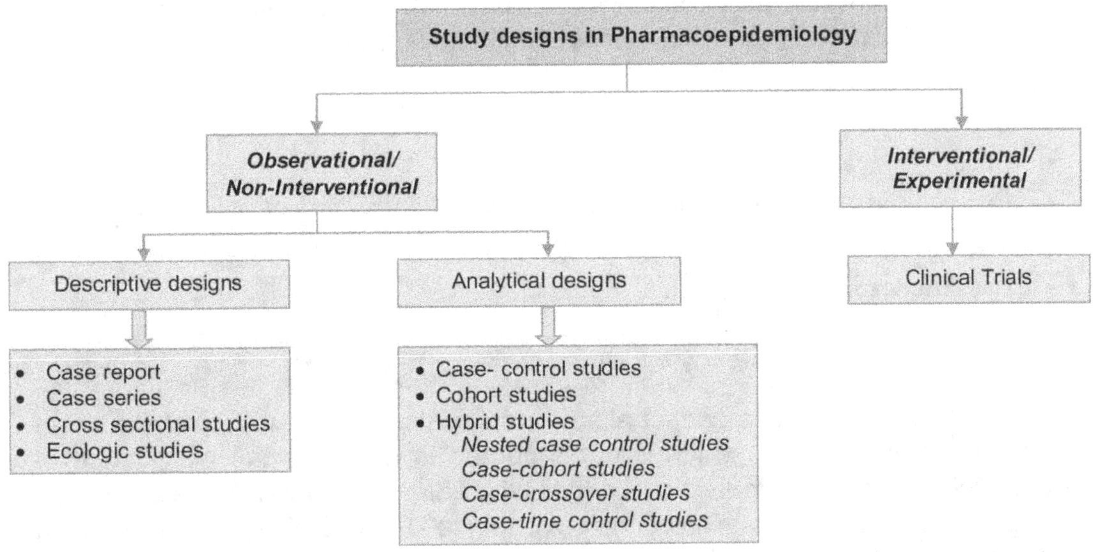

Figure 39.1 Types of study designs in Pharmacoepidemiology.

❖ Descriptive designs/ studies

The main aim of descriptive studies is to generate hypothesis. These mainly involve recognition or characterization of a new problem in the population. Passive monitoring of events and reports is an important method for collecting data included in these studies. For example, the objective of these studies may be to recognize new or unknown adverse events, to gain knowledge on drug usage patterns in specific populations, or estimating the number of people at risk of developing an adverse event/ adverse drug reaction. Hence, these studies do not serve to measure associations; instead, they use frequency/ distribution measures e.g. proportions, rate, risk and prevalence.

Case reports. Case reports include an elaborative explanation of a specific and unexpected event (favorable or adverse) occurring in a single patient after exposure to a medicine/ intervention. These hold crucial importance in PE as they can serve as the first signal of an event with a drug or identification of a new unapproved indication of the drug. Case reports also constitute a crucial component for spontaneous reporting systems in pharmacovigilance.

Case series. Case series is basically an assemblage of 'case reports' sharing some common features e.g. exposure to same drug; and, occurrence of same outcome. Case series describe a particular medicine-event association and help to gain better understanding of the clinico-pathological patterns related to an adverse event. The main limitation, however, is absence of a control group which complicates the determination of causality.

Cross sectional study (Survey or Prevalence study). Cross-sectional study is based on collection of data at a single point of time with no follow-up, hence, these provide a "snapshot" of the disease prevalence/ its attributes in the population being studied at a given point of time. In this study, a random sample from the target population/ population under consideration is selected by the use of statistical techniques and data is collected as planned, the obtained data are then classified depending on exposure to drugs and outcomes observed (Box 39.1).

Advantages
- ✓ Quick.
- ✓ Cheap.
- ✓ Can be used to explore associations between certain factors or outcomes.

Disadvantages
- ✓ Causality cannot be established

Box 39.1 Cross-sectional study.

An example of the cross-sectional study is the **National Health and Nutrition Examination Survey** which was conducted to measure the prevalence of overweight and obese individuals in the United States. Children in the age group of 2 to 19 years and adults more than or equal to 20 years of age were identified as the study population. The conclusion of the study was that there was an increase in the prevalence of overweight children and obese men in the period from 1999 to 2004 while no such increase was observed in women during the same time period.

Ecologic studies. These studies assess the secular trends and generally focus on evaluating the trends observed in drug related outcomes over time or across different geographical regions. These studies usually encompass the analysis of data from a single region over different time points to estimate any changes or trends over time or analysis of data at a single time period from different regions to compare regional trends. However, since data from individuals is not gathered in ecologic studies (as group based data is analyzed) hence confounding factors are not adjusted. Another limitation is ecologic fallacy i.e. these do not provide information on actual intake of drug by the individual with disease under consideration. Hence, these studies do not provide evidence of association of a drug with an outcome.

❖ Analytical studies

Analytical studies, as defined, include a control group for making comparisons and hence possess the ability to evaluate the causal association between exposure and an event of interest. These observational studies involve quantification of beneficial or harmful drug effects in terms of measures of association such as rate, risk, odds ratios, rate ratios, or risk difference.

Case-control study (Case-referent study). In these studies, a group of patients with a particular outcome e.g. adverse event (cases) are matched with a control group without the outcome (controls) and their exposure to a risk factor such as a drug is compared. To reduce bias, the controls should be matched to cases as closely as possible for all factors other than the outcome. This design is especially applicable when more than one risk factor or determinant of a single outcome are studied (Box 39.2).

Advantages

- ✓ Efficient for rare diseases and diseases with long induction and latent period.
- ✓ Can evaluate many risk factors for the same disease so good for diseases about which little is known.
- ✓ Conducted quickly.
- ✓ Low costs.

Disadvantages

- ✓ Inefficient for rare exposures.
- ✓ Vulnerable to bias because of retrospective nature of study.
- ✓ May have poor information on exposure.
- ✓ Difficult to infer temporal relationship between exposure and disease.
- ✓ Cannot determine the incidence of an outcome, but give a measure of relative risk compared to the control group; known as odds ratio.

Box 39.2 Case-control study.

One well-known case-control study was conducted by Sir Richard Doll, a distinguished epidemiologist in London, England who demonstrated the ***causative link between cigarette smoking and lung cancer***. In 1948, a recent increase in lung cancer deaths was observed. At that time, smoking was considered as a routine habit causing no harm. Doll and his associates assumed the most likely causative factor of increase in lung cancer incidence to be environmental pollution from coal fires, automobiles etc. They conducted

Box 39.2 *Contd...*

interviews on more than 600 male patients with suspected lung, hepatocellular or bowel carcinoma in various hospitals in London. Patients admitted in hospitals having other ailments were also interviewed. The results were quite obvious and convincing: patients diagnosed with lung cancers were smokers and those not having lung cancer were non-smokers.

Cohort study. In cohort studies, a group of patients receiving a drug are identified and observed over time to determine the rate of occurrence of outcomes or adverse events. Another group of patients not receiving the drug or possibly receiving another similar drug is usually identified for comparison (control group). Cohort studies are particularly desirable for drugs not used commonly, or when single exposure is associated with more than one events or outcomes (Box 39.3).

Advantages

✓ Less recall bias.

✓ Can generate new adverse drug reaction (ADR) hypothesis.

✓ Give information about temporal association of exposure and outcome.

✓ Helpful in the calculation of time dependence of events (true incidence rates, relative risks, and attributable risks) and frequency of outcome in a defined population.

Disadvantages

✓ Require large sample sizes.

✓ Expensive and time consuming.

✓ Not efficient in detecting rare outcomes, particularly those occurring after long term exposure or having a delayed presentation.

✓ Susceptible to bias if large number of subjects are lost to follow-up (high drop-out rate).

Box 39.3 Cohort study.

One famous cohort study is the **Framingham Heart Study**, conducted by the National Heart, Lung, and Blood Institute (NHLBI) under National Institutes of Health (NIH). This study was designed with an objective to identify various variables or factors contributing to the causation of cardiovascular disease (CVD), a leading cause of death in United States. The study began in 1948 by recruiting an *Original cohort* of 5209 males and females in the age group of 30 to 62 years living in Framingham and Massachusetts, who did not have any present or past history of overt symptoms of cardiovascular disease or myocardial infarction or stroke. Since that time the study has added an *Offspring cohort* in 1971, the *Omni cohort* in 1994, a *Third generation cohort* in 2002, a *New Offspring spouse cohort* in 2003, and a *Second generation Omni cohort* in 2003. Over the years, careful observation and monitoring of the population enrolled in this study has been helpful in identifying some major risk factors for development of CVD like blood pressure, blood cholesterol and triglyceride levels, age, gender and psychological issues etc.

Hybrid studies. These designs encompass the combination of several standard epidemiologic designs leading to a higher quality and efficiency. In these studies, cases are identified on the basis of a particular outcome; and drug use is compared among several different types of comparison groups.

Various types of hybrid studies include:

- *Nested Case-Control study.* This is a type of case-control study which is nested in a cohort study or randomized clinical trial. In nested case-control studies, the target population is observed prospectively till the time there occur a defined number of new cases of a disease of interest or an adverse outcome to a treatment. Subjects in the same cohort without the case condition serve as controls. This type of study design is more commonly used to gather some additional information related to use of a particular drug and to study confounding factors. Generally, when it is impractical to collect the desired data for entire cohort (a common occurrence), a nested case-control study is the design of choice.

- *Case-Cohort study.* The design of this study resembles a nested case-control study, however the difference is that in a case-cohort study the information on exposure and coexisting variables/ confounders is gathered from all selected cases, whereas controls represent a randomly selected sample from the original cohort. The proportion of persons exposed to drug in cases is compared to the proportion of persons exposed to drug in the reference cohort (which may include cases).

- *Case-Crossover study.* In this study, only those subjects are included in evaluation which exhibit the outcome of interest (considered as cases); control subjects are selected from the same group of subjects identified as cases, but at an earlier point of time, so that the cases serve as their own controls like in cross-over studies. This study design is especially desirable when the disease of interest does not show any variation over time and when the exposure is acute, short-lasting and transient. The case-crossover design helps in eliminating selection bias and any issues in selection and enrolment of controls. However, this design is not preferred when the disease under consideration is chronic. In case-crossover studies, the odds of taking a drug near the time of onset of an outcome is compared with odds of taking the drug at a remote time.

- *Case-Time-Control study.* This type of design is an extension of the case-crossover study, however it also takes into consideration the period effect or time effect, with emphasis on any changes in drug use pattern over a period of time. This design is recommended when
  ✓ there is variation in the presence or degree of exposure over time,
  ✓ two or more variables of interest are evaluated at different times,
  ✓ drug effect is distinctly isolated from disease severity.

ADVANTAGES OF PHARMACOEPIDEMIOLOGICAL METHODS

- ✓ Allow examination of groups not included in trials.
- ✓ Useful to study people over time and effects that the drugs have on these people and effects of compliance.
- ✓ Can generate effectiveness data.
- ✓ Generate signals.
- ✓ Can indicate new areas of research.
- ✓ Compare patterns of drug use.
- ✓ Monitoring prescribing behavior.
- ✓ Great deal of flexibility due to data from variety of sources.

DISADVANTAGES OF PHARMACOEPIDEMIOLOGICAL METHODS

- ✓ Causation difficult to establish.
- ✓ Incomplete records and missing data.
- ✓ In rare diseases confirmation is difficult.
- ✓ Bias and confounding (Table 39.3).

Table 39.3 Biases in Pharmacoepidemiology.	
Selection bias	Misrepresentation of the assessment of a variable/ outcome of interest, which is due to inclusion/ selection in the study of groups of subjects having an uncommon and dissimilar relationship with drug. It is of 4 types:
Referral bias	This can occur if drug-related reasons are responsible for referring a patient to a tertiary care institute, for instance.
Self-Selection bias	This type of bias arises when patients decide themselves regarding their participation in a study or withdrawing from it depending on factors like drug exposure or change in state of health.
Prevalence Bias	May be seen in case–control study when prevalent cases with a condition are selected instead of the newly identified cases.
Protopathic Bias	This may occur if a particular therapeutic intervention or procedure is started, removed or altered in response to the initial manifestation of disease , which is however undiagnosed at that time.
Information bias	It is related to the accuracy/ fallacy in information gathered on exposure, disease state and other variables like confounding factors.
Confounding	This is defined as the influence of other associated factors related to both drug exposure and the outcome, and may lead to occurrence of partial or whole of the observed effect, absence of effect, or a reversal of the effect.

CHAPTER 40

Pharmacoeconomics

OVERVIEW

Introduction
PE and Outcomes Research
Perspectives in PE
Components of Costs
Cost Models
Discounting of Costs and Benefits
Types of Pharmacoeconomic Analysis
   Cost Minimization Analysis (CMA)

Cost Effectiveness Analysis (CEA)
Cost Benefit Analysis (CBA)
Cost Utility Analysis (CUA)
Methods for Performing PE Analysis
Decision Analysis as a Tool for PE
Sensitivity Analysis
Steps for Conducting a PE Analysis
Applications of Pharmacoeconomics

INTRODUCTION

Pharmacoeconomics (PE): The scientific discipline that deals with study and evaluation of costs and outcomes (consequences) of pharmacological interventions and associated services and their effect on stakeholders including individuals, systems involved in providing health care services and society as a whole.

Applied Pharmacoeconomics: The application of pharmacoeconomic principles, strategies and methodologies to specify net worth of pharmaceutical products and services utilized in real-world scenario.

Why the need of Pharmacoeconomics?

- Pharmacoeconomics assists in making clinical decisions by providing information about costs and consequences of alternative methods of treatment.
- As the costs of healthcare are rising, decision makers demand the best value in healthcare (i.e. optimizing healthcare results) for the money they spend.
- The concepts and principles of PE help in utilization of the limited resources (budget) in the best possible and most efficient manner.
- PE analyses are relevant for pharmaceutical industry for strategic planning, both in early drug development and in determining the likely price of future drugs.

PE AND OUTCOMES RESEARCH

PE and Outcomes research are two related disciplines. Outcomes research refers to broader consideration of the measurement of the efficacy or effectiveness of treatment. To help decision making regarding a pharmacological intervention and/or associated health care services, the pharmacoeconomic evaluation takes into consideration an integrated assessment of the economic, clinical, and/or humanistic outcomes. (i.e. ECHO model) (Figure 40.1).

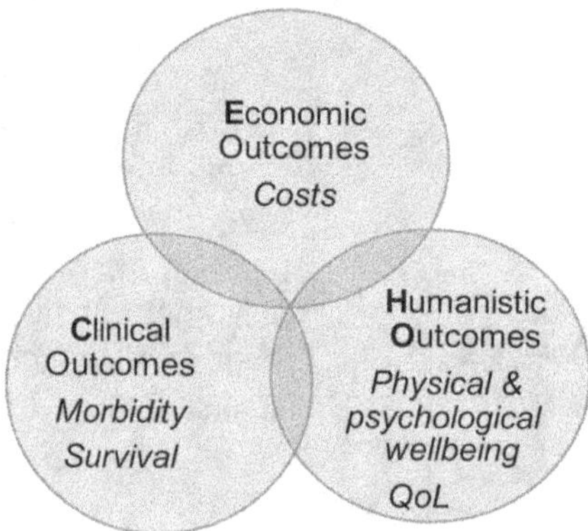

Figure 40.1 ECHO model: The 3 Outcomes Research parameters for decision making.

PERSPECTIVES IN PE

The specific costs and benefits that are included in any economic evaluation depend on the *perspective* that has been chosen for the analysis (Figure 40.2).

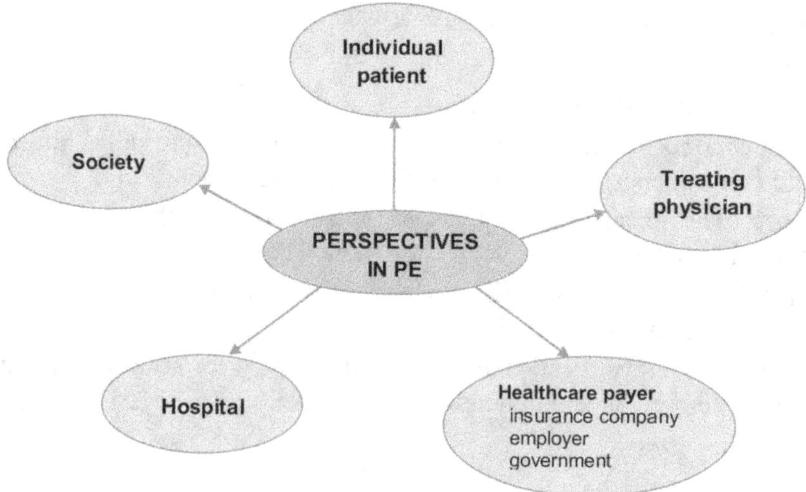

Figure 40.2 Different perspectives in PE.

COMPONENTS OF COSTS (FIGURE 40.3)

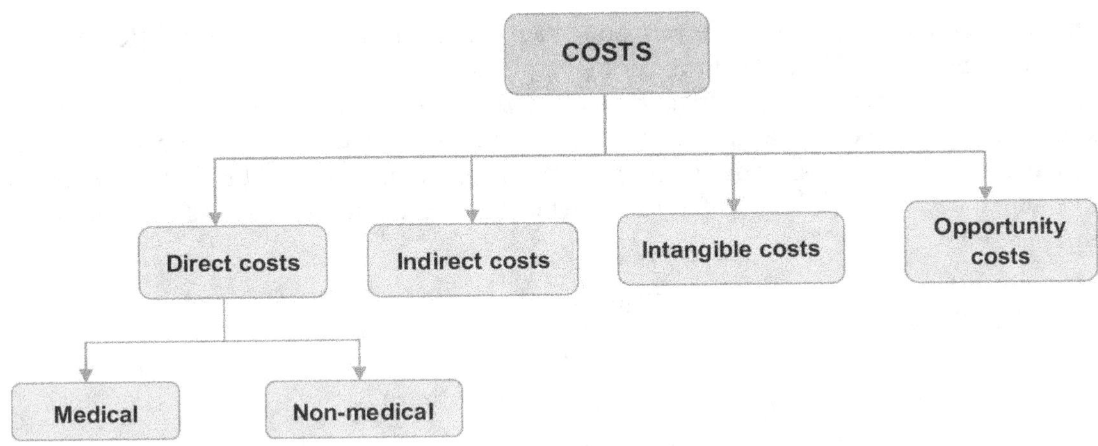

Figure 40.3 Various components of costs.

- **Direct Costs.** *Fixed* (building, equipment and staff salaries) and *variable* (drug costs, needles, syringes etc) costs of medical/nonmedical care and services associated directly with a medical condition or healthcare intervention.
    - ♦ *Direct medical costs* e.g. Drug acquisition costs, treatment costs (hospital, physician visits), monitoring (laboratory tests, physician visits), management of adverse events.
    - ♦ *Direct non-medical costs* e.g. Home modifications (e.g., wheelchair ramp), travel to hospital costs.
- **Indirect Costs.** Cost of lost or diminished productivity as a result of morbidity or early mortality associated with a medical condition or treatment e.g. lost productivity (time off work), value of lost productivity (lost income), caregiver time.
- **Intangible Costs.** Costs assigned to amount of suffering that occurs because of the disease or healthcare intervention e.g. pain, suffering, inconvenience.
- **Opportunity Costs.** These represent the economic benefit forgone when using one therapy instead of the next best alternative therapy.

COST MODELS

- **Top-down model** - These estimate the overall burden of diseases and are referred as *"cost of illness"* studies. The most commonly used method is based on an estimate of the prevalence of a particular disease in a given year and estimates of costs accrued during that year.
- **Bottom-up model** - These are based on the prospective collection of data about individual patients.

DISCOUNTING OF COSTS AND BENEFITS

Discounting, a procedure used in economic analysis, is used to standardize different cost-benefit- time profiles in order to make a comparison of total costs involved and benefits accrued. Discounting rests on *"time preference principle"* which states that costs incurred and benefits received in near future are of higher significance than costs and benefits in the distant future. The process of discounting involves determining the Net Present Value (NPV) of future costs and benefits of alternative methods of treatment by choosing an appropriate discount rate.

$$\textit{Net Present Value (NPV)} = \frac{\text{Future value}}{(1+r)^n}$$

where   r = discount rate (typically ranges from .03 to .06)

       n = the number of years in the future

Distribution of Costs and benefits	Example	Effect of applying discounting to both cost and benefits
Costs occur at different times	Surgery vs drug treatment of peptic ulcer	Makes drug treatment more attractive
Benefits occur at different times	Drug treatment of hypertension vs established hypertensive heart failure	Makes treatment of established hypertensive heart failure more attractive
Costs and benefits occur at different times	Screening and treatment of hyperlipidemia vs CABG for coronary artery disease	Discounting future costs favors screening and treatment; Discounting future benefits favors CABG as benefits occur immediately.

Impact of discounting on economic analysis.

TYPES OF PHARMACOECONOMIC ANALYSIS (FIGURE 40.4)

❖ **Cost minimization analysis (CMA)**

Simplest of the pharmacoeconomics tools.

Compares the costs of two or more alternatives that have a demonstrated equivalence in therapeutic outcome (i.e. *therapeutically equivalent alternatives*). Once therapeutic equivalence is demonstrated, the focus is on choosing the one with the smallest total costs. Although the 2 alternatives must achieve the major outcome of interest equally, they may still have different other outcomes.

E.g. brand vs. generic products, minor surgery as inpatient or outpatient procedure, different routes of administration of the same drug.

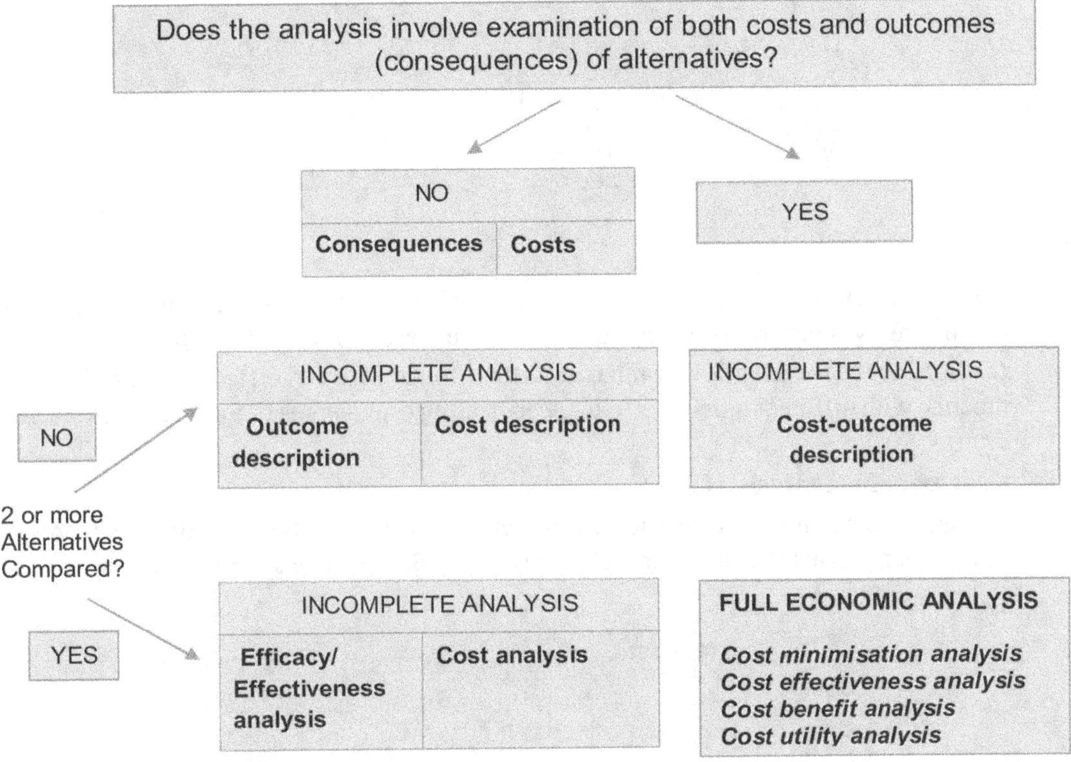

Figure 40.4 Different types of PE analyses.

❖ **Cost effectiveness analysis (CEA)**

In this type of analysis, the major outcome of interest is single and common to all alternatives but different treatments/programmes have *different success rates* in achieving this common outcome. Treatments are then compared in terms of the cost per unit of success e.g. cost per life year saved, cost per ulcer healed or cost per extra mmHg blood pressure reduction etc.

For making comparisons, ***marginal or incremental analysis*** is employed which is useful to assess the comparative efficiency of interventions providing greater benefit at high cost or lesser benefit at low cost than the available ones.

Results are expressed as ***Cost-Effectiveness Ratio (CER)*** and/or ***Incremental CER (ICER)***

Example of CEA:

Treatments	A	B
Cost	X	Y
Outcome: Life years gained	M	N
Cost effectiveness ratio (CER); Cost per life yrs gained	X / M	Y / N
Incremental CER; Cost per additional life yrs gained by A*	(X – Y) / (M – N)	

*assuming A is both more expensive and more effective than B

CEA is frequently used to compare interventions within a single disease area e.g. comparing two programs designed to prevent excess mortality (cost per life saved).
Limitation: it does not allow comparisons to be made between different areas of clinical practice with different outcomes (e.g. ulcer-healing drug versus blood-pressure lowering drug).

❖ **Cost benefit analysis (CBA)**

In this, all costs (inputs) and benefits (outcomes) of different interventions are expressed in monetary terms. Results can be expressed as ***Benefit to cost ratio*** or ***Net benefit***
Example of CBA:

Treatment	A	B
Cost ($)	X	Y
Outcome: Life years gained ($)	C	D
*Benefit to cost ratio**	C / X	D / Y
*Net benefit**	C – X ($)	D – Y ($)

*choose alternative with the largest value

The most controversial aspect of CBA is putting a value on items that are perceived to be inherently unsuitable for valuation e.g. loss of vision, suffering, death etc. Few techniques used to obtain value of the health state include

♦ ***Human capital approach.*** Human beings are considered as equivalent to capital equipment in the context of working lives concerned so that they are assumed to deliver a course of productivity in future years.

♦ ***Willingness to pay.*** Hypothetical examples are used to ask individuals how much they would be willing to pay to secure improvements in treatment.

♦ ***Standard gamble technique.*** Respondents are asked to imagine being in the health state being valued and are then told that there is a treatment which could restore them to full health; however, the treatment also has the possibility of causing immediate death. They are asked to indicate how much risk of dying they would be ready to acquire in order to be 'cured', a readiness to accept a greater risk of immediate death leading to the value on the current health state being lower.

❖ **Cost utility analysis (CUA)**

This is the most difficult economic analysis; compares treatment alternatives or programs where costs are calculated in financial/ monetary terms and outcomes evaluated in terms of subject preferences or quality of life.

Utility based units i.e. QALY (Quality adjusted life years) or **QTWIST** (Quality-Adjusted Time Without Symptoms of disease and Toxicity) are used as outcome measures.

$$QALY = Q \times Y$$

Q = Quality of life (utility)

Y = Quantity (years) of life

QALYs have the advantage of being able to capture gains in quality of life and quantity of life (= survival) in a single measure. The QALY adjusts the duration of life for its quality by allocating a value (known as a *utility value*) between 0 and 1 (where 0 represents death or health states considered as bad as being dead and 1 represents perfectly healthy state) for every year of life. Negative utility values are also possible for some conditions that are considered to be worse than being dead, such as the end stage of a degenerative illness.

In CUA, results are expressed as *Cost utility ratio (CUR)* i.e. extra cost per one QALY gained when switching between alternatives, which is based on marginal or incremental analysis.

Example of CUA:

Treatment	A	B
Cost	X	Y
QALY gained	Q1	Q2
Cost utility ratio (CUR)	$(X - Y) / (Q1 - Q2)$	

QALY League Tables rank various interventions according to cost per QALY. These are used as lead to make decisions on how to assign the resources; to seek to move resources from endeavours expensive in context of health benefits generated and towards endeavours relatively cheaper in cost.

Methods for utility assessment

♦ **Direct methods**

o *Time trade off.* Individuals are asked to choose between living for a given time in a state of poor health and living for a shorter time in full health. They are then asked to decide how many years they would be ready to surrender in order to achieve a perfect state of health. If a respondent indicates they would be willing to give up 2 of the 10 years to be 'cured', this would translate into a utility value of 0.8. A worse health state, in which a respondent would give up 5 years to be free of the condition, would result in a utility value of 0.5.

o   *Visual Analogue Scale.* Respondents are asked to mark a line (usually labeled 0–100) with an 'X' to indicate their valuation of the health state. The distance from 0 to X is measured and divided by 100 to give the utility value. This is a simple technique but has the disadvantage that the respondent is not asked to make any sort of trade-off or sacrifice in valuing the health state. It is therefore considered an inferior technique by economists.

o   *Standard gamble technique.* As described above.

♦ **Indirect methods**. Quality of life scales e.g SF-36, EQ-5D

METHODS FOR PERFORMING PE ANALYSIS

- *Clinical Trial.*
- *Piggyback Study:* A study in which economic analysis is grafted or added onto a designed clinical study/protocol.
- *Observational Study.*
- *Modeling.* An analytic technique used to project real-world processes and events from actual events observed in studies. Generally used to project beyond the time-frame of the study.

DECISION ANALYSIS AS A TOOL FOR PE

Decision analysis. A formal model for describing and analyzing a decision; also called medical decision taking. This technique is particularly relevant to decisions about inclusion of drugs in formularies.

Decision Tree: A diagram of a set of actions, with their probabilities and the values of the outcomes listed. It is used to analyze a decision. There are 2 types of decision models.

- *Simple decision trees.* Used to model outcomes occurring in short-term and having a definite conclusion e.g acute illness.
- *Recursive decision trees.* Used to model chronic illnesses and are cyclical in nature e.g. Markov model.

Figure 40.5 depicts example of decision tree analysis.

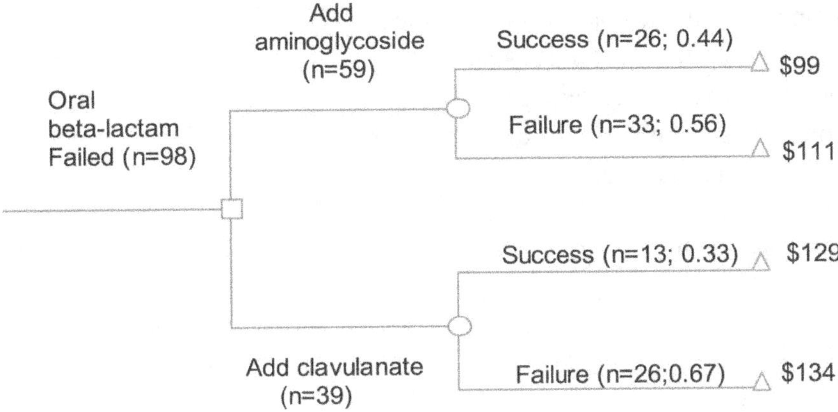

Figure 40.5 An example of decision tree analysis.

Determining which option is the least costly, most effective or produces the highest return is called **rolling back the tree.**

The **expected value of a treatment option** in a decision tree is a weighted average of all the potential costs that may be incurred by people receiving that therapy. The expected value is calculated by multiplying the amount to be paid at the right of every branch by probabilities of that payoff happening and adding them to the subsequent calculations of all weighted payoffs for the option.

e.g. in the given case;

Expected value of aminoglycoside = ($99 × 0.44) + ($111 × 0.56) = $105.72

Expected value of clavulanate = ($129 × 0.33) + ($134 × 0.67) = $132.35

Since we are modeling the costs of therapy, the preferred option would be one with lower cost i.e. aminoglycoside.

SENSITIVITY ANALYSIS

This is a technique to assess the robustness of results of the study. It demonstrates dependence/independence of a result on a particular assumption. By altering important variables and then recalculating results, sensitivity analysis tests the validity of conclusions.

STEPS FOR CONDUCTING A PE ANALYSIS

1. Defining the study problem.
2. Determining from whose perspective it is conducted.
3. Determining the alternative options and consequences.

4. Choosing the suitable pharmacoeconomic method.
5. Perform discounting on future benefits.
6. Recognize the resources required.
7. Demonstrate the probabilities of outcome events.
8. Employ decision analysis.
9. Execute sensitivity analysis.
10. Display the results.

APPLICATIONS OF PHARMACOECONOMICS

- ✓ Assist in decision making and allocating scarce resources.
- ✓ Assessing the value of a new agent.
- ✓ Justify the addition of new clinical service.
- ✓ Pharmaceutical companies use it to evaluate pricing of a drug and also to make decisions to pursue or not to pursue particular development program.
- ✓ Third-party payers use such information to decide whether to pay for a particular treatment, or to determine what price they are willing to pay.
- ✓ Re-pricing of an already marketed medicine.
- ✓ Convincing a formulary committee to place the medicine on their approved list.
- ✓ Helping to convince one or more regulatory authorities to approve a medicine.
- ✓ Developing clinical strategies.

SECTION – J

CLINICAL RESEARCH: SPECIAL AREAS

Contents

Oncology Clinical Trials

INTRODUCTION

Oncology research and clinical trials in oncology are increasing very rapidly. The drug development process of anti-cancer drugs involves general steps similar to other therapeutic areas although there are several unique aspects associated with oncology research. Also, drug development in the field of oncology is quite challenging due to a number of reasons (Table 41.1).

Table 41.1 Challenges in the way of oncology clinical trials.

✓ Inter- individual heterogeneity in the tumor biological processes.

✓ High lethality or life threatening nature of most of the malignancies.

✓ Narrow therapeutic indices of many available anticancer drugs.

✓ Complex protocols often involving multiple therapeutic approaches and /or drugs.

✓ Frequent association of cancers with other co-morbidities and concomitant medications which can affect the occurrence and/ severity of adverse events.

✓ Complex disease presentation in different patients with varied signs and symptoms.

TYPES OF CLINICAL TRIALS IN ONCOLOGY

1. **Natural history trials**

   These are generally conducted as prospective studies aiming to determine the natural disease course when treated with standard therapy or left untreated.

2. **Prevention trials**

   The aim of these trials is to evaluate the cancer risk and effectiveness of methods to decrease or prevent the occurrence of cancer. The participants in these trials can be healthy individuals not having cancer but with risk factors for developing cancer or individuals who have had a cancer and are at high risk of developing a new cancer.

   These trials can be:

   Action studies (doing something): focus on determining whether actions like lifestyle measures (exercise, avoiding smoking or alcohol etc.) can influence the incidence of cancer.

   Agent studies (taking something): these are called *"Chemoprevention trials"* as here the focus is on determining whether intake of some agents like drugs, vitamin supplements etc. may decrease the risk of a certain cancer.

3. **Screening and early-detection trials**

   Screening is a type of diagnostic testing conducted on population at risk of developing a disease/ cancer, as an attempt for earlier diagnosis relative to manifestation as per natural history. The principle of screening is that a disease if diagnosed at an earlier stage is relatively more treatable or curable.

   The *objective* of these trials is to assess the effectiveness of screening test/s for detecting cancer at an earlier stage and their effect on mortality or complications.

   The *outcome measures* in these trials are survival (most common), incidence of advanced disease and stage shifts.

   A drawback of these trials is introduction of *"lead time bias"* i.e. screen –detected cases appear to have longer survival due to early detection; such bias needs to be corrected to evaluate the true benefit of screening.

   While designing such trials, the number and interval of screenings is an important aspect which needs to be taken into account.

   Various *tools* employed in cancer screening trials include tissue sampling, laboratory tests like genetic testing and tumor markers, imaging tests, physical examination, family history (pedigree charting) etc.

4. **Treatment/ Interventional trials**

   These trials are conducted in patients with cancer to evaluate newer treatment options such as:

   - New drugs/ combination of drugs.
   - Vaccines.
   - Radiotherapy.
   - Surgical approaches.
   - Combination of treatments.

5. **Quality of life trials/ Palliative trials or supportive care trials**

   Such trials evaluate improvement in the quality of life (QOL) of cancer patients, especially those with advanced disease and experiencing adverse effects of chemotherapy. They are also designed to assess the effectiveness of palliative measures like drugs to alleviate associated co-morbidities e.g. pain, depression, sleep disorders;

psychosocial interventions, exercising, talking with counselor etc. The focus of these trials is not only the patients but also their families and care-givers.

SALIENT FEATURES OF ONCOLOGY CLINICAL TRIALS

PHASE 1 TRIALS

In oncology, phase 1 studies are conducted in cancer patients who are refractory to standard therapy and there are no more treatment options available; and ideally possess adequate organ system functions and performance status. Practical difficulties may be encountered in finding such fairly healthy advanced cancer patients thereby slowing recruitment process and increasing trial duration.

In determining DLT, only first cycle/course of treatment is taken into consideration, hence minimal data on cumulative toxicity can be obtained.

Starting dose is calculated from one-third of the toxic dose low (1/3 TDL) in a large animal species or one-tenth of the lethal dose in mice (1/10 LD_{10}); for dose escalation, Modified Fibonacci scheme is followed.

PHASE 2 AND 3 TRIALS

Nature of Trial Population

The overall population of cancer patients is very heterogenous including many factors having significant influence on the conduct of clinical trials. Various points need to be considered while determining the inclusion and exclusion criteria for enrolment in oncology trials (Table 41.2).

Table 41.2 Important points to consider while determining subject eligibility criteria for inclusion in oncology clinical trials.
• Define an adequate life expectancy e.g. 6 months; need to have sufficient time to demonstrate safety and efficacy of test compound/ intervention.
• Documentation of malignancy on the basis of histological or cytological evidence prior to administering intervention.
• Define the individual performance status, an important prognostic factor in oncology.
• Define clearly the primary malignancy, stage, molecular and radiological features, any progression or metastasis.
• Identify all types of previous treatments received whether chemotherapy, radiotherapy, surgery, immunotherapy, hormonal agents etc.
• Define organ function parameters, medical history, concomitant disease or medications to minimize the risk of adverse effects.
• Documentation of genotype may be required in some studies depending on the agent under investigation.

Choice of Comparator

Placebos are almost never used in oncology clinical trials when a standard treatment exists. If however, the protocol demands the administration of placebo as comparator, it should always be done in conjunction with other approved treatment/s.

Outcome Parameters in Oncology Clinical Trials

Efficacy outcomes/ end points

♦ An important efficacy outcome in solid tumor studies is *RECIST (response evaluation criteria in solid tumors)* criteria. In RECIST criteria, data analysis is done in relation to target (primary) lesions, non-target (secondary) lesions, and new lesions to determine an overall response (OR). The response categories are:
  - Complete response (CR).
  - Partial response (PR).
  - Stable disease (SD).
  - Progressive disease (PD).
  - Non-evaluable.

♦ Another outcome measure used in oncology trials is *time to event* e.g. survival, disease progression and failure. Endpoints used are:
  - Overall survival (OS): time from randomization till death.
  - Disease free survival (DFS): time from randomization till recurrence of tumor or death from any cause.
  - Progression free survival (PFS): time from randomization till objective tumor progression or death.
  - Time to progression (TTP): time from randomization till objective tumor progression excluding deaths.
  - Time to treatment failure (TTF): time from randomization to discontinuation of treatment for any reason e.g. toxicity, no efficacy, death.
  - Time to progression of cancer symptoms.

♦ *Patient reported outcomes* (PROs) e.g. health related quality of life (HRQOL) are generally included as secondary end points in cancer clinical trials.

♦ In case of liquid malignancies e.g. hematological malignancies like leukemias, efficacy parameters can be
  - reduction in cancer cells count
  - increase in the proportion of cancer free cells

Safety outcomes/ endpoints

In oncology clinical trials, adverse events are conventionally graded according to some standard guidelines e.g. CTCAE (Common Terminology Criteria for Adverse Events) grading developed by National Cancer Institute (NCI). The latest version of CTCAE (v 5.0) was published in 2017 and classifies adverse events into 5 grades viz. grade 1 (mild), grade 2 (moderate), grade 3 (severe), grade 4 (life-threatening) and grade 5 (death related to adverse event). However, all the grades may not be applicable for certain adverse events e.g. for iron overload the lowest grade is 2 (asymptomatic, intervention not needed); highest grade for tinnitus and vertigo is 3.

NCI has also developed the patient reported outcomes version of CTCAE i.e PRO-CTCAE which provides a standard method to assess symptomatic adverse events from the patient's perspective.

DIFFERENCES BETWEEN ONCOLOGY AND NON ONCOLOGY CLINICAL TRIALS

Table 41.3 highlights some major points that distinguish the clinical trials in oncology from the non oncology trials.

Table 41.3 Key differentiating features between oncology and non oncology clinical trials		
Features	**Non oncology trials**	**Oncology trials**
Trial population	healthy volunteers in phase 1	cancer patients in phase 1
Comparator	generally placebo controlled	placebo never used if standard therapy exists/ placebo in addition to approved therapies
Efficacy parameters	depending on investigational agent	tumor response, survival, quality of life
Adverse event grading	mild, moderate, severe	grade 1 to 5 (CTCAE guidelines)

SPECIAL DESIGNS USED IN ONCOLOGY CLINICAL TRIALS

1. **Basket trials.**

   These trials aim to test the efficacy of a new drug (targeted anti-cancer therapy)/ drug combination in patients presenting with different types of cancers having a common genetic/ molecular mutation or biomarker (Figure 41.1). Using this design, new drug can also be evaluated across varied cancer populations such as those defined by histology, disease stage, demographic characteristics of patients or prior therapies etc. These trials hold special utility in rare cancer types and cancers having rare gene mutations. Another name for these trials is "Bucket trials".

   Few examples of basket trials:

   - In 2006, imatinib mesylate got FDA approval for 5 different types of cancers (non-gastrointestinal stromal tumors) having a common KIT mutation on the basis of a single-phase II basket trial (Imatinib Target Exploration Consortium Study B2225). The trial tested the drug across 40 tumor subtypes and 24 indications/ subgroups.

- In 2011, vemurafenib was approved for treatment of melanoma with a specific BRAF V600 mutation. Later, in 2017, the drug's approval was extended to Erdheim-Chester disease, a rare blood cancer on the basis of results of a phase -II VE-basket trial.

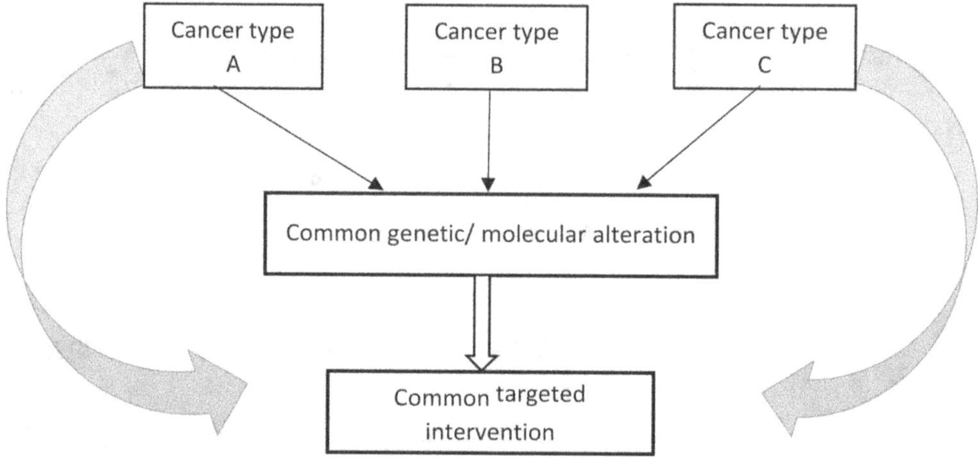

Figure 41.1 Design of a basket (bucket) trial.

2. Umbrella trials.

In these trials, multiple drugs (targeted therapies) are tested simultaneously under one large trial in patients with one type of cancer but with different molecular/ genetic mutations (Figure 41.2). The term "umbrella" denotes stratification of one proposed cancer type into different molecular/ genetic subtypes.

An example of umbrella trial is the BATTLE (Biomarker-integrated Approaches of Targeted Therapy for Lung Cancer Elimination) trial which tested the efficacy of erlotinib, vandetanib, erlotinib plus bexarotene, or sorafenib in non-small cell lung cancer patients having different corresponding biomarkers.

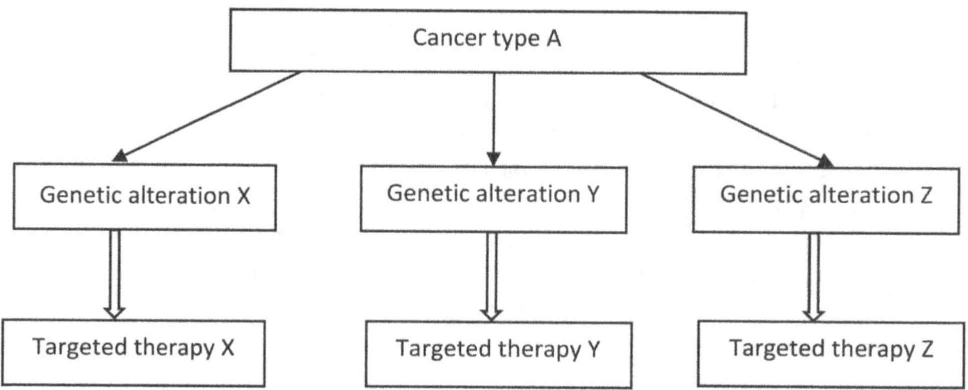

Figure 41.2 Design of an umbrella trial.

3. **Super umbrella trials.**

These include the combination of basket and umbrella trials.

4. **Platform trials.**

These trials test multiple interventions against a single control group and incorporate adaptation rules specified *a priori* in the protocol like ability to drop ineffective arms early and flexibility to add new arms during the trial conduct (Figure 41.3). These are also known as multi-arm, multi-stage (MAMS) design trials. An example is the STAMPEDE (Systemic Therapy in Advancing or Metastatic Prostate Cancer: Evaluation of Drug Efficacy) trial evaluating multiple therapeutic options in hormone naïve prostate cancer.

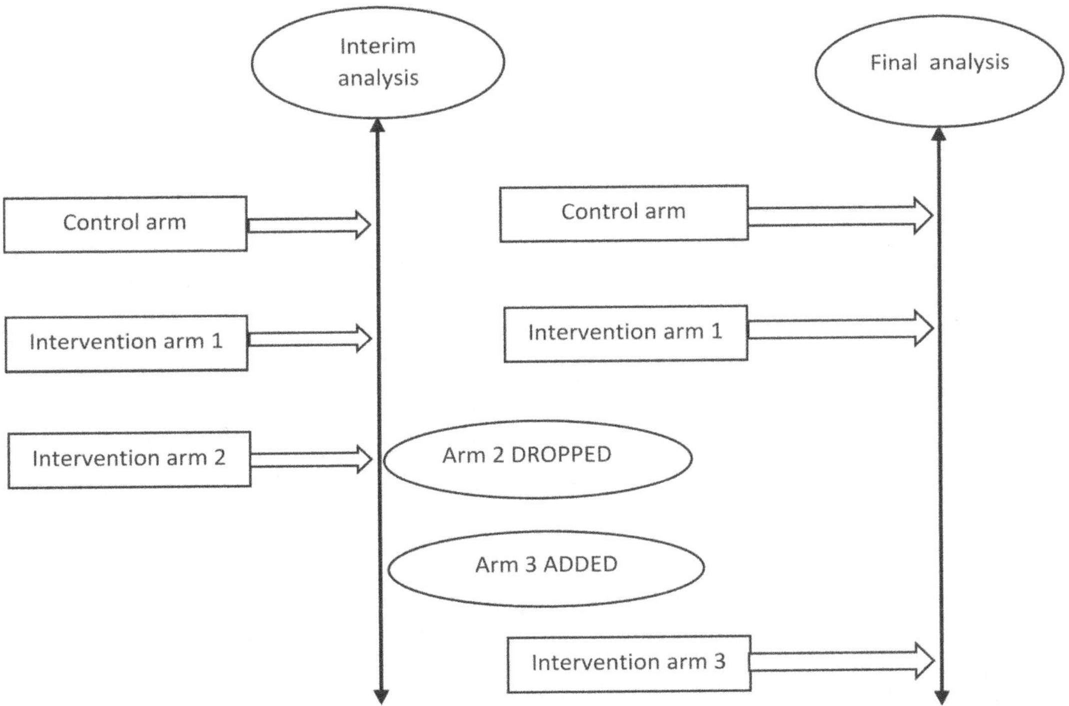

Figure 41.3 Design of a platform trial.

CHAPTER 42

Clinical Research on Vaccines

OVERVIEW

Introduction
Evaluation of Vaccines
  Preclinical Studies
  Clinical Studies

Salient Features of Vaccine Trials
Special Considerations

INTRODUCTION

Unlike the industrialized nations, there are no distinct regulations for vaccines in India. The clinical trials of vaccines fall under the purview of the New Drugs and Clinical Trials Rules, 2019. Under the act, all vaccines come under the category of new drugs. Also, concurrent phase 2 or 3 trials can be conducted in India for vaccines developed outside India.

EVALUATION OF VACCINES

PRECLINICAL STUDIES

- ✓ Animal pharmacology studies to establish the action of vaccines i.e. immunogenicity should be conducted. According to WHO guidelines on non-clinical evaluation of vaccines, immunogenicity studies should be conducted in animal models as they may provide valuable "proof of concept" information to further plan the clinical phase of vaccine development program.
- ✓ Animal toxicology studies should be conducted as single and repeat dose studies in two animal species. The dose, route and duration of exposure should justify the intended human dose. For recombinant vaccines, studies with two routes of administration may be needed.
- ✓ The studies should be carried out in appropriate animal models having sensitivity to the pathogenic organism or toxin. Ideally, the animal model selected should be able to elicit an immune response to the vaccine antigen.

CLINICAL STUDIES

The guidelines to conduct clinical trials on investigational vaccines are identical to those regulating drug trials. Formal regulatory approval from DCGI is required. For clinical trials on recombinant vaccines, an additional approval needs to be obtained from the Department of Biotechnology (DBT) and its advisory committees like the Institutional Biosafety Committee (IBSC), Recombinant Committee on Genetic Manipulation (RCGM) and Genetic Engineering Approval Committee (GEAC). For serological testing from overseas, an additional approval is required from Directorate General of Foreign Trade (DGFT).

Characteristics of clinical trial phases of vaccines

Phase I : This involves introduction of a vaccine into human subjects for the first time with an aim to determine its safety and biological effects including immunogenicity. The dose and route of administration of investigational vaccine is evaluated. During this phase, low risk participants are conventionally involved e.g. trial aiming to study immunogenicity to hepatitis B vaccine should involve low risk subjects.

Pharmacokinetic studies are usually not necessary to identify properties of the immune response to known or assumed action of vaccine. The class, subclass and function of particular antibody released, the time lag for appearance of antibody and duration of adequate antibody titer is estimated. Additional information usually gathered includes status of cell-mediated immunity, presence of any cross reactive antibodies and/or interaction with pre-existing antibodies that can influence immune system.

Phase II : These are the initial trials conducted in a restricted number of volunteers from target populations like children, adults or those at risk of exposure to pathogens. The main aim of these trials is to evaluate the efficacy (immunogenicity) and dose range of investigational vaccines; although pharmacokinetics and safety can also be studied. Early Phase II is generally an exploratory trial while late Phase II is usually a pivotal efficacy study.

Phase III : The trials conducted during this phase aim to assess the safety and effectiveness of vaccine in disease prevention. These are usually carried out as multi-centric studies involving large number of volunteers (up to thousands). For new vaccines, in phase 3 trials, clinical protection needs to be measured. The studies should preferably be performed in an area with low endemicity to avoid confounding due to protection given by natural exposure.

SALIENT FEATURES OF VACCINE TRIALS

- The protocols for vaccine trials should include a detailed description of various aspects like subject selection criteria, regimen for administering test and reference vaccine, validation of techniques employed to detect antibody titer levels etc. Additionally, protocols of studies evaluating new vaccine should include a section on details of manufacturing process, quality control measures, storage conditions, stability data etc.

- The protection provided by vaccines is measured as vaccine efficacy and /or vaccine effectiveness. Efficacy in vaccine trials refers to a decrease in incidence of disease after vaccination compared to the incidence before vaccination. Effectiveness refers to protective rate conferred in a given population.

- For vaccines containing a known antigen for which the level of protective antibody is well established, immunogenicity studies may be sufficient to demonstrate clinical efficacy.

- Immunogenicity can be expressed as *seroconversion* (predefined increase in antibody concentration), *seroprotection* (proportion of subjects achieving antibody titres over a certain protective level) and *geometric mean titre* (average titre for a group of subjects calculated by taking antilog of the mean of log antibody titres).

- The pharmacodynamic studies are conducted to gather information when other routes of administration are claimed for the investigational vaccine e.g. oral vaccine, or when vaccine consists of novel adjuvants or excipients. These are also conducted to assess additional parameters e.g. age at vaccination, effect of concomitantly administered vaccines, effect of changes in vaccine strain on efficacy and safety, and interchangeability of vaccine.

- Bridging studies can be conducted to strengthen evidence on clinical comparability of efficacy, safety and immunogenicity of new formulation when there is a modification in vaccine composition with respect to adjuvant, preservative, or change in manufacturing process, site or scale.

- In RCTs, the use of placebo as comparator is justified in cases where no approved effective vaccine exists. The opinion from community can also be sought regarding the choice of comparator. The subjects in control groups when administered placebo or ineffective vaccines are exposed to a risk of contracting the disease; in case of occurrence of such an event, free medical management should be provided as long as required.

- Vaccine trials should be conducted by investigator/s having adequate and requisite infrastructure for evaluation of sero-conversion. The investigator should be provided with quality control data of the test batch of vaccine manufactured for clinical trials.

- Children being a vulnerable group, due consideration should be given in selecting age, gender, ethnicity and health status for enrolling them in vaccine clinical trials particularly if they belong to an over-researched community.

- Post Marketing Surveillance (PMS) needs to be carried out following sero-conversion studies. PMS data should be obtained in a significant sample of population sensitive enough to identify adverse effects and other safety concerns.

- Arrangements should be made for post trial access of vaccine to the control group. However, in cases where the investigational vaccine is for pediatric age group; by the time trial is completed children in the control arm may cross the age when vaccine is proposed to have efficacy in terms of protection from disease. Under such circumstances, control arm could be given some other alternative effective vaccine for that particular age group although this does not restore clinical equipoise. EC may assess the viability and ethical considerations for each case individually. Post trial access to the vaccine should be initially provided to the community from which trial subjects were drawn.

SPECIAL CONSIDERATIONS

- **Combination vaccines.** The efficacy of each antigenic component needs to be evaluated. In cases where each individual component is validated for correlates of protection; immunogenicity studies need to be carried out. However, when validation has not been done for each component, controlled clinical trials should be conducted. Also, there is requirement for non-inferiority trials demonstrating the non- inferiority of combination vaccine in terms of immunogenicity or efficacy, compared to vaccines with individual components.
- **Active or live - attenuated vaccines.** The subject to be administered the vaccine should be duly informed of the possible small risk of producing that particular infection.
- **Recombinant vaccines.** There is little existing knowledge regarding the risks associated with vaccines produced by recombinant DNA technology. However, for all the recombinant vaccines/ products the guidelines issued by the department of biotechnology should be strictly adhered to.
- **HIV preventive vaccine.** During the conduct of trials with HIV preventive vaccine, serology results may become positive after vaccination. Although this does not stipulate presence of active infection but may lead to issues with employment and travel. To avoid any complication, a certificate expressing the subject's participation in HIV vaccine trial may be issued.
- **Generic vaccines.** The generic version of new vaccines already launched in other markets after favorable data from extensive Phase III trials should be compared with the reference vaccine with respect to sero-conversion in an adequately sized study sample.

Orphan Drug Research

INTRODUCTION

Orphan/ rare disease is defined by WHO as a disease or condition with a prevalence of $< 1/1000$ population. The definition criteria, however, differ across different parts of world e.g. in US, it is defined as any disorder affecting $<200,000$ population at a single time point; in European Union (EU) as disorders affecting $<1/2000$ population; in India as disorder affecting not more than five lac persons in India. Hence, a disorder may be considered as rare in one geographical area but not in another e.g. IgA nephropathy is rare in EU but common in Asia and Africa.

An orphan drug can be defined as the drug which is used to treat an orphan disease/ disorder (Box 43.1).

> **Box 43.1** The New Drugs and Clinical Trials Rules, 2019.
>
> **Orphan drug**: a drug indicated for a condition which affects not more than five lac persons in India.

DRUG DEVELOPMENT PROCESS IN ORPHAN DISEASES

CHALLENGES IN DRUG DEVELOPMENT PROCESS OF ORPHAN DISEASES

The drug development process in orphan diseases is complicated by a lot of issues. Table 43.1 includes the various challenges faced in this area and potential strategies to overcome them.

REGULATORY REQUIREMENTS

The regulatory requirements for marketing approval of new drugs are common for all disorders, irrespective of their prevalence. This requirement is the demonstration of 'significant evidence' that the drug is able to produce its affirmed efficacy; which is based on two statistically significant trials at a type 1 error rate of 5%. However, the standard principle of evidence of efficacy may not be rigorously pertinent to orphan/ rare disorders.

INCREASING ACCESSIBILITY OF ORPHAN DRUGS

The methodological constraints encountered during various stages of drug development in orphan diseases, however, demand flexibilities in the drug approval process to increase their accessibility at the patient end. For example,

- Judicious use of innovative trial designs, biomarker-based end points and appropriate analytical techniques in order to combat the methodological challenges encountered during execution of trials in the field of orphan diseases.
- Provisions for accelerated pathways and fast track designation to overcome time concerns and hasten the approval process.
- Not being subservient to statistical significance only e.g. USFDA approval of Xuriden (uridine triacetate) for treating a rare disorder, hereditary orotic aciduria was based on the demonstration of clinical significance in an open label trial enrolling four patients in the absence of an appropriate control group.
- Provision of *progressive licensing* pathway aiming to switch the focus from premarket evaluation to that of recurrent/constant learning. In this, drug is granted early approval for higher risk population; approval is revisited at additional points as the data from approved as well as broadened candidate population is assessed.

Table 43.1 Challenges in the drug development process of orphan diseases and potential strategies to handle them.

Challenges	Potential strategies to handle
Patient recruitment • Small number of patients • Geographical dispersion of potential participants	• multicenter/ multinational collaboration • collaboration with patient organizations • patient contact registries • technologies such as telemedicine • more active search of patients (e.g. call reminders) • open–label designs • adoption of drop-out strategies • monetary incentives to participants
Study outcomes • Poorly defined clinical parameters • Lack of standard measures of assessing the disorder activity or progression	Need to develop validated biomarkers/ surrogate end points to support the clinical outcomes
Study duration Difficulty in deciding the appropriate duration of study due to incomplete knowledge about the natural course of rare diseases	Improve the understanding of natural history of disorder and its pathophysiology and preclinical models
Study design Randomised trials difficult to execute due to small and heterogenous population available for rare/ orphan diseases.	Adoption of alternative trial designs • within- patient designs (e.g. cross-over, n of 1) • adaptive designs
Choice of control group • ethical issues with the use of placebo, • lack of standard treatment to serve as active control	Use of external controls (e.g. historical controls) usually recommended
Statistical issues Low power of study due to • small sample size and • high inter-individual variability	Appropriate statistical methods to obtain maximal data from limited number of subjects showing heterogeneity e.g. acceptance of a greater type 1 error rate
Limited researchers Lack of clinical researchers having adequate qualifications and expertise in designing and executing trials for orphan disorders	• Educational programs to spread awareness and knowledge in orphan disease area • training of researchers in the area of rare diseases

Limited R and D in orphan disease area
• Less interest of pharmaceutical industry in drug development for rare diseases due to relatively lesser financial benefits on investment
• Lack of funding
	• Providing incentives to boost new drug development for orphan disorders e.g. The **Orphan Drug Act (1983)** in USA laid provisions for providing incentives in the form of
	    protocol assistance from the FDA,
	    tax benefits,
	    providing waivers for regulatory fee
	    granting exclusive marketing rights for 7 years.

Surgical Clinical Trials

INTRODUCTION

The role of randomized controlled clinical trials in surgery and other skill-dependent therapies has been a matter of debate for many years. There is always the need of a strong justification to give precedence to societal benefits over exposure of a number of patients to sham surgery or a less than state-of-the-art surgery to evaluate a new surgical technical or procedure. Compared to many medical disciplines, the clinical trials in surgery are conducted less frequently and with diminished rigor. Because of the absence of rigorous evaluation, many widely used surgical procedures in the past have probably been ineffective, suboptimal or unsafe. Many of such procedures have eventually been discarded and rejected in recent decades on the basis of randomized controlled trials e.g. internal mammary artery ligation for angina pectoris, prefrontal lobotomies for schizophrenia, kidney decapsulation for hypertension etc. Hence, the crucial role of clinical trials in providing a conclusive evidence on efficacy and safety of surgical procedures cannot be denied.

TYPES OF SURGICAL CLINICAL TRIALS

Table 44.1 depicts a broad overview of the various types of clinical trials involving surgical procedures.

Table 44.1 Types of surgical clinical trials.
1. Evaluation of treatment of a particular disease by surgery compared to medical treatment.
2. Evaluation of treatment of a particular disease by surgery compared to non-medical treatment modalities e.g. hyperthermia, radiation therapy.
3. Comparison of two or more surgical procedures e.g. modified versus conventional procedure, new versus old procedure.
4. Comparison of a surgical procedure performed with and without adjunct medical or other therapy.
5. Evaluation of drugs administered during surgical procedures e.g. neuromuscular blocking drugs, anesthetic agents etc.
6. Evaluation of surgical materials used during surgical procedures e.g. suture materials, adhesives etc.

UNIQUE NATURE OF SURGICAL TRIALS

The process of conducting clinical trials in surgery may be different in a number of ways as compared to trials in medical disciplines. Some salient and distinguishing features of surgical trials are as mentioned below:

1. The development of new surgical procedures does not necessarily follow the different developmental phases as described with pharmaceutical agents. Generally, new surgical methods can be quickly and readily compared with standard methods in clinical trials after demonstration of feasibility.

2. In contrast to drugs or other medical interventions, surgical techniques are generally developed by a single or small subset of surgeons with relatively low expenditure.

3. Unlike pharmacologic agents, surgical procedures often function on physical principles and are associated with a high degree of determinism.

4. Surgical procedures are associated with a powerful placebo response. Hence, evaluation of surgical procedures in comparison to placebo is quite needed. However, the use of true placebo in surgery, such as sham surgery is always a matter of ethical concern and has to be justified on the basis of sound scientific principles.

5. Surgical methods inherently have strong potential for selection bias i.e. procedures are generally developed in and applied to patients with good prognosis. Although this practice exposes the surgical patients to short term risks, the long term risks may be less than in non surgical group.

6. Study design in surgical trials may be quite different from medical trials due to one-time and irreversible nature of most surgical procedures while on the other hand medicines need to be administered at multiple times to treat a disorder.

7. The outcomes in surgical procedures are also influenced to a greater degree by the technical skill of operating surgeons. This is in contrast to medical trials where the technical skill of investigators plays a less critical role in determining outcomes.

8. Most of the medical trials have clearly defined measurable end points and trials are usually completed within a defined period of time; long term follow up of patients after trial completion is generally not done. In surgical trials, however, patients are generally followed up for some period after completion of surgery as end points usually refer to a certain event occurring after surgery (e.g. re-hospitalization for same problem, occurrence of a new episode) or observation till a certain defined time.

BARRIERS TO CLINICAL TRIALS IN SURGERY

The designing and conduct of clinical trials in surgical disciplines is associated with many barriers (Table 44.2).

Table 44.2   Barriers to surgical clinical trials.

- Reluctance of many surgeons in applying randomization to studies of patient outcomes, making the process of comparing surgical procedures quite tedious.
- Practical issues in blinding patients and/or surgeons.
- Lack of any specific regulations governing surgical trials in contrast to trials evaluating drugs and medical devices.
- Ethical issues with the use of a true placebo or sham surgery
- Higher chances of encountering immediate risks in surgical patients
- Practical issues in efficacy assessment due to inherent and unavoidable confounding factors like technical skill of the surgeon, ancillary care, selection bias etc.

SECTION – K

ANNEXURES

CONTENTS

Common Technical Document

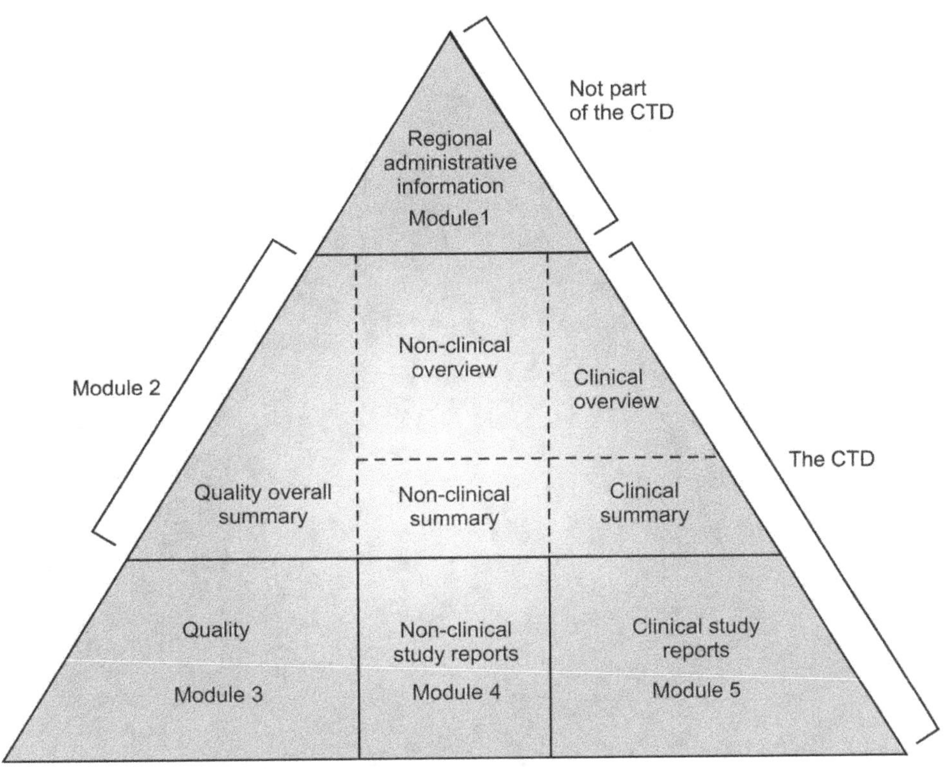

The CTD triangle.

The CTD is organized into 5 modules: Module 1 is region specific; Modules 2,3,4 and 5 are intended to be common for all regions.

Source: https://www.ich.org/fileadmin/Public_Web_Site/ICH_Products/CTD/CTD_triangle.pdf

Clinical Trial Registration

ANNEXURE II (a)

PROCESS OF CLINICAL TRIAL REGISTRATION WITH CTRI

Clinical trial registration with CTRI can be done by a TRIALIST (one who wishes to register clinical trial in CTRI) / REGISTRANT (an individual who is authorized to submit trial data for registration in order to register a trial).

Various steps involved in the registration process are as detailed below.

- Go to the CTRI website: www.ctri.nic.in. The home page will be displayed.
- If registering a trial for the first time, the trialist/ registrant need to obtain username and password.
- On the left side of the home page, in the window "SIGN IN TO CTRI"; click on "**New applicant**". This will open a page showing instructions for new applicants and a form.
- Please fill the details in the form after reading instructions as provided. Click on "SUBMIT".
- A message is displayed showing successful submission of the registration request to the CTRI. Mail regarding successful registration and username/ password would be sent to email id (filled in form).
- Username/password would be activated after a second confirmatory mail from CTRI.
- Upon activation of username/ password, the trialist/ registrant would be able to login to CTRI.
- Go to home page, in the window "SIGN IN TO CTRI" enter username/password and login. (As a security measure, wrong entries of username/ password for >10 consecutive times would lead to automatic locking.)
- On successful login, you would be directed to your personal "WELCOME PAGE" showing a table of "Total trials" registered by you including the trials under entry stage, under review stage, registered trials and terminated/ suspended trials.
- To upload a trial, click on "MAIN PAGE" in the welcome page.

- Then click on "ADD NEW TRIAL".

- Enter the "PUBLIC TITLE", "SCIENTIFIC TITLE" and "Acronym (optional)". For any assistance regarding the titles, click on the information icon. Click on "PROCEED".

- Now, the trial would appear under the heading "TRIALS UNDER ENTRY/ REVIEW".

- Subsequently, the other parts of trial registration form may be filled in any sequence by clicking on "UPDATE" link.

- The trial registration form is divided into 8 parts with multiple sub-parts. Click on each part individually and upload the information after entering part 1 (already entered by now). (For any assistance required, download the "TRIAL REGISTRATION DATASET" given in the login box containing detailed instructions on how to enter information in all individual parts).

- Once all the trial details are entered in form, please check for completeness and accuracy in all fields by generating the PDF file/ go to "main page"---------- click "FULL DETAILS".

- If any modification required, click on "UPDATE" ---------- click on "PROCEED" to save changes.

- On satisfaction, click on "SUBMIT TRIAL TO CTRI".

  After submission, if all the mandatory information is adequately filled a "TRIAL ACKNOWLEDGEMENT NUMBER" will be displayed which should be quoted in all trial related communications.

NOTE: In case of **postgraduate thesis**; please enter the MD student details under "Principal Investigator" and the Guide/ Professor details under "Contact person".

ANNEXURE II (b)

PROCESS OF CLINICAL TRIAL REGISTRATION WITH CLINICALTRIALS.GOV

Clinicaltrials.gov is a registry of clinical trials provided by the U.S. National Library of Medicine (NLM). It is the largest database of clinical trials.

Clinical studies involving human subjects assessing biomedical and/or health outcomes can be registered with clinicaltrials.gov provided they conform to

- any applicable human subject or ethics review regulations (or equivalent) and
- any applicable regulations of the national or regional health authority (or equivalent).

Steps to register a clinical study with clinicaltrials.gov

1. Determination of the person responsible for registering the clinical study and which Protocol Registration and Results System (PRS) account should be used.

   (PRS is a web-based data entry system to register a clinical study or to submit results information for an already registered study).

2. Go through the submission requirements.

   Description of the items to be submitted may be obtained from Protocol Registration Data Elements Definitions.

   The Interventional Study Protocol Registration Template is a useful tool to understand and gather the data needed to complete each registration module.

3. Login to PRS.
4. Enter the required and optional data elements.
5. Preview, inspect and release (submit) the record.

Common Forms for Ethics Committee Review

In order to harmonize and unify the submission of various documents to ECs across the country, ICMR Bioethics unit at NCDIR (National Centre for Disease Informatics and Research), Bangalore with funding support by THSTI (Translational Health Science and Technology Institute) prepared the "Common forms for ethics committee review" in 2019. These forms provide a common EC format to improve the ethical review of biomedical and health research in the country.

Advantages of "Common forms for ethics committee review"

- Simplification of the process of submission to EC.
- In case of multi-centric studies, due to the use of standardized forms, the ethical review process will be streamlined and less time and effort demanding.
- The forms have been made comprehensively to gather all relevant information about study protocol and provide assistance to EC in its review procedures.

The "Common forms for ethics committee review" comprise of:

- ✓ an application form for initial review which gathers details pertaining to basic information, research and participant related information, declarations and checklists;
- ✓ 13 annexures providing formats for other types of EC reviews, adverse events, protocol violations and reporting formats;
- ✓ additional forms focusing on clinical trials, socio-behavioral, public health research and human genetics testing research.

The forms are available in both word and PDF formats and can be freely downloaded from ICMR and ICMR Bioethics Unit web page with the help of links as:

http://ethics.ncdirindia.org/Tools_and_Instruments.aspx

https://www.icmr.nic.in/sites/default/files/guiddelines

Hard copy of the forms is also available and can be requested from ICMR Bioethics Unit, NCDIR, Bangalore.

Conflict of Interest (COI) Form/Declaration Form for IEC Members

(TEMPLATE)

I am familiar with the COI policy of IEC according to which no IEC member may participate in the initial or continuing review or decision making process of any project in which he/ she has an actual or potential conflict of interest except to provide information as requested by the IEC.

I declare that I have a _______________ (type of COI: financial or non-financial) in relation to the project entitled _______________ submitted for review to the IEC. The reason for my COI is _______________.

I assure to refrain from the review or decision making process of this project.

Signature of IEC member

Date:

Signature of Chairperson

Date:

NABH Standards for Accreditation of Ethics Committees

Standard 1. Authority for formation of EC.
Objective elements • Procedures to specify the authority under which the EC is established and administratively governed. • Documented policy to ensure the independence of the EC. • Functioning of EC as per applicable rules and regulations.
Standard 2. Standard Operating Procedures (SOPs)
Objective elements • Adequate procedures for development, review and revision of SOPs. • List of mandatory procedures for Ethics Committee ✓ terms of reference for EC; ✓ protocol submission; ✓ ethical review, ✓ decision making, minutes recording, post meeting activities including monitoring; ✓ documentation and archiving
Standard 3. EC composition
Objective elements • Multidisciplinary and multi-sectorial composition. • Subject experts and representatives of vulnerable subjects shall be invited as required with prior intimation.

Table *Contd...*

- Terms of reference for membership, appointment, reconstitution and resignation.
- Well defined roles and responsibilities of EC members.
- Training of members in applicable rules and regulations and EC SOPs.

Conflict of interest and confidentiality addressed.

Standard 4. Protection of subject rights, safety and well-being

Objective elements

- Documentation and specification of rights and responsibilities of subjects.
- Subject's participation and withdrawal from the trial to be voluntary and with prior intimation.
- Information and comprehension (initial and ongoing)of the subjects of the associated risks and benefits of the trial.
- Protection of subject confidentiality and privacy.
- Trial monitoring to ensure equitable selection of subjects, with special emphasis on vulnerable and high risk subjects.
- Appropriate compensation for trial participation provided to subjects as per the rules and regulation.
- Serious adverse events to be addressed, adequate medical care provided and an appropriate reporting mechanism to be followed as per applicable rules and regulations.
- Compensation for injury to the subject to be as per rules and regulations and monitored for noncompliance.
- Complaints and concerns of subjects to be addressed and managed adequately.

Standard 5. Administrative support

Objective elements

- Ensuring adequate finance, human resource and secretariat for administrative work and record keeping, with due care and confidentiality.
- Financial transparency of EC activities and functioning.
- Procedure for communication between EC, investigator/ relevant site staff, institution and regulatory authority.

Standard 6. Review process

Objective elements

- Formal meetings to be conducted for review by EC within a reasonable time.
- Initial review of proposed clinical trial on scientific and ethical grounds.

Table *Contd...*

- Review of informed consent document, assent form (as applicable) and translations for appropriateness of language, accuracy and completeness of information.
- Review of the informed consent processes proposed to be followed at the site for a particular trial.
- Evaluation of recruitment strategies.
- Evaluation of proposals involving special groups and vulnerable population.
- Evaluation of contract and budget for indemnity, compensation, roles and responsibilities.
- Formal meetings to review any of the protocol, consent forms and investigators brochure

Periodic review of trial for continuation, risk evaluation and adverse event monitoring.

Standard 7. Decision making and post-meeting activities

Objective elements

- Decision making process (approval/disapproval/pending/revoking) to be as per applicable rules and regulations
- Subject recruitment in the trial only after approval from EC and regulatory authority.
- Declaration of conflict of interest, if any, prior to the review and voluntary withdrawal during decision making process.
- Approvals to be based on risk assessment, scientific validity and adherence to ethical principles.
- Deliberations and decisions made during the meetings to be documented, approved, signed and maintained as minutes of meeting.
- Evaluation of protocol deviations and non-compliances and appropriate actions taken.
- Analyses of serious adverse events and compensation amount assessed and reported to regulatory authority.
- Written notification of all decisions/opinions to the investigator.

Standard 8. Monitoring

Objective elements

- Monitoring of subject's rights, safety and wellbeing.
- Ensuring adequacy of informed consent process.

Table *Contd...*

<table>
<tr><td>

- Conduct of for-cause assessments in cases of non-compliance and/or any trial related complaints.
- Identification of any opportunities for improvement and initiation of appropriate actions.

</td></tr>
<tr><td>

Standard 9. Self-assessment

</td></tr>
<tr><td>

Objective elements

- Conduct of periodic self-assessments.
- Implementation of corrective and preventive actions (as required).

</td></tr>
<tr><td>

Standard 10. Record keeping and archival

</td></tr>
<tr><td>

Objective elements

- Periodic review of security, confidentiality and integrity of all proposals and associated documents.
- Archival of documents and records after completion /termination of trial as per applicable rules and regulations.
- Appropriate record retrieval policies and procedures to be in place.

</td></tr>
</table>

Source: www.nabh.co/Images/PDF/EC_Standard.pdf

Participant/Patient Information Sheet

(TEMPLATE)

Name of the participant:

Study title:

You are being invited to participate in this research study being conducted at… (name of the trial site)…as you have been found eligible for inclusion in this study. This document contains all the pertinent information regarding the study. Please read this thoroughly and feel free to raise any queries.

Purpose of research

This is a research study conducted in subjects having… (disease condition)….

(A brief description of disease condition including its etiology, symptoms, prevalence, prognosis, alternative procedures or treatment options available).

(A brief information on investigational drug especially efficacy and safety aspects and the rationale for testing it in the current study).

The results of this study may prove beneficial to society in terms of improvement in medical knowledge and providing treatment options to patients in future.

Study design and procedures

We plan to enroll ……. (number) ….. subjects in this study and you will be one of them.

Subjects/ patients in this study will be randomly divided into … (number)….……groups i.e. …… (name of groups) …… and you will receive the respective treatment.

In case of placebo controlled trial, a brief description of placebo for example; you may receive a placebo treatment which is an inactive or a dummy medication devoid of any therapeutic effect, given to increase scientific validity of study. Also, a placebo is needed to implement blinding i.e. both you and the investigator are unaware of the treatment assigned to you which is important for an unbiased evaluation of the study drug.

In case of randomized study, a statement stating "The assignment to a particular group will be done randomly i.e. purely determined by chance".

In case of blinded study, a statement stating the personnel who will be blinded e.g. ………….. (blinded personnel) ….will not be aware of the treatment allotted to you.

The expected duration of your participation in this study is……… After randomization, you need to come to the … (name of the clinic/trial site) ……..(frequency of visits, total duration). During each visit, ………… (procedures done) …..

Your Responsibilities

You need to provide your personal and health status related details as required. You should follow the instructions given to you by study personnel and take the medications as advised. Besides the scheduled follow up visits, you may also need to report at other times when called upon.

Possible Risks/Discomforts to you

The drug which you will be given is known to cause ………… (common and rare reported adverse events)…..Due measures will be taken to prevent the occurrence of such symptoms. If you encounter any adverse event, adequate medical management will be provided to you free of cost in the hospital. Also, though rare, some new adverse event may occur which has not been reported with this drug so far in literature.

Possible Benefits to you

You may experience improvement in your clinical condition with this treatment. However, it is also possible that the investigational product given to you may fail to provide intended therapeutic effect.

Apart from reporting to the clinical site as and when required, you will have no other expenditure. You will not be required to pay for medications or any investigations related to the study.

Confidentiality of your information

All the information related to you including your personal details, medical history, results of investigations etc. will be kept strictly confidential and no one except the research team personnel, sponsors, ethics committee and regulatory authorities will have access to your data. The information from this study, if published in scientific journals or presented at scientific meetings, will not disclose your identity.

Financial compensation and medical management

If you suffer any injury during the clinical trial, you will be provided free medical management as long as required or till it is established to be not related to the trial per se, whichever is earlier.

In the event of a trial related injury or death, you shall be provided financial compensation.

Payment for Participation in Study

Apart from free medical management and financial compensation in case of trial related injury or death, you will not receive any payment in the form of money for participation in this study.

Termination of your Participation

Your participation in the study may be terminated without your consent if you do not follow the instructions properly or the investigator anticipates any harm in your further participation in the study.

Decision to Withdraw

The participation in this research is purely voluntary and you have right to withdraw at any time during the course of study without giving any reasons although it is advisable to talk to research team prior to stopping the treatment. Your withdrawal from the study will not affect your medical care or legal rights.

Right to new Information

You will be notified in a timely manner if any significant information, good or bad, comes to our knowledge regarding the study drug, after that you can decide about your further continuation in the study.

Contact Person

If, at anytime, you have queries related to the trial or in the event of any injury you are free to contact any of the persons listed below:

Principal Investigator

Name:

Address:

Contact number:

Co-Investigator

Name:

Address:

Contact number:

Informed Consent Form to Participate in A Clinical Trial

(TEMPLATE)

Study title:

Study number:

Subject's initials/ Name:

Age of subject/ Date of birth:

Subject's address:

Subject's Qualification:

Subject's Occupation: Student/ Self-employed/ Service/ House wife/ Others (Tick as appropriate)

Subject's annual income:

Subject's nominee (for compensation in case of trial related death)

    Name:

    Address:

    Relation with subject:

	Place initials in the box (Subject)
1. I have read and understood the information sheet dated…..for the above mentioned study and was given the opportunity to raise queries.	
2. I am participating in the study voluntarily and understand my freedom to withdraw at any time without giving any reason,	
3. I agree to give access of my health records pertaining to current study and any further related study to the study sponsor, others working on his behalf, ethics committee and the regulatory authorities even after my withdrawal from the study. However, my identity should not be revealed to third parties or in any publication.	
4. I will not restrict the use of any data or results arising from this study for scientific purposes.	
5. I give my consent to participate in the above mentioned study.	

Signature (thumb impression)   Date: DD/MM/YY

[Subject/ Legally Acceptable Representative]

Signatory's name:

Signature of the study Investigator: Date: DD/MM/YY

Name of the study Investigator:

Signature of witness: Date: DD/MM/YY

Name of witness:

A copy of duly filled informed consent form and patient information sheet shall be handed over to the subject or his/her attendant.

Child Assent Document

(TEMPLATE)

(To be read aloud to the child)

My name is … (identify yourself to the child by your name)…… I am doing a research study on……. (disease condition of interest)……… A research study is when we collect a lot of information to know about something. I would like to tell you about this study and ask if you will take part in it.

Why are we doing this study?

We are doing this study to find out ……whether a new medicine will help children like you who have (disease condition of interest)…..OR….we want to understand why children get (disease condition being studied)……OR ……as the case may be………

What will happen if you participate in this study?

Only if you agree, …..(explain the study procedures, when to come for follow up visits, what will be done during follow up, etc. in easily understandable language depending upon the age of child)…….

What benefit you will have by being part of this study?

A benefit means that something good happens to you. The benefits may be …..(brief description about effect of intervention being studied)……. However, it is not necessary that everyone who takes part in this study will get some benefit.

What discomfort there might be and what will be done to minimize it?

If the study involves taking blood samples…..At (time of taking blood sample e.g. at baseline, during follow up visits;)…we will insert a needle in your arm and take a teaspoonful of blood. It will hurt as much as a pin prick and the pain will subside within 5 minutes. The area of needle prick may appear red for some time. Your blood sample will be taken….(total number of times during the course of study)…..

If any other anticipated discomfort,…(explain accordingly)…..

What are the risks of being part of this study?

We don't think that any big problem will happen to you as part of this study, but you might …(brief about side effects) ….If you have any problem, please tell your parents who can contact…..(contact person)…. at any time.

Do you wish to participate in this study?

You will be included in this study only if you agree to participate. If you do not want to take part in this study, you can say "NO"; no one will be angry with you. Also if you say "YES" and change your mind later any time, it will be OK too. No one will scold you.

Do you have any questions?

If you want to ask any questions, please feel free to ask ……..(details of contact person)….

NOTE:

❖ **FOR CHILDREN <12 YEARS**

Signature of child is not required, but documentation of assent is required on this form as:

I have explained the study to ________________________(*print name of child here*) in language he/she can understand, and the child has agreed to be in the study.

____   _____________________

Signature of person conducting assent discussion   Date

Name of person conducting assent discussion *(Print name)*

❖ **FOR ADOLESCENTS (12-<18 YEARS)**

The child would be provided a copy of this form to keep with him.

_________________________________   _________________________   ________

Adolescent's Signature   Date   Age

____

Adolescent's Name (*print*)

_________________________________   _________________________

Signature of person conducting assent discussion   Date

____

Name of person conducting assent discussion (*print*)

Age Factor (F) for the Calculation of Quantum of Compensation

(Based on Workmen Compensation ACT)

Age (in years)	Factor	Age (in years)	Factor
upto 16	228.54	41	181.37
17	227.49	42	178.49
18	226.38	43	175.54
19	225.22	44	172.52
20	224.00	45	169.44
21	222.71	46	166.29
22	221.37	47	163.07
23	219.95	48	159.80
24	218.47	49	156.47
25	216.91	50	153.09
26	215.28	51	149.67
27	213.57	52	146.20
28	211.79	53	142.68
29	209.92	54	139.13
30	207.98	55	135.56
31	205.95	56	131.95
32	203.85	57	128.33
33	201.66	58	124.70
34	199.40	59	121.05
35	197.06	60	117.41
36	194.64	61	113.77
37	192.14	62	110.14
38	189.56	63	106.52
39	186.90	64	102.93
40	184.17	>65	99.37

Source: New Drugs and Clinical Trials Rules 2019 G.S.R. 227(E) accessible at: https://cdsco.gov.in/opencms/opencms/system/modules/CDSCO.WEB/elements/download_file_division.jsp?num_id=NDI2MQ==

Serious Adverse Event (SAE) Reporting Form

(TEMPLATE)

Important note: As per the current regulations, it is required that the Investigator sends SAE report to Sponsor, IEC and CDSCO within 24 hours of the event occurrence.

Country where the SAE has occurred.	
SAE report of death (Yes/No)	
Study protocol title	
Study protocol ID/ No.	
Copy of IEC permission	
Copy of permission from CDSCO	
CTRI Registration no.	
Sponsor details (Address, contact no., email)	
Details of CRO (Address, contact no., email)	
Type of report (tick as appropriate)	**Initial / Follow up**
In case of follow up, date and no. of initial or last submitted report	

1. SUBJECT/ PATIENT DETAILS				
Initials*				
ID No.*				
Gender **(Tick as appropriate)**	Male ☐	Female ☐	Others ☐	Unknown ☐
Age / Date of birth				
Weight (kg)				
Height (cm)				

2. SUSPECTED DRUG (S)				
Generic name*				
Indication(s)				
Dosage form & strength				
Daily dose & regimen				
Route of administration				
Starting date (DD/MM/YY) & time of day				
Stopping date (DD/MM/YY) and time				
Duration of treatment				

3. OTHER DRUG(S) (including non-prescription/OTC drugs and non-drug therapies)				
Generic name				
Indication(s)				
Dosage form & strength				
Daily dose & regimen				
Route of administration				
Starting date (DD/MM/YY) & time of day				
Stopping date (DD/MM/YY) and time				
Duration of treatment				

4. DETAILS OF SAE
Specific diagnosis for the event* ____
Full description of the event including reported symptoms, signs, body site and severity

Seriousness criterion/criteria (tick as appropriate)

☐	Fatal	☐	Life threatening
☐	In-patient hospitalization (out-patient study)	☐	Prolongation of hospitalization (in-patient study)
☐	Persistent or significant disability	☐	Congenital anomaly/ birth defect
☐	Any significant medical event		

Start date (and time) of event onset (DD/MM/YY) : ☐☐☐☐☐☐

Stop date (and time) or duration of treatment (DD/MM/YY) : ☐☐☐☐☐☐

Dechallenge (tick as appropriate)

	Positive
	Negative
	Not done
	Done but response not known
	Not known

Rechallenge (tick as appropriate)

	Positive
	Negative
	Not done
	Done but response not known
	Not known

Setting (tick as appropriate)

	Hospital
	Nursing home
	Out patient clinic
	Home
	Others

5. OUTCOME	
	Resolved
	Resolved with sequel
	Ongoing
	Stable chronic condition
	Continuing at death
	Death

Results of any specific test(s)		
For fatal outcome	Cause of death	
	Relation to suspected reaction	
	Autopsy findings (if any)	

Other information	
Any significant medical history	
Any significant family history	
H/O drug or alcohol abuse	
Any special investigations (if done); findings	
Causality assessment by Investigator	
Causality assessment by Sponsor/CRO	
Causality assessment method used as per protocol	

6. INVESTIGATOR DETAILS*	
Name and address of Investigator	
Telephone no.	
Profession (Specialty)	
Date of reporting the event to Central Licencing Authority	
Date of reporting the event to ethics committee overseeing the site	
Signature of the Investigator or Sponsor	

*Mandatory fields

Case Report Form

(TEMPLATE)

Protocol ID/No. (version)............   Subject ID: ....

Study title	
Study protocol ID/No. (version)	
Investigator/ Site	
Subject ID	
Instructions to fill the CRF	

- Use ball point refill filled pen to fill the form.
- Mention the date (DD/MM/YY) while appending the signature.
- Any corrections should be made by striking off the data entered with a single line.
- Corrections made should be appended with signature and date.
- Fill all the sections of CRF; no section should be left blank.

INCLUSION CRITERIA	
1. Age	Yes/ No
2.	Yes/ No
3. Willing to give written informed consent	Yes/ No
Response to all the above criteria should be "YES"; if any "NO" selected, the subject is ineligible for participation.	
EXCLUSION CRITERIA	
1.....	Yes/ No
2.....	Yes/ No
Response to all the above criteria should be "NO"; if any "YES" selected, the subject is ineligible for participation.	

Page no.   Filled by.............   Checked by..............

Protocol ID/No. (version)............   Subject ID: ....

SUBJECT/ PATIENT CHARACTERISTICS

Subject initials	
Randomised (Yes/ No); If no, reason	
Randomization code	
Age/ Gender	
Height (cm) / weight (kg)	
BMI (kg/m^2)	
H/O smoking	
H/O alcohol consumption	

DISEASE CHARACTERISTICS

Clinical diagnosis	
Duration of….(disease condition)	
Signs and symptoms…..	
Other relevant points of consideration depending on disease condition of interest	

MEDICAL HISTORY

Presence of any conditions relevant to the study including their duration, control, any associated complication etc.	

TREATMENT HISTORY

Concomitant medications		
Drug	Start date (DD/MM/YY) or duration of intake	Daily dose
Any past medical treatments		
Drug	Duration of intake	When stopped

Page no.   Filled by.............   Checked by..............

Protocol ID/No. (version)............   Subject ID: ....

TREATMENT DISPENSED

Visit no.				
Quantity (number)				
Date (DD/MM/YY)				
Date of next visit (DD/MM/YY)				
Instructions:				

CLINICAL EXAMINATION

Parameter	Screening (DD/MM/YY)	Baseline (DD/MM/YY)	Visit 1.... (DD/MM/YY) (..... day/ week ...)
.... (specific for the study) ...			
Any positive medical history since last visit; if yes, fill AE reporting form			
Any intake of medications other than specified in protocol; if yes, fill concomitant medications section			
Compliance; number of remaining pills in the medicine container (as mentioned in study protocol)			
Remarks			

OUTCOMES ASSESSMENT

Parameter	Baseline (0 day/week...)	Visit 1 (..... day/ week...)	Visit 2... (..... day/ week...)
Outcome parameters/ End points specific for the study			

Page no.   Filled by.............   Checked by.............

Protocol ID/No. (version)............   Subject ID: ....

UNSCHEDULED VISIT

Date (DD/MM/YY)	
Reason of visit	
Clinical examination	
......	
Any positive medical history since last visit; if yes, fill AE reporting form	
Any intake of medications other than specified in protocol; if yes, fill concomitant medications section	
Compliance; number of remaining pills in the medicine container	
Outcome parameters	
......	
Remarks	

Page no.   Filled by.............   Checked by..............

Common Terminology Criteria for Adverse Events (CTCAE)

VERSION: 5.0; PUBLISHED: NOVEMBER 2017

Grading of Adverse Event	Clinical Description
Grade 1	Mild; asymptomatic or mild symptoms; clinical or diagnostic observations only; intervention not indicated.
Grade 2	Moderate; minimal, local or noninvasive intervention indicated; limiting age appropriate instrumental ADL*.
Grade 3	Severe or medically significant but not immediately life-threatening; hospitalization or prolongation of hospitalization indicated; disabling; limiting self care ADL**.
Grade 4	Life-threatening consequences; urgent intervention indicated
Grade 5	Death related to AE.

Activities of Daily Living (ADL):

*Instrumental ADL refer to preparing meals, shopping for groceries or clothes, using the telephone, managing money, etc.

**Self care ADL refer to bathing, dressing and undressing, feeding self, using the toilet, taking medications, and not bedridden.

Source: Common terminology criteria for adverse events (CTCAE). https://ctep.cancer.gov/protocoldevelopment/electronic_applications/docs/ctcae_v5_quick_reference_8.5x11.pdf

Naranjo's Scale/Algorithm for Causality Assessment of Adverse Events

Questions	Yes	No	Don't know
Presence of previous conclusive report on adverse reaction.	+1	0	0
Did adverse event appear subsequent to administration of suspected drug?	+2	−1	0
Did adverse event improve on drug discontinuation or on administration of specific antagonist?	+1	0	0
Did the adverse event reappear when the drug was re-administered?	+2	−1	0
Are there any alternative causes other than the suspected drug that could have caused the reaction on their own?	−1	+2	0
Did the adverse event reappear when a placebo was administered?	−1	+1	0
Was the incriminated drug detected in toxic concentration in blood (fluids)?	+1	0	0
Did the Adverse event worsen on increasing the dose or decreased in severity with lower doses?	+1	0	0
Past history of any similar reaction to the same or similar drugs.	+1	0	0
Was the adverse event confirmed by objective evidence?	+1	0	0
Total score 0- Doubtful 1-4 Possible, 5-8 Probable, ≥ 9 Definite			

Index